WD 456   HHH7844   22.99

WD 456

Vol. 67, Supplement 1

RESUSCITATION

December 2005

CONTENTS

Abstracts/contents list published in: Biological Abstracts, Cambridge Scientific Abstracts, Current Contents, EMBASE, Index Medicus

RESUSCITATION

Volume 67 (2005)

Official Journal of the European Resuscitation Council

also affiliated with the
American Heart Association, the Australian Resuscitation Council,
the New Zealand Resuscitation Council and the Resuscitation Council of Southern Africa

Also available on

SCIENCE DIRECT®

www.sciencedirect.com

for online access via your library

RESUSCITATION

Official Journal of the European Resuscitation Council

also affiliated with the American Heart Association, the Australian Resuscitation Council, the New Zealand Resuscitation Council, the Resuscitation Council of Southern Africa and the Japan Resuscitation Council

Volume 67 (2005)

ELSEVIER

AMSTERDAM—LONDON—NEW YORK—OXFORD—PARIS—SHANNON—TOKYO

ELSEVIER

ISBN-13: 9780080448701
ISBN-10: 0-08-044870-4

British Library Cataloguing in Publication Data
A catalogue record for this book is available from the British Library.

Library of Congress Cataloguing in Publication Data
A catalogue record for this book is available from the Library of Congress.

Note
Knowledge and best practice in this field are constantly changing. As new research and experience broaden our knowledge, changes in practice, treatment and drug therapy may become necessary or appropriate. Readers are advised to check the most current information provided (i) on procedures featured or (ii) by the manufacturer of each product to be administered, to verify the recommended dose or formula, the method and duration of administration, and contraindications. It is the responsibility of the practitioner, relying on their own experience and knowledge of the patient, to make diagnoses, to determine dosages and the best treatment for each individual patient, and to take all appropriate safety precautions. To the fullest extent of the law, neither the Publisher nor the [Editors/Authors] [delete as appropriate] assumes any liability for any injury and/or damage to persons or property arising out or related to any use of the material contained in this book.

www.elsevierhealth.com

The Publisher's Policy is to use Paper manufactured from sustainable forests.

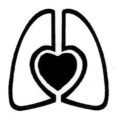

EUROPEAN RESUSCITATION COUNCIL

Interdisciplinary Council for Resuscitation Medicine and Emergency Medical Care

The European Resuscitation Council (ERC) is a multidisciplinary advisory medical body for coordinating the activities of European organisations with a legitimate interest in cardiopulmonary resuscitation medicine and for improving the standards of resuscitation throughout Europe.

Officers (2004 – 2005)

Chairman:
D. Zideman (United Kingdom)

Executive Director:
L. Bossaert (Belgium)

Chairman Elect
Bernd Böttiger (Germany)

Hon. Secretary:
K. Monsieurs (Belgium)

Hon. Treasurer:
J. Bahr (Germany)

Journal Editor:
P. Baskett (United Kingdom)

ILCOR Liaison Officer:
J. Nolan (United Kingdom)

Representatives of European Societies
ESC: D. Ferreira (Portugal)
ESICM: B. Walden (Switzerland)
EuSEM: H. Askitopoulou (Greece)
Red Cross EU: P. Cassan

Coordinators of Working Groups
BLS & AED: P. Cassan (France)
ALS: C. Deakin (United Kingdom)
ALS: E. Soreide (Norway)
PLS: D. Biarent (Belgium)
Research: J. Herlitz (Sweden)

Members (2004 – 2005)
J. Andres (Poland)
M. Baubin (Austria)
A. Carneiro (Portugal)
E. Cerchiari (Italy)
A. Certug (Turkey)
M. Colquhoun (United Kingdom)
C. Dioszeghy (Hungary)
B. Dirks (Germany)
D. Fishman (Switzerland)
M. Georgiou (Cyprus)
A. Handley (United Kingdom)
S. Holmberg (Sweden)
S. Hunyadi-Antevecic (Croatia)
G. Abbas Khalifa (Egypt)
K. Lexow (Norway)
F. Lippert (Denmark)
V. Marecek (Czech Republic)
P. Mols (Belgium)
V. Moroz (Russia)
L. Papadimitriou (Greece)
PENDING (UAE)
T. Silfvast (Finland)
C. Urkia Mieres (Spain)
A. Van Drenth (Netherlands)
D. Vlahovic (Slovenia)

More information about ERC can be obtained from the Secretariat, European Resuscitation Council, PO Box 113, BE-2610 Antwerp, Belgium. Tel.: +32 3 826 9321; Fax: +32 3 826 9323 (secretariat); e-mail: info@erc.edu; www.erc.edu

The European Resuscitation Council was founded in 1989 and includes representatives of the major European countries, the major European organisations with interest in CPR, e.g. the European Academy of Anesthesiology (EAA), the European Society for Cardiology (ESC), the European Society for Intensive Care Medicine (ESICM), the European Society for Emergency Medicine (EuSEM), the Red Cross of the EU Countries, and other national and/or multinational organisations that are active in the field of resuscitation.

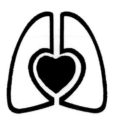

EUROPEAN RESUSCITATION COUNCIL

Interdisciplinary Council for Resuscitation Medicine and Emergency Medical Care

The **primary** objective of the ERC is to save human life by improving standards of resuscitation in Europe, and by coordinating the activities of European organisations with a legitimate interest in cardiopulmonary resuscitation.

The **secondary objectives are:**

1. to produce guidelines and recommendations appropriate to Europe for practice of Basic and Advanced Cardiopulmonary and Cerebral Resuscitation
2. to design teaching programmes suitable for all trainees, ranging from the lay public to the qualified physician
3. to conduct a critical review of CPR practice and to advise on updating guidelines
4. to promote and encourage appropriate research
5. to promote audit of resuscitation practice including standardisation of records of resuscitation attempts
6. to organise relevant scientific meetings in Europe
7. to promote political and public awareness of resuscitation requirements and practice

The work of the European Resuscitation Council is undertaken by Working Groups:

1. Basic Life Support
2. Advanced Life Support
3. Pediatric Life Support
4. Training and Education Working Group

There are the following categories of membership:

1. *Active members*
    (a) *National representatives:* Representatives of European and national organisations with an interest in or active in the field of CPR, for example Anaesthetic, Cardiac, Intensive Care, Emergency Medicine and Resuscitation Societies, and relevant academic bodies
    (b) *Individual members:* Medically qualified individuals making a special contribution to the field of CPR, approved by the Executive Committee.
2. *Associate members*
    Medical non-European and non-medical individuals willing to participate in the activities of the Association
3. *Corresponding members*
    Individuals wishing to be informed of the activities of the Association
4. *Honorary members*
    May be appointed by the Executive Committee who will be individuals who have displayed outstanding merit in promoting the objectives of the Association
5. *Patron members*
    May be nominated by the Executive Committee from among the principal and major sponsors

The national or European Societies are encouraged to apply for an institutional subscription to the journal Resuscitation.

ERC MEMBERS AND RESUSCITATION

All ERC members are cordially encouraged to take an active interest in the journal Resuscitation. Members are therefore invited:
(a) to seek and encourage the submission of high quality research and clinical papers which are within the scope of the journal.
(b) to discuss with the editors and ERC officers whether the contents of the journal fulfil their needs.
(c) to help the editors and publisher in seeking the best way in which potential readers can be informed about the journal.
Individual ERC members are offered the journal Resuscitation as part of the membership of the ERC.

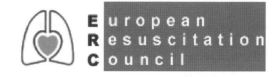
European
Resuscitation
Council

MEMBERSHIP FORM

PLEASE COMPLETE THIS FORM AND SEND TO:

ERC SECRETARIAT   PHONE + 32 3 8213616
PO BOX 113   EMAIL info@erc.edu
B-2610 WILRIJK, BELGIUM WEB   www.erc.edu
FAX + 32 3 821 4983

PLEASE TYPE OR PRINT IN CAPITALS

1. PERSONAL INFORMATION

First Name (*)					
Last Name (*)					
Date of Birth	[dd/mm/yy]				
Title	O Mr	O Mrs	O Ms	O Dr	O Prof

2. ADDRESS INFORMATION
[complete either or both columns]

	Office Address	Home Address
Organisation		
Department		
Address (*)		
Zip (*)		
City (*)		
Country (*)		
Phone (*)		
Fax		
Email (*)		
Mobile		
Send ERC Mail to (*)	O above office address	O above home address

(*) = required

3. MEMBERSHIP TYPE

Select	Type	Membership Fee (EUR)
O	Full Member	140
O	Active ERC Instructor (1)	125
O	Instructor joining ERC for first time (2)	90
O	Membership without Journal (3)	90

(1): for certified ERC instructors, having given minimal 3 courses during 2004 (include list of given courses during 2004).
(2): for certified ERC instructors only, joining for first time.
(3): for members from Central- and Eastern European countries, Russian Federation AND for students, all countries. Includes electronic access to the Journal.

4. PAYMENT

I want to pay by:

O	VISA / MASTERCARD Card Holder: Card Number: Expiry Date (mm/yy):
O	Bank Transfer (1)
O	Cheque (2)

(1) Please submit your payment order to:

Fortis Bank
Wilrijkstraat 10
BE-2650 Edegem, Belgium

Account 001-3097088-51
ERC Secretariat VZW

IBAN BE: 75 0013 0970 8851
BIC CODE: GEBA BE BB

Reference: ERC Membership + your name

Please note to add a bank charge of EUR 15 when paying from bank outside the EU-15 countries.

(2) Please send double-crossed cheque, together with copy of this form, to

ERC Secretariat VZW
PO Box 113
BE-2610 Wilrijk, Belgium

Make cheque payable to ERC Secretariat VZW

Please note to add a bank charge of EUR 15 when issuing a non-Belgian cheque.

DATE: **SIGNATURE:**

European Resuscitation Council Guidelines for Resuscitation 2005

Edited by Jerry Nolan and Peter Baskett

Resuscitation (2005) 67S1, S1—S2

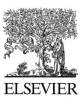

ELSEVIER

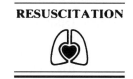

www.elsevier.com/locate/resuscitation

Preface

This supplement of *Resuscitation* contains the European Resuscitation Council (ERC) Guidelines for Resuscitation 2005. It is derived from the 2005 International Consensus Conference on Cardiopulmonary Resuscitation and Emergency Cardiovascular Care Science with Treatment Recommendations produced by the International Liaison Committee on Resuscitation (ILCOR) published simultaneously in an issue of *Resuscitation*.

The European representatives at that Conference, held in Dallas in January 2005, more than pulled their weight in the process of producing the Consensus on Science conclusions arising as a result of presentations and debate. Their names are listed at the end of this Foreword, and the resuscitation community in Europe and beyond is most grateful to them for their talent, dedication and selfless hard work. In addition, they, and many others from Europe, also produced worksheets addressing the evidence for and against every conceivable detail of resuscitation theory and practice.

The ERC Guidelines contain recommendations that, by consensus of the European representatives, are suitable for European practice in the light of today's conclusions agreed in the Consensus on Science. As with the Consensus on Science document, they represent an enormous amount of work by many people who have worked against the clock to produce the Guidelines for Europe. Each section of the Guidelines has been masterminded and coordinated by the leaders of the ERC working groups and areas of special interest.

Such ventures do not happen without leadership, and we are grateful to Vinay Nadkarni, Bill Montgomery, Peter Morley, Mary Fran Hazinski, Arno Zaritsky, and Jerry Nolan for guiding the Consensus on Science process through to completion. It would not be invidious to single out Jerry Nolan, the ILCOR

co-chairman, for thanks and praise. He is universally respected and popular, and has proved to be a wonderful ambassador for Europe. His scientific credibility and understanding are beyond doubt and his integrity, dedication, sheer hard work, patience and meticulous attention to detail and sensitivities have won the admiration of all. He has led the Consensus on Science process on our behalf, and has been the lead co-ordinator in producing the European Guidelines.

Finally we thank our publishers, Elsevier, through the Publishing Editor for *Resuscitation*, Anne Lloyd and her colleagues, for their professionalism, tolerance and patience in these endeavours.

Representatives from Europe at the International Consensus Conference held in Dallas, USA, in January 2005

Hans-Richard Arntz (Germany), Dennis Azzopardi (UK), Jan Bahr (Germany), Gad Bar-Joseph (Israel), Peter Baskett (UK), Michael Baubin (Austria), Dominique Biarent (Belgium), Bob Bingham (UK), Bernd Böttiger (Germany), Leo Bossaert (Belgium), Steven Byrne (UK), Pierre Carli (France), Pascal Cassan (France), Sian Davies (UK), Charles Deakin (UK), Burkhard Dirks (Germany), Volker Doerges (Germany), Hans Domanovits (Austria), Christoph Eich (Germany), Lars Ekstrom (Sweden), Peter Fenici (Italy), F. Javier Garcia-Vega (Spain), Henrik Gervais (Germany) Anthony Handley (UK), Johan Herlitz (Sweden), Fulvio Kette (Italy), Rudolph Koster (Netherlands), Kristian Lexow (Norway), Perttu Lindsberg (Finland), Freddy Lippert (Denmark), Vit Marecek (Czech Republic), Koenraad Monsieurs (Belgium), Jerry Nolan (UK), Narcisco

doi:10.1016/j.resuscitation.2005.10.001

Perales (Spain), Gavin Perkins (UK), Sam Richmond (UK), Antonio Rodriquez Nunez (Spain), Sten Rubertsson (Sweden), Sebastian Russo (Germany), Jas Soar (UK), Eldar Soreide (Norway), Petter Steen (Norway), Benjamin Stenson (UK), Kjetil Sunde (Norway), Caroline Telion (France), Andreas Thierbach (Germany), Christian Torp Pederson (Denmark), Volker Wenzel (Austria), Lars Wik (Norway), Benno Wolke (Germany), Jonathan Wyllie (UK), David Zideman (UK).

Peter Baskett
David Zideman

Resuscitation (2005) **67S1**, S3—S6

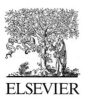

RESUSCITATION

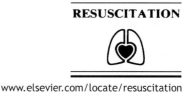

www.elsevier.com/locate/resuscitation

European Resuscitation Council Guidelines for Resuscitation 2005
Section 1. Introduction

Jerry Nolan

It is five years since publication of the Guidelines 2000 for Cardiopulmonary Resuscitation (CPR) and Emergency Cardiovascular Care (ECC).[1] The European Resuscitation Council (ERC) based its own resuscitation guidelines on this document, and these were published as a series of papers in 2001.[2–7] Resuscitation science continues to advance, and clinical guidelines must be updated regularly to reflect these developments and advise healthcare providers on best practice. In between major guideline updates (about every five years), interim advisory statements can inform the healthcare provider about new therapies that might influence outcome significantly;[8] we anticipate that further advisory statements will be published in response to important research findings.

The guidelines that follow do not define the only way that resuscitation should be achieved; they merely represent a widely accepted view of how resuscitation can be undertaken both safely and effectively. The publication of new and revised treatment recommendations does not imply that current clinical care is either unsafe or ineffective.

Consensus on science

The International Liaison Committee on Resuscitation (ILCOR) was formed in 1993.[9] Its mission is to identify and review international science and knowledge relevant to CPR, and to offer consensus on treatment recommendations. The process for the latest resuscitation guideline update began in 2003, when ILCOR representatives established six task forces: basic life support; advanced cardiac life support; acute coronary syndromes; paediatric life support; neonatal life support; and an interdisciplinary task force to address overlapping topics, such as educational issues. Each task force identified topics requiring evidence evaluation, and appointed international experts to review them. To ensure a consistent and thorough approach, a worksheet template was created containing step-by-step directions to help the experts document their literature review, evaluate studies, determine levels of evidence and develop recommendations.[10] A total of 281 experts completed 403 worksheets on 276 topics; 380 people from 18 countries attended the 2005 International Consensus Conference on ECC and CPR Science with Treatment Recommendations (C2005), which took place in Dallas in January 2005.[11] Worksheet authors presented the results of their evidence evaluations and proposed summary scientific statements. After discussion among all participants, these statements were refined and, whenever possible, supported by treatment recommendations. These summary science statements and treatment recommendations have been published in the 2005 International Consensus on Cardiopulmonary Resuscitation and Emergency Cardiovascular Care Science with Treatment Recommendations (CoSTR).[12]

doi:10.1016/j.resuscitation.2005.10.002

From science to guidelines

The resuscitation organisations forming ILCOR will publish individual resuscitation guidelines that are consistent with the science in the consensus document, but will also consider geographic, economic and system differences in practice, and the availability of medical devices and drugs. These 2005 ERC Resuscitation Guidelines are derived from the CoSTR document but represent consensus among members of the ERC Executive Committee. The ERC Executive Committee considers these new recommendations to be the most effective and easily learned interventions that can be supported by current knowledge, research and experience. Inevitably, even within Europe, differences in the availability of drugs, equipment, and personnel will necessitate local, regional and national adaptation of these guidelines.

Demographics

Ischaemic heart disease is the leading cause of death in the world.[13-17] Sudden cardiac arrest is responsible for more than 60% of adult deaths from coronary heart disease.[18] Based on data from Scotland and from five cities in other parts of Europe, the annual incidence of resuscitation for out-of-hospital cardiopulmonary arrest of cardiac aetiology is 49.5—66 per 100,000 population.[19,20] The Scottish study includes data on 21,175 out-of-hospital cardiac arrests, and provides valuable information on aetiology (Table 1.1). The incidence of in-hospital cardiac arrest is difficult to assess because it is influenced heavily by factors such as the criteria for hospital admission and implementation of a do-not-attempt-resuscitation (DNAR) policy. In a general hospital in the UK, the incidence of primary cardiac arrest (excluding those with DNAR and those arresting in the emergency department) was 3.3/1000 admissions;[21] using the same exclusion criteria, the incidence of cardiac arrest in a Norwegian University hospital was 1.5/1000 admissions.[22]

The Chain of Survival

The actions linking the victim of sudden cardiac arrest with survival are called the Chain of Survival. They include early recognition of the emergency and activation of the emergency services, early CPR, early defibrillation and early advanced life support. The infant-and-child Chain of Survival

Table 1.1 Out-of-hospital cardiopulmonary arrests (21,175) by aetiology.[19]

Aetiology	Number (%)
Presumed cardiac disease	17451 (82.4)
Non-cardiac internal aetiologies	1814 (8.6)
Lung disease	901 (4.3)
Cerebrovascular disease	457 (2.2)
Cancer	190 (0.9)
Gastrointestinal haemorrhage	71 (0.3)
Obstetric/paediatric	50 (0.2)
Pulmonary embolism	38 (0.2)
Epilepsy	36 (0.2)
Diabetes mellitus	30 (0.1)
Renal disease	23 (0.1)
Non-cardiac external aetiologies	1910 (9.0)
Trauma	657 (3.1)
Asphyxia	465 (2.2)
Drug overdose	411 (1.9)
Drowning	105 (0.5)
Other suicide	194 (0.9)
Other external	50 (0.2)
Electric shock/lightning	28 (0.1)

includes prevention of conditions leading to the cardiopulmonary arrest, early CPR, early activation of the emergency services and early advanced life support. In hospital, the importance of early recognition of the critically ill patient and activation of a medical emergency team (MET) is now well accepted.[23] Previous resuscitation guidelines have provided relatively little information on treatment of the patient during the post-resuscitation care phase. There is substantial variability in the way comatose survivors of cardiac arrest are treated in the initial hours and first few days after return of spontaneous circulation (ROSC). Differences in treatment at this stage may account for some of the interhospital variability in outcome after cardiac arrest.[24] The importance of recognising critical illness and/or angina and preventing cardiac arrest (in- or out-of-hospital), and post resuscitation care has been highlighted by the inclusion of these elements in a new four-ring Chain of Survival. The first link indicates the importance of recognising those at risk of cardiac arrest and calling for help in the hope that early treatment can prevent arrest. The central links in this new chain depict the integration of CPR and defibrillation as the fundamental components of early resuscitation in an attempt to restore life. The final link, effective post resuscitation care, is targeted at preserving function, particularly of the brain and heart (Figure 1.1).[25,26]

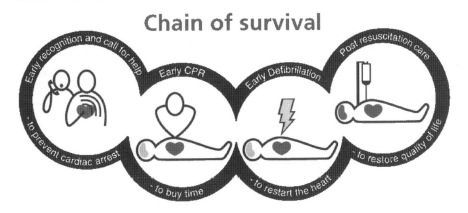

Figure 1.1   ERC Chain of Survival.

The universal algorithm

The adult basic, adult advanced and paediatric resuscitation algorithms have been updated to reflect changes in the ERC Guidelines. Every effort has been made to keep these algorithms simple yet applicable to cardiac arrest victims in most circumstances. Rescuers begin CPR if the victim is unconscious or unresponsive, and not breathing normally (ignoring occasional gasps). A single compression—ventilation (CV) ratio of 30:2 is used for the single rescuer of an adult or child (excluding neonates) out of hospital, and for all adult CPR. This single ratio is designed to simplify teaching, promote skill retention, increase the number of compressions given and decrease interruption to compressions. Once a defibrillator is attached, if a shockable rhythm is confirmed, a single shock is delivered. Irrespective of the resultant rhythm, chest compressions and ventilations (2 min with a CV ratio of 30:2) are resumed immediately after the shock to minimise the 'no-flow' time. Advanced life support interventions are outlined in a box at the centre of the ALS algorithm (see Section 4). Once the airway is secured with a tracheal tube, laryngeal mask airway (LMA) or Combitube, the lungs are ventilated at a rate of 10 min^{-1} without pausing during chest compressions.

Quality of CPR

Interruptions to chest compressions must be minimised. On stopping chest compressions, the coronary flow decreases substantially; on resuming chest compressions, several compressions are necessary before the coronary flow recovers to its previous level.[27] Recent evidence indicates that unnecessary interruptions to chest compressions

occur frequently both in and out of hospital.[28—31] Resuscitation instructors must emphasise the importance of minimising interruptions to chest compressions.

Summary

It is intended that these new guidelines will improve the practice of resuscitation and, ultimately, the outcome from cardiac arrest. The universal ratio of 30 compressions to two ventilations should decrease the number of interruptions in compression, reduce the likelihood of hyperventilation, simplify instruction for teaching and improve skill retention. The single-shock strategy should minimise 'no-flow' time. Resuscitation course materials are being updated to reflect these new guidelines.

References

1. American Heart Association, In collaboration with International Liaison Committee on Resuscitation. Guidelines for cardiopulmonary resuscitation and emergency cardiovascular care—an international consensus on science. Resuscitation 2000;46:3—430.
2. Handley AJ, Monsieurs KG, Bossaert LL, European Resuscitation Council Guidelines 2000 for Adult Basic Life Support. A statement from the Basic Life Support and Automated External Defibrillation Working Group. Resuscitation 2001;48:199—205.
3. Monsieurs KG, Handley AJ, Bossaert LL, European Resuscitation Council Guidelines 2000 for Automated External Defibrillation. A statement from the Basic Life Support and Automated External Defibrillation Working Group. Resuscitation 2001;48:207—9.
4. de Latorre F, Nolan J, Robertson C, Chamberlain D, Baskett P, European Resuscitation Council Guidelines 2000 for Adult Advanced Life Support. A statement from the Advanced Life Support Working Group. Resuscitation 2001;48:211—21.

5. Phillips B, Zideman D, Garcia-Castrillo L, Felix M, Shwarz-Schwierin U, European Resuscitation Council Guidelines 2000 for Basic Paediatric Life Support. A statement from the Paediatric Life Support Working Group. Resuscitation 2001;48:223—9.

6. Phillips B, Zideman D, Garcia-Castrillo L, Felix M, Shwarz-Schwierin V, European Resuscitation Council Guidelines 2000 for Advanced Paediatric Life Support. A statement from Paediatric Life Support Working Group. Resuscitation 2001;48:231—4.

7. Phillips B, Zideman D, Wyllie J, Richmond S, van Reempts P, European Resuscitation Council Guidelines 2000 for Newly Born Life Support. A statement from the Paediatric Life Support Working Group. Resuscitation 2001;48:235—9.

8. Nolan JP, Morley PT, Vanden Hoek TL, Hickey RW. Therapeutic hypothermia after cardiac arrest. An advisory statement by the Advancement Life support Task Force of the International Liaison committee on Resuscitation. Resuscitation 2003;57:231—5.

9. The Founding Members of the International Liaison Committee on Resuscitation. The International Liaison Committee on Resuscitation (ILCOR)—past, present and future. Resuscitation 2005;67:157—61.

10. Morley P, Zaritsky A. The evidence evaluation process for the 2005 International Consensus on Cardiopulmonary Resuscitation and Emergency Cardiovascular Care Science With Treatment Recommendations. Resuscitation 2005;67:167—70.

11. Nolan JP, Hazinski MF, Steen PA, Becker LB. Controversial topics from the 2005 International Consensus Conference on Cardiopulmonary Resuscitation and Emergency Cardiovascular Care Science with treatment recommendations. Resuscitation 2005;67:175—9.

12. International Liaison Committee on Resuscitation. 2005 International Consensus on Cardiopulmonary Resuscitation and Emergency Cardiovascular Care Science with Treatment Recommendations. Resuscitation 2005;67:157—341.

13. Murray CJ, Lopez AD. Mortality by cause for eight regions of the world: global burden of disease study. Lancet 1997;349:1269—76.

14. Sans S, Kesteloot H, Kromhout D. The burden of cardiovascular diseases mortality in Europe. Task Force of the European Society of Cardiology on Cardiovascular Mortality and Morbidity Statistics in Europe. Eur Heart J 1997;18:1231—48.

15. Kesteloot H, Sans S, Kromhout D. Evolution of all-causes and cardiovascular mortality in the age-group 75—84 years in Europe during the period 1970—1996; a comparison with worldwide changes. Eur Heart J 2002;23:384—98.

16. Fox R. Trends in cardiovascular mortality in Europe. Circulation 1997;96:3817.

17. Levi F, Lucchini F, Negri E, La Vecchia C. Trends in mortality from cardiovascular and cerebrovascular diseases in Europe and other areas of the world. Heart 2002;88:119—24.

18. Zheng ZJ, Croft JB, Giles WH, Mensah GA. Sudden cardiac death in the United States, 1989 to 1998. Circulation 2001;104:2158—63.

19. Pell JP, Sirel JM, Marsden AK, Ford I, Walker NL, Cobbe SM. Presentation, management, and outcome of out of hospital cardiopulmonary arrest: comparison by underlying aetiology. Heart 2003;89:839—42.

20. Herlitz J, Bahr J, Fischer M, Kuisma M, Lexow K, Thorgeirsson G. Resuscitation in Europe: a tale of five European regions. Resuscitation 1999;41:121—31.

21. Hodgetts TJ, Kenward G, Vlackonikolis I, et al. Incidence, location and reasons for avoidable in-hospital cardiac arrest in a district general hospital. Resuscitation 2002;54:115—23.

22. Skogvoll E, Isern E, Sangolt GK, Gisvold SE. In-hospital cardiopulmonary resuscitation. 5 years' incidence and survival according to the Utstein template. Acta Anaesthesiol Scand 1999;43:177—84.

23. The MERIT study investigators. Introduction of the medical emergency team (MET) system: a cluster-randomised controlled trial. Lancet 2005;365:2091—7.

24. Langhelle A, Tyvold SS, Lexow K, Hapnes SA, Sunde K, Steen PA. In-hospital factors associated with improved outcome after out-of-hospital cardiac arrest. A comparison between four regions in Norway. Resuscitation 2003;56:247—63.

25. Langhelle A, Nolan J, Herlitz J, et al. Recommended guidelines for reviewing, reporting, and conducting research on post-resuscitation care: The Utstein style. Resuscitation 2005;66:271—83.

26. Perkins GD, Soar J. In hospital cardiac arrest: missing links in the chain of survival. Resuscitation 2005;66:253—5.

27. Kern KB, Hilwig RW, Berg RA, Ewy GA. Efficacy of chest compression-only BLS CPR in the presence of an occluded airway. Resuscitation 1998;39:179—88.

28. Wik L, Kramer-Johansen J, Myklebust H, et al. Quality of cardiopulmonary resuscitation during out-of-hospital cardiac arrest. JAMA 2005;293:299—304.

29. Abella BS, Alvarado JP, Myklebust H, et al. Quality of cardiopulmonary resuscitation during in-hospital cardiac arrest. JAMA 2005;293:305—10.

30. Abella BS, Sandbo N, Vassilatos P, et al. Chest compression rates during cardiopulmonary resuscitation are suboptimal: a prospective study during in-hospital cardiac arrest. Circulation 2005;111:428—34.

31. Valenzuela TD, Kern KB, Clark LL, et al. Interruptions of chest compressions during emergency medical systems resuscitation. Circulation 2005;112:1259—65.

Resuscitation (2005) **67S1**, S7—S23

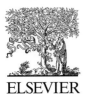

RESUSCITATION

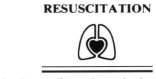

www.elsevier.com/locate/resuscitation

European Resuscitation Council Guidelines for Resuscitation 2005
Section 2. Adult basic life support and use of automated external defibrillators

Anthony J. Handley, Rudolph Koster, Koen Monsieurs, Gavin D. Perkins, Sian Davies, Leo Bossaert

Basic life support (BLS) refers to maintaining airway patency and supporting breathing and the circulation, without the use of equipment other than a protective device.[1] This section contains the guidelines for adult BLS by lay rescuers and for the use of an automated external defibrillator (AED). It also includes recognition of sudden cardiac arrest, the recovery position and management of choking (foreign-body airway obstruction). Guidelines for in-hospital BLS and the use of manual defibrillators may be found in Sections 3 and 4b.

Introduction

Sudden cardiac arrest (SCA) is a leading cause of death in Europe, affecting about 700,000 individuals a year.[2] At the time of the first heart rhythm analysis, about 40% of SCA victims have ventricular fibrillation (VF).[3–6] It is likely that many more victims have VF or rapid ventricular tachycardia (VT) at the time of collapse but, by the time the first ECG is recorded, their rhythm has deteriorated to asystole.[7,8] VF is characterized by chaotic, rapid depolarisation and repolarisation. The heart loses its coordinated function and stops pumping blood

effectively.[9] Many victims of SCA can survive if bystanders act immediately while VF is still present, but successful resuscitation is unlikely once the rhythm has deteriorated to asystole.[10] The optimum treatment for VF cardiac arrest is immediate bystander CPR (combined chest compression and rescue breathing) plus electrical defibrillation. The predominant mechanism of cardiac arrest in victims of trauma, drug overdose, drowning, and in many children is asphyxia; rescue breaths are critical for resuscitation of these victims.

The following concept of the Chain of Survival summarises the vital steps needed for successful resuscitation (Figure 1.1). Most of these links are relevant for victims of both VF and asphyxial arrest.[11]

1. Early recognition of the emergency and calling for help: activate the emergency medical services (EMS) or local emergency response system, e.g. ''phone 112''.[12,13] An early, effective response may prevent cardiac arrest.
2. Early bystander CPR: immediate CPR can double or triple survival from VF SCA.[10,14–17]
3. Early defibrillation: CPR plus defibrillation within 3—5 min of collapse can produce survival rates as high as 49—75%.[18–25] Each minute of

delay in defibrillation reduces the probability of survival to discharge by 10—15%.[14,17]

4. Early advanced life support and post-resuscitation care: the quality of treatment during the post-resuscitation phase affects outcome.[26]

In most communities, the time from EMS call to EMS arrival (response interval) is 8 min or longer.[27] During this time the victim's survival is dependent on early initiation by bystanders of the first three of the links of the Chain of Survival.

Victims of cardiac arrest need immediate CPR. This provides a small but critical blood flow to the heart and brain. It also increases the likelihood that a defibrillatory shock will terminate VF and enable the heart to resume an effective rhythm and effective systemic perfusion. Chest compression is especially important if a shock cannot be delivered sooner than 4 or 5 min after collapse.[28,29] Defibrillation interrupts the uncoordinated depolarisation-repolarisation process that occurs during VF. If the heart is still viable, its normal pacemakers then resume their function and produce an effective rhythm and resumption of circulation. In the first few minutes after successful defibrillation, the rhythm may be slow and ineffective; chest compressions may be needed until adequate cardiac function returns.[30]

Lay rescuers can be trained to use an automated external defibrillator (AED) to analyse the victim's cardiac rhythm and deliver a shock if VF is present. An AED uses voice prompts to guide the rescuer. It analyses the ECG rhythm and informs the rescuer if a shock is needed. AEDs are extremely accurate and will deliver a shock only when VF (or its precursor, rapid ventricular tachycardia) is present.[31] AED function and operation are discussed in Section 3.

Several studies have shown the benefit on survival of immediate CPR, and the detrimental effect of delay before defibrillation. For every minute without CPR, survival from witnessed VF decreases by 7—10%.[10] When bystander CPR is provided, the decline in survival is more gradual and averages 3—4% min^{-1}.[10,14,17] Overall, bystander CPR doubles or triples survival from witnessed cardiac arrest.[10,14,32]

Adult BLS sequence

BLS consists of the following sequence of actions (Figure 2.1).

1 Make sure you, the victim and any bystanders are safe.
2 Check the victim for a response (Figure 2.2).

Adult basic life support

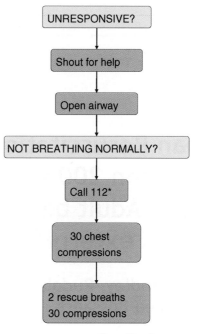

*or national emergency number

Figure 2.1 Adult basic life support algorithm.

- gently shake his shoulders and ask loudly: ''Are you all right?''
3a If he responds
  - leave him in the position in which you find him provided there is no further danger
  - try to find out what is wrong with him and get help if needed
  - reassess him regularly

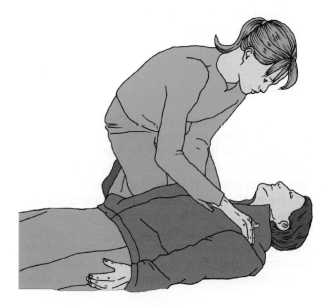

Figure 2.2 Check the victim for a response. © 2005 European Resuscitation Council.

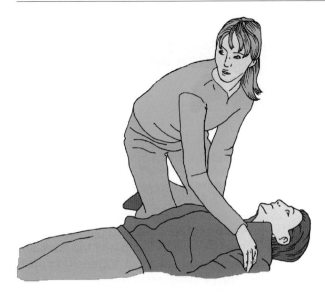

Figure 2.3 Shout for help. © 2005 European Resuscitation Council.

3b If he does not respond
- shout for help (Figure 2.3)
- turn the victim onto his back and then open the airway using head tilt and chin lift (Figure 2.4)
  - ○ place your hand on his forehead and gently tilt his head back keeping your thumb and

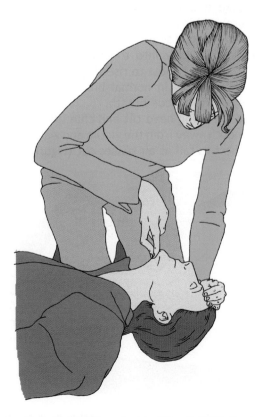

Figure 2.4 Head tilt and chin lift. © 2005 European Resuscitation Council.

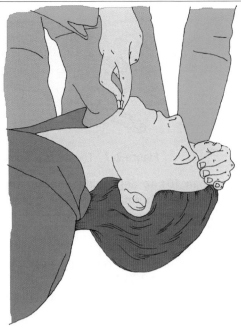

Figure 2.5 Head tilt and chin lift in detail. © 2005 European Resuscitation Council.

index finger free to close his nose if rescue breathing is required (Figure 2.5)
  - ○ with your fingertips under the point of the victim's chin, lift the chin to open the airway
4 Keeping the airway open, look, listen and feel for normal breathing (Figure 2.6).
- Look for chest movement.
- Listen at the victim's mouth for breath sounds.
- Feel for air on your cheek.

In the first few minutes after cardiac arrest, a victim may be barely breathing, or taking infrequent, noisy gasps. Do not confuse this with normal breathing. Look, listen, and feel for no

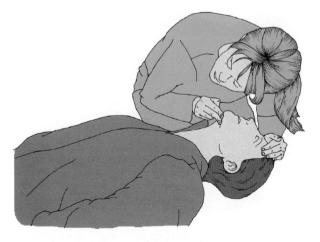

Figure 2.6 Look listen and feel for normal breathing. © 2005 European Resuscitation Council.

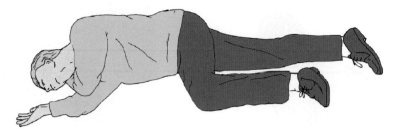

Figure 2.7 The recovery position. © 2005 European Resuscitation Council.

more than 10 s to determine whether the victim is breathing normally. If you have any doubt whether breathing is normal, act as if it is not normal.

5a If he is breathing normally
- turn him into the recovery position (see below) (Figure 2.7)
- send or go for help/call for an ambulance
- check for continued breathing

5b If he is not breathing normally
- send someone for help or, if you are on your own, leave the victim and alert the ambulance service; return and start chest compression as follows:
  - kneel by the side of the victim
  - place the heel of one hand in the centre of the victim's chest (Figure 2.8)
  - place the heel of your other hand on top of the first hand (Figure 2.9)
  - interlock the fingers of your hands and ensure that pressure is not applied over the victim's ribs (Figure 2.10). Do not apply any pressure over the upper abdomen or the bottom end of the bony sternum (breastbone)
  - position yourself vertically above the victim's chest and, with your arms straight, press down on the sternum 4—5 cm (Figure 2.11)
  - after each compression, release all the pressure on the chest without losing contact between your hands and the sternum; repeat at a rate of about 100 min^{-1} (a little less than 2 compressions s^{-1})
  - compression and release should take equal amounts of time

6a Combine chest compression with rescue breaths.
- After 30 compressions open the airway again using head tilt and chin lift (Figure 2.12).
- Pinch the soft part of the nose closed, using the index finger and thumb of your hand on the forehead.
- Allow the mouth to open, but maintain chin lift.
- Take a normal breath and place your lips around his the mouth, making sure that you have a good seal.
- Blow steadily into the mouth while watching for the chest to rise (Figure 2.13), taking about 1 s as in normal breathing; this is an effective rescue breath.
- Maintaining head tilt and chin lift, take your mouth away from the victim and watch for the chest to fall as air passes out (Figure 2.14).

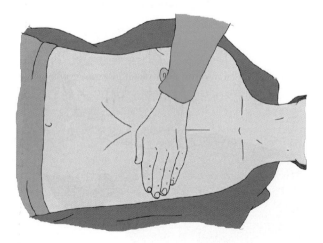

Figure 2.8 Place the heel of one hand in the centre of the victim's chest. © 2005 European Resuscitation Council.

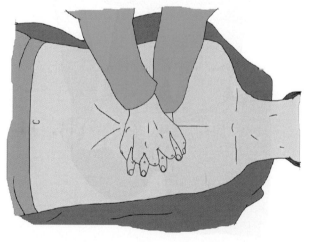

Figure 2.9 Place the heel of your other hand on top of the first hand. © 2005 European Resuscitation Council.

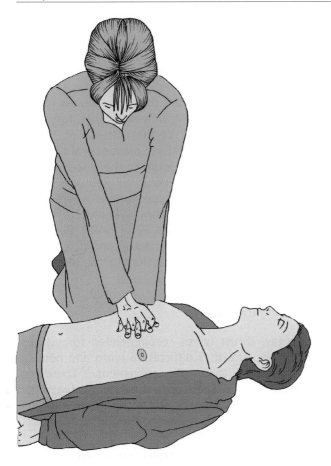

Figure 2.10 Interlock the fingers of your hands. © 2005 European Resuscitation Council.

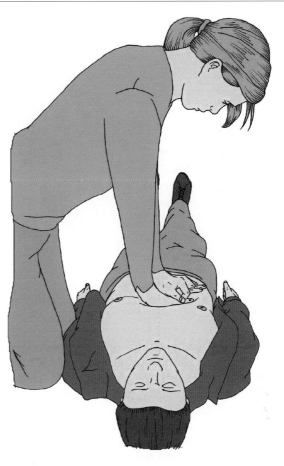

Figure 2.11 Press down on the sternum 4—5 cm. © 2005 European Resuscitation Council.

- Take another normal breath and blow into the victim's mouth once more, to achieve a total of two effective rescue breaths. Then return your hands without delay to the correct position on the sternum and give a further 30 chest compressions.
- Continue with chest compressions and rescue breaths in a ratio of 30:2.
- Stop to recheck the victim only if he starts breathing normally; otherwise do not interrupt resuscitation.

  If your initial rescue breath does not make the chest rise as in normal breathing, then before your next attempt:
- check the victim's mouth and remove any obstruction
- recheck that there is adequate head tilt and chin lift
- do not attempt more than two breaths each time before returning to chest compressions

  If there is more than one rescuer present, another should take over CPR every 1—2 min to prevent fatigue. Ensure the minimum of delay during the changeover of rescuers.

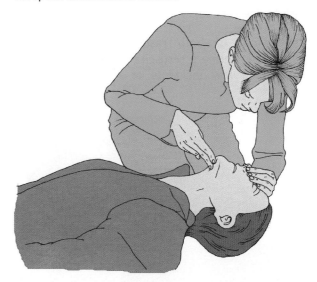

Figure 2.12 After 30 compressions open the airway again using head tilt and chin lift. © 2005 European Resuscitation Council.

6b Chest-compression-only CPR may be used as follows.
- If you are not able or are unwilling to give rescue breaths, give chest compressions only.

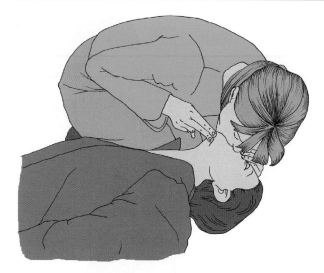

Figure 2.13 Blow steadily into his mouth whilst watching for his chest to rise. © 2005 European Resuscitation Council.

- If chest compressions only are given, these should be continuous, at a rate of $100\,min^{-1}$.
- Stop to recheck the victim only if he starts breathing normally; otherwise do not interrupt resuscitation.

7 Continue resuscitation until
- qualified help arrives and takes over
- the victim starts breathing normally
- you become exhausted

Risk to the rescuer

The safety of both rescuer and victim are paramount during a resuscitation attempt. There have been few incidents of rescuers suffering

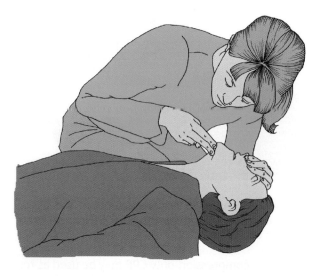

Figure 2.14 Take your mouth away from the victim and watch for his chest to fall as air comes out. © 2005 European Resuscitation Council.

adverse effects from undertaking CPR, with only isolated reports of infections such as tuberculosis (TB)[33] and severe acute respiratory distress syndrome (SARS).[34] Transmission of HIV during CPR has never been reported. There have been no human studies to address the effectiveness of barrier devices during CPR; however, laboratory studies have shown that certain filters, or barrier devices with one-way valves, prevent oral bacterial transmission from the victim to the rescuer during mouth-to-mouth ventilation.[35,36] Rescuers should take appropriate safety precautions where feasible, especially if the victim is known to have a serious infection, such as TB or SARS. During an outbreak of a highly infectious condition such as SARS, full protective precautions for the rescuer are essential.

Opening the airway

The jaw thrust is not recommended for lay rescuers because it is difficult to learn and perform and may itself cause spinal movement.[37] Therefore, the lay rescuer should open the airway using a head tilt-chin lift manoeuvre for both injured and non-injured victims.

Recognition of cardiorespiratory arrest

Checking the carotid pulse is an inaccurate method of confirming the presence or absence of circulation.[38] However, there is no evidence that checking for movement, breathing or coughing ('signs of a circulation') is diagnostically superior. Healthcare professionals as well as lay rescuers have difficulty determining the presence or absence of adequate or normal breathing in unresponsive victims.[39,40] This may be because the airway is not open[41] or because the victim is making occasional (agonal) gasps. When bystanders are asked by ambulance dispatchers over the telephone if breathing is present, they often misinterpret agonal gasps as normal breathing. This erroneous information can result in the bystander withholding CPR from a cardiac arrest victim.[42] Agonal gasps are present in up to 40% of cardiac arrest victims. Bystanders describe agonal gasps as barely breathing, heavy or laboured breathing, or noisy or gasping breathing.[43]

Laypeople should, therefore, be taught to begin CPR if the victim is unconscious (unresponsive) and not breathing normally. It should be emphasised during training that agonal gasps occur commonly in the first few minutes after SCA. They are an indication for starting CPR immediately and should not be confused with normal breathing.

Initial rescue breaths

During the first few min after non-asphyxial cardiac arrest the blood oxygen content remains high, and myocardial and cerebral oxygen delivery is limited more by the diminished cardiac output than a lack of oxygen in the lungs. Ventilation is, therefore, initially less important than chest compression.[44]

It is well recognised that skill acquisition and retention is aided by simplification of the BLS sequence of actions.[45] It is also recognized that rescuers are frequently unwilling to carry out mouth-to-mouth ventilation for a variety of reasons, including fear of infection and distaste for the procedure.[46–48] For these reasons, and to emphasise the priority of chest compressions, it is recommended that in adults CPR should start with chest compression rather than initial ventilation.

Ventilation

During CPR the purpose of ventilation is to maintain adequate oxygenation. The optimal tidal volume, respiratory rate and inspired oxygen concentration to achieve this, however, are not fully known. The current recommendations are based on the following evidence:

1. During CPR, blood flow to the lungs is substantially reduced, so an adequate ventilation-perfusion ratio can be maintained with lower tidal volumes and respiratory rates than normal.[49]
2. Not only is hyperventilation (too many breaths or too large a volume) unnecessary, but it is harmful because it increases intrathoracic pressure, thus decreasing venous return to the heart and diminishing cardiac output. Survival is consequently reduced.[50]
3. When the airway is unprotected, a tidal volume of 1 l produces significantly more gastric distention than a tidal volume of 500 ml.[51]
4. Low minute-ventilation (lower than normal tidal volume and respiratory rate) can maintain effective oxygenation and ventilation during CPR.[52–55] During adult CPR, tidal volumes of approximately 500–600 ml (6–7 ml kg^{-1}) should be adequate.
5. Interruptions in chest compression (for example to give rescue breaths) have a detrimental effect on survival.[56] Giving rescue breaths over a shorter time will help to reduce the duration of essential interruptions.

The current recommendation is, therefore, for rescuers to give each rescue breath over about 1 s, with enough volume to make the victim's chest rise, but to avoid rapid or forceful breaths This recommendation applies to all forms of ventilation during CPR, including mouth-to-mouth and bag-valve-mask (BVM) with and without supplementary oxygen.

Mouth-to-nose ventilation is an effective alternative to mouth-to-mouth ventilation.[57] It may be considered if the victim's mouth is seriously injured or cannot be opened, the rescuer is assisting a victim in the water, or a mouth-to-mouth seal is difficult to achieve.

There is no published evidence on the safety, effectiveness or feasibility of mouth-to-tracheostomy ventilation, but it may be used for a victim with a tracheostomy tube or tracheal stoma who requires rescue breathing.

To use bag-mask ventilation requires considerable practice and skill.[58,59] The lone rescuer has to be able to open the airway with a jaw thrust while simultaneously holding the mask to the victim's face. It is a technique that is appropriate only for lay rescuers who work in highly specialised areas, such as where there is a risk of cyanide poisoning or exposure to other toxic agents. There are other specific circumstances in which non-healthcare providers receive extended training in first aid which could include training, and retraining, in the use of bag-mask ventilation. The same strict training that applies to healthcare professionals should be followed.

Chest compression

Chest compressions produce blood flow by increasing the intrathoracic pressure and by directly compressing the heart. Although chest compressions performed properly can produce systolic arterial pressure peaks of 60–80 mmHg, diastolic pressure remains low and mean arterial pressure in the carotid artery seldom exceeds 40 mmHg.[60] Chest compressions generate a small but critical amount of blood flow to the brain and myocardium and increase the likelihood that defibrillation will be successful. They are especially important if the first shock is delivered more than 5 min after collapse.[61]

Much of the information about the physiology of chest compression and the effects of varying the compression rate, compression-to-ventilation ratio and duty cycle (ratio of time chest is compressed to total time from one compression to the next) is derived from animal models. However, the conclusions of the 2005 Consensus Conference[62] included the following:

(1) Each time compressions are resumed, the rescuer should place his hands without delay ''in the centre of the chest''.[63]

(2) Compress the chest at a rate of about 100 min^{-1}.[64–66]

(3) Pay attention to achieving the full compression depth of 4–5 cm (for an adult).[67,68]

(4) Allow the chest to recoil completely after each compression.[69,70]

(5) Take approximately the same amount of time for compression and relaxation.

(6) Minimise interruptions in chest compression.

(7) Do not rely on a palpable carotid or femoral pulse as a gauge of effective arterial flow.[38,71]

There is insufficient evidence to support a specific hand position for chest compression during CPR in adults. Previous guidelines have recommended a method of finding the middle of the lower half of the sternum by placing one finger on the lower end of the sternum and sliding the other hand down to it.[72] It has been shown that for healthcare professionals the same hand position can be found more quickly if rescuers are taught to ''place the heel of your hand in the centre of the chest with the other hand on top'', provided the teaching includes a demonstration of placing the hands in the middle of the lower half of the sternum.[63] It is reasonable to extend this to laypeople.

Compression rate refers to the speed at which compressions are given, not the total number delivered in each minute. The number delivered is determined by the rate, but also by the number of interruptions to open the airway, deliver rescue breaths and allow AED analysis. In one out-of-hospital study rescuers recorded compression rates of 100–120 min^{-1} but, the mean number of compressions was reduced to 64 min^{-1} by frequent interruptions.[68]

Compression—ventilation ratio

Insufficient evidence from human outcome studies exists to support any given compression:ventilation ratio. Animal data support an increase in the ratio above 15:2.[73–75] A mathematical model suggests that a ratio of 30:2 would provide the best compromise between blood flow and oxygen delivery.[76,77] A ratio of 30 compressions to two ventilations is recommended for the single rescuer attempting resuscitation on an adult or child out of hospital. This should decrease the number of interruptions in compression, reduce the likelihood of hyperventilation,[50,78] simplify instruction for teaching and improve skill retention.

Compression-only CPR

Healthcare professionals as well as lay rescuers admit to being reluctant to perform mouth-to-mouth ventilation in unknown victims of cardiac arrest.[46,48] Animal studies have shown that chest compression-only CPR may be as effective as combined ventilation and compression in the first few minutes after non-asphyxial arrest.[44,79] In adults, the outcome of chest compression without ventilation is significantly better than the outcome of giving no CPR.[80] If the airway is open, occasional gasps and passive chest recoil may provide some air exchange.[81,82] A low minute-ventilation may be all that is necessary to maintain a normal ventilation-perfusion ratio during CPR.

Laypeople should, therefore, be encouraged to perform compression-only CPR if they are unable or unwilling to provide rescue breaths, although combined chest compression and ventilation is the better method of CPR.

CPR in confined spaces

Over-the-head CPR for single rescuers and straddle CPR for two rescuers may be considered for resuscitation in confined spaces.[83,84]

Recovery position

There are several variations of the recovery position, each with its own advantages. No single position is perfect for all victims.[85,86] The position should be stable, near a true lateral position with the head dependent, and with no pressure on the chest to impair breathing.[87]

The ERC recommends the following sequence of actions to place a victim in the recovery position:

- Remove the victim's spectacles.
- Kneel beside the victim and make sure that both legs are straight.
- Place the arm nearest to you out at right angles to the body, elbow bent with the hand palm uppermost (Figure 2.15).
- Bring the far arm across the chest, and hold the back of the hand against the victim's cheek nearest to you (Figure 2.16).
- With your other hand, grasp the far leg just above the knee and pull it up, keeping the foot on the ground (Figure 2.17).
- Keeping his hand pressed against his cheek, pull on the far leg to roll the victim towards you onto his side.
- Adjust the upper leg so that both hip and knee are bent at right angles.
- Tilt the head back to make sure the airway remains open.

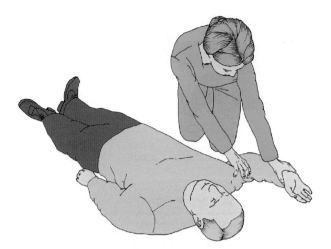

Figure 2.15 Place the arm nearest to you out at right angles to his body, elbow bent with the hand palm uppermost. © 2005 European Resuscitation Council.

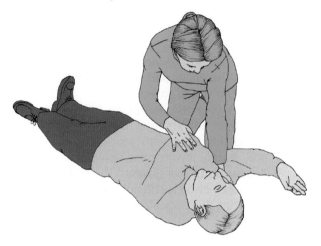

Figure 2.16 Bring the far arm across the chest, and hold the back of the hand against the victim's cheek nearest to you. © 2005 European Resuscitation Council.

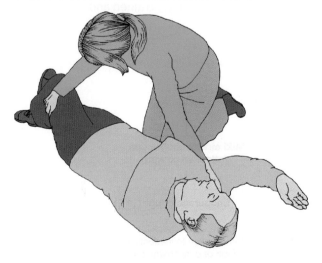

Figure 2.17 With your other hand, grasp the far leg just above the knee and pull it up, keeping the foot on the ground. © 2005 European Resuscitation Council.

- Adjust the hand under the cheek, if necessary, to keep the head tilted (Figure 2.18).
- Check breathing regularly.

If the victim has to be kept in the recovery position for more than 30 min turn him to the opposite side to relieve the pressure on the lower arm.

Foreign-body airway obstruction (choking)

Foreign-body airway obstruction (FBAO) is an uncommon but potentially treatable cause of accidental death.[88] Each year approximately 16,000 adults and children in the UK receive treatment in an emergency department for FBAO. Fortunately, less than 1% of these incidents are fatal.[89] The commonest cause of choking in adults is airway obstruction caused by food such as fish, meat or poultry.[89] In infants and children, half the reported episodes of choking occur while eating (mostly confectionery), and the remaining choking episodes occur with non-food items such as coins or toys.[90] Deaths from choking are rare in infants and children; 24 deaths a year on average were reported in the UK between 1986 and 1995, and over half of these children were under 1 year.[90]

As most choking events are associated with eating, they are commonly witnessed. Thus, there is often the opportunity for early intervention while the victim is still responsive.

Recognition

Because recognition of airway obstruction is the key to successful outcome, it is important not to confuse this emergency with fainting, heart attack, seizure or other conditions that may cause sudden respiratory distress, cyanosis or loss of consciousness. Foreign bodies may cause either mild or severe airway obstruction. The signs and symptoms enabling differentiation between mild and severe airway obstruction are summarised in Table 2.1. It is important to ask the conscious victim 'Are you choking?'

Adult FBAO (choking) sequence

(This sequence is also suitable for use in children over the age of 1 year) (Figure 2.19).

1 If the victim shows signs of mild airway obstruction
  - Encourage him to continue coughing but do nothing else
2 If the victim shows signs of severe airway obstruction and is conscious

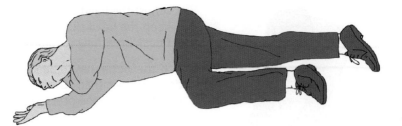

Figure 2.18 The recovery position. © 2005 European Resuscitation Council.

Table 2.1 Differentiation between mild and severe foreign body airway obstruction (FBAO)[a]

Sign	Mild obstruction	Severe obstruction
''Are you choking?''	''Yes''	Unable to speak, may nod
Other signs	Can speak, cough, breathe	Cannot breathe/wheezy breathing/silent attempts to cough/unconsciousness

[a] General signs of FBAO: attack occurs while eating; victim may clutch at neck.

- Apply up to five back blows as follows.
  - Stand to the side and slightly behind the victim.
  - Support the chest with one hand and lean the victim well forwards so that when the obstructing object is dislodged it comes out of the mouth rather than goes further down the airway.
  - Give up to five sharp blows between the shoulder blades with the heel of your other hand
- Check to see if each back blow has relieved the airway obstruction. The aim is to relieve the obstruction with each slap rather than necessarily to give all five.
- If five back blows fail to relieve the airway obstruction, give up to five abdominal thrusts as follows:
  - Stand behind the victim and put both arms round the upper part of his abdomen.
  - Lean the victim forwards.
  - Clench your fist and place it between the umbilicus and xiphisternum.
  - Grasp this hand with your other hand and pull sharply inwards and upwards.
  - Repeat up to five times.
- If the obstruction is still not relieved, continue alternating five back blows with five abdominal thrusts.

3 If the victim at any time becomes unconscious.
- Support the victim carefully to the ground.
- Immediately activate EMS.
- Begin CPR (from 5b of the adult BLS sequence). Healthcare providers, trained and experienced

Adult FBAO Treatment

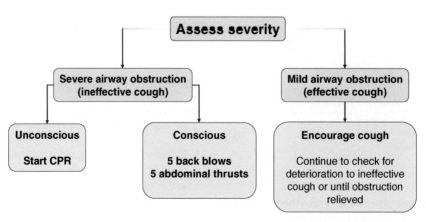

Figure 2.19 Adult foreign body airway obstruction treatment algorithm.

in feeling for a carotid pulse, should initiate chest compressions, even if a pulse is present in the unconscious choking victim.

FBAO causing mild airway obstruction

Coughing generates high and sustained airway pressures and may expel the foreign body. Aggressive treatment, with back blows, abdominal thrusts and chest compression, may cause potentially serious complications and could worsen the airway obstruction. It should be reserved for victims who have signs of severe airway obstruction. Victims with mild airway obstruction should remain under continuous observation until they improve, as severe airway obstruction may develop.

FBAO with severe airway obstruction

The clinical data on choking are largely retrospective and anecdotal. For conscious adults and children over 1 year with a complete FBAO, case reports demonstrate the effectiveness of back blows or 'slaps', abdominal thrusts and chest thrusts.[91] Approximately 50% of episodes of airway obstruction are not relieved by a single technique.[92] The likelihood of success is increased when combinations of back blows or slaps, and abdominal and chest thrusts are used.[91]

A randomised trial in cadavers[93] and two prospective studies in anaesthetised volunteers[94,95] showed that higher airway pressures can be generated using chest thrusts compared with abdominal thrusts. Since chest thrusts are virtually identical to chest compressions, rescuers should be taught to start CPR if a victim of known or suspected FBAO becomes unconscious. During CPR, each time the airway is opened the victim's mouth should be quickly checked for any foreign body that has been partly expelled. The incidence of unsuspected choking as a cause of unconsciousness or cardiac arrest is low; therefore, during CPR routinely checking the mouth for foreign bodies is not necessary.

The finger sweep

No studies have evaluated the routine use of a finger sweep to clear the airway in the absence of visible airway obstruction,[96–98] and four case reports have documented harm to the victim[96,99] or rescuer.[91] Therefore, avoid use of a blind finger sweep and manually remove solid material in the airway only if it can be seen.

Aftercare and referral for medical review

Following successful treatment for FBAO, foreign material may nevertheless remain in the upper or lower respiratory tract and cause complications later. Victims with a persistent cough, difficulty swallowing or the sensation of an object being still stuck in the throat, should therefore be referred for a medical opinion.

Abdominal thrusts can cause serious internal injuries, and all victims treated with abdominal thrusts should be examined for injury by a doctor.[91]

Resuscitation of children (see also Section 6) and victims of drowning (see also Section 7c)

Both ventilation and compression are important for victims of cardiac arrest when the oxygen stores become depleted—about 4–6 min after collapse from VF and immediately after collapse from asphyxial arrest. Previous guidelines tried to take into account the difference in pathophysiology, and recommended that victims of identifiable asphyxia (drowning; trauma; intoxication) and children should receive 1 min of CPR before the lone rescuer left the victim to get help. The majority of cases of SCA out of hospital, however, occur in adults, and are of cardiac origin due to VF. These additional recommendations, therefore, added to the complexity of the guidelines while affecting only a minority of victims.

It is important to be aware that many children do not receive resuscitation because potential rescuers fear causing harm. This fear is unfounded; it is far better to use the adult BLS sequence for resuscitation of a child than to do nothing. For ease of teaching and retention, therefore, laypeople should be taught that the adult sequence may also be used for children who are not responsive and not breathing.

The following minor modifications to the adult sequence will, however, make it even more suitable for use in children.

• Give five initial rescue breaths before starting chest compressions (adult sequence of actions, 5b).

- A lone rescuer should perform CPR for approximately 1 min before going for help.
- Compress the chest by approximately one third of its depth; use two fingers for an infant under 1 year; use one or two hands for a child over 1 year as needed to achieve an adequate depth of compression.

The same modifications of five initial breaths, and 1 min of CPR by the lone rescuer before getting help, may improve outcome for victims of drowning. This modification should be taught only to those who have a specific duty of care to potential drowning victims (e.g. lifeguards). Drowning is easily identified. It can be difficult, on the other hand, for a layperson to determine whether cardiorespiratory arrest is a direct result of trauma or intoxication. These victims should, therefore, be managed according to the standard protocol.

Use of an automated external defibrillator

Section 3 discusses the guidelines for defibrillation using both automated external defibrillators (AEDs) and manual defibrillators. However, there are some special considerations when an AED is to be used by lay or non-healthcare rescuers.

Standard AEDs are suitable for use in children older than 8 years. For children between 1 and 8 years use paediatric pads or a paediatric mode if available; if these are not available, use the AED as it is. Use of AEDs is not recommended for children less than 1 year.

Sequence for use of an AED

See Figure 2.20.

(1) Make sure you, the victim, and any bystanders are safe.
(2) If the victim is unresponsive and not breathing normally, send someone for the AED and to call for an ambulance.
(3) Start CPR according to the guidelines for BLS.
(4) As soon as the defibrillator arrives
- switch on the defibrillator and attach the electrode pads. If more than one rescuer is present, CPR should be continued while this is carried out
- follow the spoken/visual directions
- ensure that nobody touches the victim while the AED is analysing the rhythm
5a If a shock is indicated
- ensure that nobody touches the victim

- push shock button as directed (fully automatic AEDs will deliver the shock automatically)
- continue as directed by the voice/visual prompts
5b If no shock indicated
- immediately resume CPR, using a ratio of 30 compressions to 2 rescue breaths
- continue as directed by the voice/visual prompts
6 Continue to follow the AED prompts until
- qualified help arrives and takes over
- the victim starts to breathe normally
- you become exhausted

CPR before defibrillation

Immediate defibrillation, as soon as an AED becomes available, has always been a key element in guidelines and teaching, and considered of paramount importance for survival from ventricular fibrillation. This concept has been challenged because evidence suggests that a period of chest compression before defibrillation may improve survival when the time between calling for the ambulance and its arrival exceeds 5 min.[28,61,100] One study[101] did not confirm this benefit, but the weight of evidence supports a period of CPR for victims of prolonged cardiac arrest before defibrillation.

In all of these studies CPR was performed by paramedics, who protected the airway by intubation and delivered 100% oxygen. Such high-quality ventilation cannot be expected from lay rescuers giving mouth-to-mouth ventilation. Secondly, the benefit from CPR occurred only when the delay from call to the availability of a defibrillator was greater than 5 min; the delay from collapse to arrival of the rescuer with an AED will rarely be known with certainty. Thirdly, if good bystander CPR is already in progress when the AED arrives, it does not seem logical to continue it any further. For these reasons these guidelines recommend an immediate shock, as soon as the AED is available. The importance of early uninterrupted external chest compression is emphasised.

Voice prompts

In several places, the sequence of actions states 'follow the voice/visual prompts'. The prompts are usually programmable, and it is recommended that they be set in accordance with the sequence of shocks and timings for CPR given in Section 2. These should include at least:

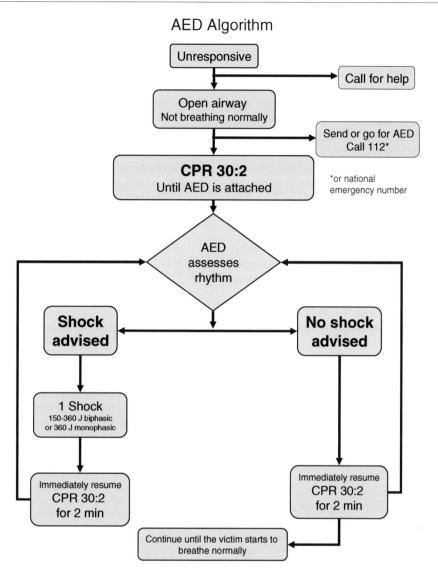

Figure 2.20 Algorithm for use of an automated external defibrillator.

(1) a single shock only, when a shockable rhythm is detected
(2) no rhythm check, or check for breathing or a pulse, after the shock
(3) a voice prompt for immediate resumption of CPR after the shock (giving chest compressions in the presence of a spontaneous circulation is not harmful)
(4) two minutes for CPR before a prompt to assess the rhythm, breathing or a pulse is given

The shock sequence and energy levels are discussed in Section 3.

Fully-automatic AEDs

Having detected a shockable rhythm, a fully-automatic AED will deliver a shock without further input from the rescuer. One manikin study showed that untrained nursing students committed fewer safety errors using a fully-automatic AED rather than a semi-automatic AED.[102] There are no human data to determine whether these findings can be applied to clinical use.

Public access defibrillation programmes

Public access defibrillation (PAD) and first responder AED programmes may increase the number of victims who receive bystander CPR and early defibrillation, thus improving survival from out-of-hospital SCA.[103] These programmes require an organised and practised response with rescuers trained and equipped to recognise emergencies, activate the EMS system, provide CPR and use the AED.[104,105] Lay rescuer AED programmes with very rapid response times in airports,[22] on aircraft[23]or in casinos,[25] and uncontrolled studies using police officers as first responders,[106,107] have achieved reported survival rates as high as 49—74%.

The logistic problem for first responder programmes is that the rescuer needs to arrive not just earlier than the traditional EMS, but within 5—6 min of the initial call, to enable attempted defibrillation in the electrical or circulatory phase of cardiac arrest.[108] With longer delays, the survival curve flattens;[10,17] a few minutes' gain in time will have little impact when the first responder arrives more than 10 min after the call[27,109] or when a first responder does not improve on an already short EMS response time.[110] However, small reductions in response intervals achieved by first-responder programmes that have an impact on many residential victims may be more cost effective than the larger reductions in response interval achieved by PAD programmes that have an impact on fewer cardiac arrest victims.[111,112]

Recommended elements for PAD programmes include:

- a planned and practised response
- training of anticipated rescuers in CPR and use of the AED
- link with the local EMS system
- programme of continuous audit (quality improvement)

Public access defibrillation programmes are most likely to improve survival from cardiac arrest if they are established in locations where witnessed cardiac arrest is likely to occur.[113] Suitable sites might include those where the probability of cardiac arrest occurring is at least once in every 2 years (e.g., airports, casinos, sports facilities).[103] Approximately 80% of out-of-hospital cardiac arrests occur in private or residential settings;[114] this fact inevitably limits the overall impact that PAD programmes can have on survival rates. There are no studies documenting effectiveness of home AED deployment.

References

1. Recommended guidelines for uniform reporting of data from out-of-hospital cardiac arrest: the 'Utstein style'. Prepared by a Task Force of Representatives from the European Resuscitation Council, American Heart Association. Heart and Stroke Foundation of Canada, Australian Resuscitation Council. Resuscitation 1991;22:1—26.
2. Sans S, Kesteloot H, Kromhout D. The burden of cardiovascular diseases mortality in Europe. Task Force of the European Society of Cardiology on Cardiovascular Mortality and Morbidity Statistics in Europe. Eur Heart J 1997;18:1231—48.
3. Cobb LA, Fahrenbruch CE, Olsufka M, Copass MK. Changing incidence of out-of-hospital ventricular fibrillation, 1980—2000. JAMA 2002;288:3008—13.
4. Rea TD, Eisenberg MS, Sinibaldi G, White RD. Incidence of EMS-treated out-of-hospital cardiac arrest in the United States. Resuscitation 2004;63:17—24.
5. Vaillancourt C, Stiell IG. Cardiac arrest care and emergency medical services in Canada. Can J Cardiol 2004;20:1081—90.
6. Waalewijn RA, de Vos R, Koster RW. Out-of-hospital cardiac arrests in Amsterdam and its surrounding areas: results from the Amsterdam resuscitation study (ARREST) in 'Utstein' style. Resuscitation 1998;38:157—67.
7. Cummins R, Thies W. Automated external defibrillators and the Advanced Cardiac Life Support Program: a new initiative from the American Heart Association. Am J Emerg Med 1991;9:91—3.
8. Waalewijn RA, Nijpels MA, Tijssen JG, Koster RW. Prevention of deterioration of ventricular fibrillation by basic life support during out-of-hospital cardiac arrest. Resuscitation 2002;54:31—6.
9. Page S, Meerabeau L. Achieving change through reflective practice: closing the loop. Nurs Educ Today 2000;20:365—72.
10. Larsen MP, Eisenberg MS, Cummins RO, Hallstrom AP. Predicting survival from out-of-hospital cardiac arrest: a graphic model. Ann Emerg Med 1993;22:1652—8.
11. Cummins RO, Ornato JP, Thies WH, Pepe PE. Improving survival from sudden cardiac arrest: the ''chain of survival'' concept. A statement for health professionals from the Advanced Cardiac Life Support Subcommittee and the Emergency Cardiac Care Committee, American Heart Association. Circulation 1991;83:1832—47.
12. Calle PA, Lagaert L, Vanhaute O, Buylaert WA. Do victims of an out-of-hospital cardiac arrest benefit from a training program for emergency medical dispatchers? Resuscitation 1997;35:213—8.
13. Curka PA, Pepe PE, Ginger VF, Sherrard RC, Ivy MV, Zachariah BS. Emergency medical services priority dispatch. Ann Emerg Med 1993;22:1688—95.
14. Valenzuela TD, Roe DJ, Cretin S, Spaite DW, Larsen MP. Estimating effectiveness of cardiac arrest interventions: a logistic regression survival model. Circulation 1997;96:3308—13.
15. Holmberg M, Holmberg S, Herlitz J. Factors modifying the effect of bystander cardiopulmonary resuscitation on survival in out-of-hospital cardiac arrest patients in Sweden. Eur Heart J 2001;22:511—9.
16. Holmberg M, Holmberg S, Herlitz J, Gardelov B. Survival after cardiac arrest outside hospital in Sweden. Swedish Cardiac Arrest Registry. Resuscitation 1998;36:29—36.
17. Waalewijn RA, De Vos R, Tijssen JGP, Koster RW. Survival models for out-of-hospital cardiopulmonary resuscitation from the perspectives of the bystander, the first responder, and the paramedic. Resuscitation 2001;51:113—22.
18. Weaver WD, Hill D, Fahrenbruch CE, et al. Use of the automatic external defibrillator in the management of out-of-hospital cardiac arrest. N Engl J Med 1988;319:661—6.
19. Auble TE, Menegazzi JJ, Paris PM. Effect of out-of-hospital defibrillation by basic life support providers on cardiac arrest mortality: a metaanalysis. Ann Emerg Med 1995;25:642—58.
20. Stiell IG, Wells GA, DeMaio VJ, et al. Modifiable factors associated with improved cardiac arrest survival in a multicenter basic life support/defibrillation system: OPALS

Study Phase I results. Ontario Prehospital Advanced Life Support. Ann Emerg Med 1999;33:44—50.

21. Stiell IG, Wells GA, Field BJ, et al. Improved out-of-hospital cardiac arrest survival through the inexpensive optimization of an existing defibrillation program: OPALS study phase II. Ontario Prehospital Advanced Life Support. JAMA 1999;281:1175—81.

22. Caffrey S. Feasibility of public access to defibrillation. Curr Opin Crit Care 2002;8:195—8.

23. O'Rourke MF, Donaldson E, Geddes JS. An airline cardiac arrest program. Circulation 1997;96:2849—53.

24. Page RL, Hamdan MH, McKenas DK. Defibrillation aboard a commercial aircraft. Circulation 1998;97:1429—30.

25. Valenzuela TD, Roe DJ, Nichol G, Clark LL, Spaite DW, Hardman RG. Outcomes of rapid defibrillation by security officers after cardiac arrest in casinos. N Engl J Med 2000;343:1206—9.

26. Langhelle A, Nolan JP, Herlitz J, et al. Recommended guidelines for reviewing, reporting, and conducting research on post-resuscitation care: the Utstein style. Resuscitation 2005;66:271—83.

27. van Alem AP, Vrenken RH, de Vos R, Tijssen JG, Koster RW. Use of automated external defibrillator by first responders in out of hospital cardiac arrest: prospective controlled trial. BMJ 2003;327:1312—7.

28. Cobb LA, Fahrenbruch CE, Walsh TR, et al. Influence of cardiopulmonary resuscitation prior to defibrillation in patients with out-of-hospital ventricular fibrillation. JAMA 1999;281:1182—8.

29. Wik L, Myklebust H, Auestad BH, Steen PA. Retention of basic life support skills 6 months after training with an automated voice advisory manikin system without instructor involvement. Resuscitation 2002;52:273—9.

30. White RD, Russell JK. Refibrillation, resuscitation and survival in out-of-hospital sudden cardiac arrest victims treated with biphasic automated external defibrillators. Resuscitation 2002;55:17—23.

31. Kerber RE, Becker LB, Bourland JD, et al. Automatic external defibrillators for public access defibrillation: recommendations for specifying and reporting arrhythmia analysis algorithm performance, incorporating new waveforms, and enhancing safety. A statement for health professionals from the American Heart Association Task Force on Automatic External Defibrillation, Subcommittee on AED Safety and Efficacy. Circulation 1997;95:1677—82.

32. Holmberg M, Holmberg S, Herlitz J. Effect of bystander cardiopulmonary resuscitation in out-of-hospital cardiac arrest patients in Sweden. Resuscitation 2000;47:59—70.

33. Heilman KM, Muschenheim C. Primary cutaneous tuberculosis resulting from mouth-to-mouth respiration. N Engl J Med 1965;273:1035—6.

34. Christian MD, Loutfy M, McDonald LC, et al. Possible SARS coronavirus transmission during cardiopulmonary resuscitation. Emerg Infect Dis 2004;10:287—93.

35. Cydulka RK, Connor PJ, Myers TF, Pavza G, Parker M. Prevention of oral bacterial flora transmission by using mouth-to-mask ventilation during CPR. J Emerg Med 1991;9:317—21.

36. Blenkharn JI, Buckingham SE, Zideman DA. Prevention of transmission of infection during mouth-to-mouth resuscitation. Resuscitation 1990;19:151—7.

37. Aprahamian C, Thompson BM, Finger WA, Darin JC. Experimental cervical spine injury model: evaluation of airway management and splinting techniques. Ann Emerg Med 1984;13:584—7.

38. Bahr J, Klingler H, Panzer W, Rode H, Kettler D. Skills of lay people in checking the carotid pulse. Resuscitation 1997;35:23—6.

39. Ruppert M, Reith MW, Widmann JH, et al. Checking for breathing: evaluation of the diagnostic capability of emergency medical services personnel, physicians, medical students, and medical laypersons. Ann Emerg Med 1999;34:720—9.

40. Perkins GD, Stephenson B, Hulme J, Monsieurs KG. Birmingham assessment of breathing study (BABS). Resuscitation 2005;64:109—13.

41. Domeier RM, Evans RW, Swor RA, Rivera-Rivera EJ, Frederiksen SM. Prospective validation of out-of-hospital spinal clearance criteria: a preliminary report. Acad Emerg Med 1997;4:643—6.

42. Hauff SR, Rea TD, Culley LL, Kerry F, Becker L, Eisenberg MS. Factors impeding dispatcher-assisted telephone cardiopulmonary resuscitation. Ann Emerg Med 2003;42:731—7.

43. Clark JJ, Larsen MP, Culley LL, Graves JR, Eisenberg MS. Incidence of agonal respirations in sudden cardiac arrest. Ann Emerg Med 1992;21:1464—7.

44. Kern KB, Hilwig RW, Berg RA, Sanders AB, Ewy GA. Importance of continuous chest compressions during cardiopulmonary resuscitation: improved outcome during a simulated single lay-rescuer scenario. Circulation 2002;105:645—9.

45. Handley JA, Handley AJ. Four-step CPR—improving skill retention. Resuscitation 1998;36:3—8.

46. Ornato JP, Hallagan LF, McMahan SB, Peeples EH, Rostafinski AG. Attitudes of BCLS instructors about mouth-to-mouth resuscitation during the AIDS epidemic. Ann Emerg Med 1990;19:151—6.

47. Brenner BE, Van DC, Cheng D, Lazar EJ. Determinants of reluctance to perform CPR among residents and applicants: the impact of experience on helping behavior. Resuscitation 1997;35:203—11.

48. Hew P, Brenner B, Kaufman J. Reluctance of paramedics and emergency medical technicians to perform mouth-to-mouth resuscitation. J Emerg Med 1997;15:279—84.

49. Baskett P, Nolan J, Parr M. Tidal volumes which are perceived to be adequate for resuscitation. Resuscitation 1996;31:231—4.

50. Aufderheide TP, Sigurdsson G, Pirrallo RG, et al. Hyperventilation-induced hypotension during cardiopulmonary resuscitation. Circulation 2004;109:1960—5.

51. Wenzel V, Idris AH, Banner MJ, Kubilis PS, Williams JLJ. Influence of tidal volume on the distribution of gas between the lungs and stomach in the nonintubated patient receiving positive-pressure ventilation. Crit Care Med 1998;26:364—8.

52. Idris A, Gabrielli A, Caruso L. Smaller tidal volume is safe and effective for bag-valve-ventilation, but not for mouth-to-mouth ventilation: an animal model for basic life support. Circulation 1999;100(Suppl. I):I-644.

53. Idris A, Wenzel V, Banner MJ, Melker RJ. Smaller tidal volumes minimize gastric inflation during CPR with an unprotected airway. Circulation 1995;92(Suppl.):I-759.

54. Dorph E, Wik L, Steen PA. Arterial blood gases with 700 ml tidal volumes during out-of-hospital CPR. Resuscitation 2004;61:23—7.

55. Winkler M, Mauritz W, Hackl W, et al. Effects of half the tidal volume during cardiopulmonary resuscitation on acid-base balance and haemodynamics in pigs. Eur J Emerg Med 1998;5:201—6.

56. Eftestol T, Sunde K, Steen PA. Effects of interrupting precordial compressions on the calculated probability of

defibrillation success during out-of-hospital cardiac arrest. Circulation 2002;105:2270—3.

57. Ruben H. The immediate treatment of respiratory failure. Br J Anaesth 1964;36:542—9.

58. Elam JO. Bag-valve-mask O$_2$ ventilation. In: Safar P, Elam JO, editors. Advances in cardiopulmonary resuscitation: the Wolf Creek Conference on Cardiopulmonary Resuscitation. New York, NY: Springer-Verlag, Inc.; 1977. p. 73—9.

59. Dailey RH. The airway: emergency management. St. Louis, MO: Mosby Year Book; 1992.

60. Paradis NA, Martin GB, Goetting MG, et al. Simultaneous aortic, jugular bulb, and right atrial pressures during cardiopulmonary resuscitation in humans. Insights into mechanisms. Circulation 1989;80:361—8.

61. Wik L, Hansen TB, Fylling F, et al. Delaying defibrillation to give basic cardiopulmonary resuscitation to patients with out-of-hospital ventricular fibrillation: a randomized trial. JAMA 2003;289:1389—95.

62. International Liaison Committee on Resuscitation. International consensus on cardiopulmonary resuscitation and emergency cardiovascular care science with treatment recommendations. Resuscitation 2005;67.

63. Handley AJ. Teaching hand placement for chest compression—a simpler technique. Resuscitation 2002;53:29—36.

64. Yu T, Weil MH, Tang W, et al. Adverse outcomes of interrupted precordial compression during automated defibrillation. Circulation 2002;106:368—72.

65. Swenson RD, Weaver WD, Niskanen RA, Martin J, Dahlberg S. Hemodynamics in humans during conventional and experimental methods of cardiopulmonary resuscitation. Circulation 1988;78:630—9.

66. Kern KB, Sanders AB, Raife J, Milander MM, Otto CW, Ewy GA. A study of chest compression rates during cardiopulmonary resuscitation in humans: the importance of rate-directed chest compressions. Arch Intern Med 1992;152:145—9.

67. Abella BS, Alvarado JP, Myklebust H, et al. Quality of cardiopulmonary resuscitation during in-hospital cardiac arrest. JAMA 2005;293:305—10.

68. Wik L, Kramer-Johansen J, Myklebust H, et al. Quality of cardiopulmonary resuscitation during out-of-hospital cardiac arrest. JAMA 2005;293:299—304.

69. Aufderheide TP, Pirrallo RG, Yannopoulos D, et al. Incomplete chest wall decompression: a clinical evaluation of CPR performance by EMS personnel and assessment of alternative manual chest compression—decompression techniques. Resuscitation 2005;64:353—62.

70. Yannopoulos D, McKnite S, Aufderheide TP, et al. Effects of incomplete chest wall decompression during cardiopulmonary resuscitation on coronary and cerebral perfusion pressures in a porcine model of cardiac arrest. Resuscitation 2005;64:363—72.

71. Ochoa FJ, Ramalle-Gomara E, Carpintero JM, Garcia A, Saralegui I. Competence of health professionals to check the carotid pulse. Resuscitation 1998;37:173—5.

72. Handley AJ, Monsieurs KG, Bossaert LL. European Resuscitation Council Guidelines 2000 for Adult Basic Life Support. A statement from the Basic Life Support and Automated External Defibrillation Working Group(1) and approved by the Executive Committee of the European Resuscitation Council. Resuscitation 2001;48:199—205.

73. Sanders AB, Kern KB, Berg RA, Hilwig RW, Heidenrich J, Ewy GA. Survival and neurologic outcome after cardiopulmonary resuscitation with four different chest compression-ventilation ratios. Ann Emerg Med 2002;40:553—62.

74. Dorph E, Wik L, Stromme TA, Eriksen M, Steen PA. Quality of CPR with three different ventilation:compression ratios. Resuscitation 2003;58:193—201.

75. Dorph E, Wik L, Stromme TA, Eriksen M, Steen PA. Oxygen delivery and return of spontaneous circulation with ventilation:compression ratio 2:30 versus chest compressions only CPR in pigs. Resuscitation 2004;60:309—18.

76. Babbs CF, Kern KB. Optimum compression to ventilation ratios in CPR under realistic, practical conditions: a physiological and mathematical analysis. Resuscitation 2002;54:147—57.

77. Fenici P, Idris AH, Lurie KG, Ursella S, Gabrielli A. What is the optimal chest compression—ventilation ratio? Curr Opin Crit Care 2005;11:204—11.

78. Aufderheide TP, Lurie KG. Death by hyperventilation: a common and life-threatening problem during cardiopulmonary resuscitation. Crit Care Med 2004;32:S345—51.

79. Chandra NC, Gruben KG, Tsitlik JE, et al. Observations of ventilation during resuscitation in a canine model. Circulation 1994;90:3070—5.

80. Becker LB, Berg RA, Pepe PE, et al. A reappraisal of mouth-to-mouth ventilation during bystander-initiated cardiopulmonary resuscitation. A statement for healthcare professionals from the Ventilation Working Group of the Basic Life Support and Pediatric Life Support Subcommittees, American Heart Association. Resuscitation 1997;35:189—201.

81. Berg RA, Kern KB, Hilwig RW, et al. Assisted ventilation does not improve outcome in a porcine model of single-rescuer bystander cardiopulmonary resuscitation. Circulation 1997;95:1635—41.

82. Berg RA, Kern KB, Hilwig RW, Ewy GA. Assisted ventilation during 'bystander' CPR in a swine acute myocardial infarction model does not improve outcome. Circulation 1997;96:4364—71.

83. Handley AJ, Handley JA. Performing chest compressions in a confined space. Resuscitation 2004;61:55—61.

84. Perkins GD, Stephenson BT, Smith CM, Gao F. A comparison between over-the-head and standard cardiopulmonary resuscitation. Resuscitation 2004;61:155—61.

85. Turner S, Turner I, Chapman D, et al. A comparative study of the 1992 and 1997 recovery positions for use in the UK. Resuscitation 1998;39:153—60.

86. Handley AJ. Recovery position. Resuscitation 1993;26:93—5.

87. Anonymous. Guidelines 2000 for cardiopulmonary resuscitation and emergency cardiovascular care—an international consensus on science. Resuscitation 2000;46:1—447.

88. Fingerhut LA, Cox CS, Warner M. International comparative analysis of injury mortality. Findings from the ICE on injury statistics. International collaborative effort on injury statistics. Adv Data 1998;12:1—20.

89. Industry DoTa. Choking. In: Home and leisure accident report. London: Department of Trade and Industry; 1998, p. 13—4.

90. Industry DoTa. Choking risks to children. London: Department of Trade and Industry; 1999.

91. International Liaison Committee on Resuscitation. Part 2. Adult basic life support. 2005 international consensus on cardiopulmonary resuscitation and emergency cardiovascular care science with treatment recommendations. Resuscitation 2005;67:187—200.

92. Redding JS. The choking controversy: critique of evidence on the Heimlich maneuver. Crit Care Med 1979;7:475—9.

93. Langhelle A, Sunde K, Wik L, Steen PA. Airway pressure with chest compressions versus Heimlich manoeuvre in recently dead adults with complete airway obstruction. Resuscitation 2000;44:105—8.

94. Guildner CW, Williams D, Subitch T. Airway obstructed by foreign material: the Heimlich maneuver. JACEP 1976;5:675—7.

95. Ruben H, Macnaughton FI. The treatment of food-choking. Practitioner 1978;221:725—9.

96. Hartrey R, Bingham RM. Pharyngeal trauma as a result of blind finger sweeps in the choking child. J Accid Emerg Med 1995;12:52—4.

97. Elam JO, Ruben AM, Greene DG. Resuscitation of drowning victims. JAMA 1960;174:13—6.

98. Ruben HM, Elam JO, Ruben AM, Greene DG. Investigation of upper airway problems in resuscitation. 1. Studies of pharyngeal X-rays and performance by laymen. Anesthesiology 1961;22:271—9.

99. Kabbani M, Goodwin SR. Traumatic epiglottis following blind finger sweep to remove a pharyngeal foreign body. Clin Pediatr (Phila) 1995;34:495—7.

100. Eftestol T, Wik L, Sunde K, Steen PA. Effects of cardiopulmonary resuscitation on predictors of ventricular fibrillation defibrillation success during out-of-hospital cardiac arrest. Circulation 2004;110:10—5.

101. Jacobs IG, Finn JC, Oxer HF, Jelinek GA. CPR before defibrillation in out-of-hospital cardiac arrest: a randomized trial. Emerg Med Australas 2005;17:39—45.

102. Monsieurs KG, Vogels C, Bossaert LL, Meert P, Calle PA. A study comparing the usability of fully automatic versus semi-automatic defibrillation by untrained nursing students. Resuscitation 2005;64:41—7.

103. The Public Access Defibrillation Trial Investigators. Public-access defibrillation and survival after out-of-hospital cardiac arrest. N Engl J Med 2004;351:637—46.

104. Priori SBL, Chamberlain D, Napolitano C, Arntz HR, Koster R, Monsieurs K, Capucci A, Wellens H. Policy Statement: ESC-ERC recommendations for the use of AEDs in Europe. Eur Heart J 2004;25:437—45.

105. Priori SG, Bossaert LL, Chamberlain DA, et al. Policy statement: ESC-ERC recommendations for the use of automated external defibrillators (AEDs) in Europe. Resuscitation 2004;60:245—52.

106. White RD, Bunch TJ, Hankins DG. Evolution of a community-wide early defibrillation programme experience over 13 years using police/fire personnel and paramedics as responders. Resuscitation 2005;65:279—83.

107. Mosesso Jr VN, Davis EA, Auble TE, Paris PM, Yealy DM. Use of automated external defibrillators by police officers for treatment of out-of-hospital cardiac arrest. Ann Emerg Med 1998;32:200—7.

108. Weisfeldt M, Becker L. Resuscitation after cardiac arrest. A 3-phase time-sensitive model. JAMA 2002;288:3035—8.

109. Groh WJ, Newman MM, Beal PE, Fineberg NS, Zipes DP. Limited response to cardiac arrest by police equipped with automated external defibrillators: lack of survival benefit in suburban and rural Indiana—the police as responder automated defibrillation evaluation (PARADE). Acad Emerg Med 2001;8:324—30.

110. Sayre M, Evans J, White L, Brennan T. Providing automated external defibrillators to urban police officers in addition to fire department rapid defibrillation program is not effective. Resuscitation 2005;66:189—96.

111. Nichol G, Hallstrom AP, Ornato JP, et al. Potential cost-effectiveness of public access defibrillation in the United States. Circulation 1998;97:1315—20.

112. Nichol G, Valenzuela T, Roe D, Clark L, Huszti E, Wells GA. Cost effectiveness of defibrillation by targeted responders in public settings. Circulation 2003;108:697—703.

113. Becker L, Eisenberg M, Fahrenbruch C, Cobb L. Public locations of cardiac arrest: implications for public access defibrillation. Circulation 1998;97:2106—9.

114. Becker DE. Assessment and management of cardiovascular urgencies and emergencies: cognitive and technical considerations. Anesth Progress 1988;35:212—7.

Resuscitation (2005) **67S1**, S25—S37

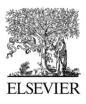

RESUSCITATION

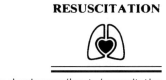

www.elsevier.com/locate/resuscitation

European Resuscitation Council Guidelines for Resuscitation 2005
Section 3. Electrical therapies: Automated external defibrillators, defibrillation, cardioversion and pacing

Charles D. Deakin, Jerry P. Nolan

Introduction

This section presents guidelines for defibrillation using both automated external defibrillators (AEDs) and manual defibrillators. All healthcare providers and lay responders can use AEDs as an integral component of basic life support. Manual defibrillation is used as part of advanced life support (ALS) therapy. In addition, synchronised cardioversion and pacing are ALS functions of many defibrillators and are also discussed in this section.

Defibrillation is the passage across the myocardium of an electrical current of sufficient magnitude to depolarise a critical mass of myocardium and enable restoration of coordinated electrical activity. Defibrillation is defined as the termination of fibrillation or, more precisely, the absence of ventricular fibrillation/ventricular tachycardia (VF/VT) at 5 s after shock delivery; however, the goal of attempted defibrillation is to restore spontaneous circulation.

Defibrillator technology is advancing rapidly. AED interaction with the rescuer through voice prompts is now established, and future technology may enable more specific instructions to be given by voice prompt. The ability of defibrillators to assess the rhythm while CPR is in progress is required to prevent unnecessary delays in CPR. Waveform analysis may also enable the defibrillator to calculate the optimal time at which to give a shock.

A vital link in the chain of survival

Defibrillation is a key link in the Chain of Survival and is one of the few interventions that have been shown to improve outcome from VF/VT cardiac arrest. The previous guidelines, published in 2000, rightly emphasised the importance of early defibrillation with minimum delay.[1]

The probability of successful defibrillation and subsequent survival to hospital discharge declines rapidly with time[2,3] and the ability to deliver early defibrillation is one of the most important factors in determining survival from cardiac arrest. For every minute that passes following collapse and defibrillation, mortality increases 7%—10% in the absence of bystander CPR.[2—4] EMS systems do not generally have the capability to deliver defibrillation through traditional paramedic responders within the first few minutes of a call, and the alternative use of trained lay responders

0300-9572/$ — see front matter © 2005 European Resuscitation Council. All Rights Reserved. Published by Elsevier Ireland Ltd.
doi:10.1016/j.resuscitation.2005.10.008

to deliver prompt defibrillation using AEDs is now widespread. EMS systems that have reduced time to defibrillation following cardiac arrest using trained lay responders have reported greatly improved survival-to-discharge rates,[5–7] some as high as 75% if defibrillation is performed within 3 min of collapse.[8] This concept has also been extended to in-hospital cardiac arrests where staff, other than doctors, are also being trained to defibrillate using an AED before arrival of the cardiac arrest team. When bystander CPR is provided, the reduction in survival rate is more gradual and averages 3%—4% per minute from collapse to defibrillation;[2–4] bystander CPR can double[2,3,9] or treble[10] survival from witnessed out-of-hospital cardiac arrest.

All healthcare providers with a duty to perform CPR should be trained, equipped, and encouraged to perform defibrillation and CPR. Early defibrillation should be available throughout all hospitals, outpatient medical facilities and public areas of mass gathering (see Section 2). Those trained in AED use should also be trained to deliver at least external chest compressions before the arrival of ALS providers, to optimise the effectiveness of early defibrillation.

Automated external defibrillators

Automated external defibrillators are sophisticated, reliable computerised devices that use voice and visual prompts to guide lay rescuers and healthcare professionals to safely attempt defibrillation in cardiac arrest victims. Automated defibrillators have been described as ''... the single greatest advance in the treatment of VF cardiac arrest since the development of CPR.''[11] Advances in technology, particularly with respect to battery capacity, and software arrhythmia analysis have enabled the mass production of relatively cheap, reliable and easily operated portable defibrillators.[12–15] Use of AEDs by lay or non-healthcare rescuers is covered in Section 2.

Automated rhythm analysis

Automated external defibrillators have microprocessors that analyse several features of the ECG, including frequency and amplitude. Some AEDs are programmed to detect spontaneous movement by the patient or others. Developing technology should soon enable AEDs to provide information about frequency and depth of chest compressions during CPR that may improve BLS performance by all rescuers.[16,17]

Automated external defibrillators have been tested extensively against libraries of recorded cardiac rhythms and in many trials in adults[18,19] and children.[20,21] They are extremely accurate in rhythm analysis. Although AEDs are not designed to deliver synchronised shocks, all AEDs will recommend shocks for VT if the rate and R-wave morphology exceed preset values.

In-hospital use of AEDs

At the time of the 2005 Consensus Conference, there were no published randomised trials comparing in-hospital use of AEDs with manual defibrillators. Two lower level studies of adults with in-hospital cardiac arrest from shockable rhythms showed higher survival-to-hospital discharge rates when defibrillation was provided through an AED programme than with manual defibrillation alone.[22,23] A manikin study showed that use of an AED significantly increased the likelihood of delivering three shocks, but increased the time to deliver the shocks when compared with manual defibrillators.[24] In contrast, a study of mock arrests in simulated patients showed that use of monitoring leads and fully automated defibrillators reduced time to defibrillation when compared with manual defibrillators.[25]

Delayed defibrillation may occur when patients sustain cardiac arrest in unmonitored hospital beds and in outpatient departments. In these areas several minutes may elapse before resuscitation teams arrive with a defibrillator and deliver shocks.[26] Despite limited evidence, AEDs should be considered for the hospital setting as a way to facilitate early defibrillation (a goal of <3 min from collapse), especially in areas where staff have no rhythm recognition skills or where they use defibrillators infrequently. An effective system for training and retraining should be in place. Adequate numbers of staff should be trained to enable achievement of the goal of providing the first shock within 3 min of collapse anywhere in the hospital. Hospitals should monitor collapse-to-first-shock intervals and resuscitation outcomes.

Strategies before defibrillation

Safe use of oxygen during defibrillation

In an oxygen-enriched atmosphere, sparking from poorly applied defibrillator paddles can cause a fire.[27–32] There are several reports of fires being caused in this way, and most have resulted in significant burns to the patient. The risk of fire during attempted defibrillation can be minimised by taking the following precautions.

- Take off any oxygen mask or nasal cannulae and place them at least 1 m away from the patient's chest.
- Leave the ventilation bag connected to the tracheal tube or other airway adjunct. Alternatively, disconnect any bag-valve device from the tracheal tube (or other airway adjunct such as the laryngeal mask airway, combitube or laryngeal tube), and remove it at least 1 m from the patient's chest during defibrillation.
- If the patient is connected to a ventilator, for example in the operating room or critical care unit, leave the ventilator tubing (breathing circuit) connected to the tracheal tube unless chest compressions prevent the ventilator from delivering adequate tidal volumes. In this case, the ventilator is usually substituted for a ventilation bag, which can itself be left connected or detached and removed to a distance of at least 1 m. If the ventilator tubing is disconnected, ensure it is kept at least 1 m from the patient or, better still, switch the ventilator off; modern ventilators generate massive oxygen flows when disconnected. During normal use, when connected to a tracheal tube, oxygen from a ventilator in the critical care unit will be vented from the main ventilator housing well away from the defibrillation zone. Patients in the critical care unit may be dependent on positive end expiratory pressure (PEEP) to maintain adequate oxygenation; during cardioversion, when the spontaneous circulation potentially enables blood to remain well oxygenated, it is particularly appropriate to leave the critically ill patient connected to the ventilator during shock delivery.
- Minimise the risk of sparks during defibrillation. Theoretically, self-adhesive defibrillation pads are less likely to cause sparks than manual paddles.

The technique for electrode contact with the chest

Optimal defibrillation technique aims to deliver current across the fibrillating myocardium in the presence of minimal transthoracic impedance. Transthoracic impedance varies considerably with body mass, but is approximately 70—80 Ω in adults.[33,34] The techniques described below aim to place external electrodes (paddles or self-adhesive pads) in an optimal position using techniques that minimise transthoracic impedance.

Shaving the chest

Patients with a hairy chest have air trapping beneath the electrode and poor electrode-to-skin electrical contact. This causes high impedance, reduced defibrillation efficacy, risk of arcing (sparks) from electrode to skin and electrode to electrode and is more likely to cause burns to the patient's chest. Rapid shaving of the area of intended electrode placement may be necessary, but do not delay defibrillation if a shaver is not immediately available. Shaving the chest per se may reduce transthoracic impedance slightly and has been recommended for elective DC cardioversion.[35]

Paddle force

If using paddles, apply them firmly to the chest wall. This reduces transthoracic impedance by improving electrical contact at the electrode—skin interface and reducing thoracic volume.[36] The defibrillator operator should always press firmly on handheld electrode paddles, the optimal force being 8 kg in adults[37] and 5 kg in children aged 1—8 years when using adult paddles[38]; 8-kg force may be attainable only by the strongest members of the cardiac arrest team, and therefore it is recommended that these individuals apply the paddles during defibrillation. Unlike self-adhesive pads, manual paddles have a bare metal plate that requires a conductive material placed between the metal and patient's skin to improve electrical contact. Use of bare metal paddles alone creates high transthoracic impedance and is likely to increase the risk of arcing and to worsen cutaneous burns from defibrillation.

Electrode position

No human studies have evaluated the electrode position as a determinant of return of spontaneous circulation (ROSC) or survival from VF/VT cardiac arrest. Transmyocardial current during defibrillation is likely to be maximal when the electrodes are placed so that the area of the heart that is fibrillating lies directly between them, i.e., ventricles in VF/VT, atria in atrial fibrillation (AF). Therefore, the optimal electrode position may not be the same for ventricular and atrial arrhythmias.

More patients are presenting with implantable medical devices (e.g., permanent pacemaker, automatic implantable cardioverter defibrillator (AICD)). MedicAlert bracelets are recommended for such patients. These devices may be damaged during defibrillation if current is discharged through electrodes placed directly over the device. Place the electrode away from the device or use an alternative electrode position as described below. On detecting VF/VT, AICD devices will discharge no more than six times. Further discharges will occur only if a new episode of VF/VT is detected. Rarely, a faulty device or broken lead may cause repeated firing; in these circumstances, the patient is likely to be conscious, with the ECG showing a relatively normal rate. A magnet placed over the AICD will disable the defibrillation function in these circumstances. AICD discharge may cause pectoral muscle contraction, but an attendant touching the patient will not receive an electric shock. AICD and pacing function should always be re-evaluated following external defibrillation, both to check the device itself and to check pacing/defibrillation thresholds of the device leads.

Transdermal drug patches may prevent good electrode contact, causing arcing and burns if the electrode is placed directly over the patch during defibrillation.[39,40] Remove medication patches and wipe the area before applying the electrode.

For ventricular arrhythmias, place electrodes (either pads or paddles) in the conventional sternal—apical position. The right (sternal) electrode is placed to the right of the sternum, below the clavicle. The apical paddle is placed in the mid-axillary line, approximately level with the V6 ECG electrode or female breast. This position should be clear of any breast tissue. It is important that this electrode is placed sufficiently laterally. Other acceptable pad positions include:

- each electrode on the lateral chest wall, one on the right and the other on the left side (bi-axillary);
- one electrode in the standard apical position and the other on the right or left upper back;
- one electrode anteriorly, over the left precordium, and the other electrode posterior to the heart just inferior to the left scapula.

It does not matter which electrode (apex/sternum) is placed in either position.

Transthoracic impedance has been shown to be minimised when the apical electrode is not placed over the female breast.[41] Asymmetrically shaped apical electrodes have a lower impedance when placed longitudinally rather than transversely.[42] The long axis of the apical paddle should therefore be orientated in a craniocaudal direction.

Atrial fibrillation is maintained by functional re-entry circuits anchored in the left atrium. As the left atrium is located posteriorly in the thorax, an anteroposterior electrode position may be more efficient for external cardioversion of atrial

fibrillation.[43] Most,[44,45] but not all,[46,47] studies have shown that anteroposterior electrode placement is more effective than the traditional antero-apical position in elective cardioversion of atrial fibrillation. Efficacy of cardioversion may be less dependent on electrode position when using biphasic impedance-compensated waveforms.[48] Either position is safe and effective for cardioversion of atrial arrhythmias.

Respiratory phase

Transthoracic impedance varies during respiration, being minimal at end expiration. If possible, defibrillation should be attempted at this phase of the respiratory cycle. Positive end-expiratory pressure (PEEP) increases transthoracic impedance and should be minimised during defibrillation. Auto-PEEP (gas trapping) may be particularly high in asthmatics and may necessitate higher than usual energy levels for defibrillation.[49]

Electrode size

The Association for the Advancement of Medical Instrumentation recommends a minimum electrode size of for individual electrodes and the sum of the electrode areas should be a minimum of 150 cm^2.[50] Larger electrodes have lower impedance, but excessively large electrodes may result in less transmyocardial current flow.[51] For adult defibrillation, both handheld paddle electrodes and self-adhesive pad electrodes 8—12 cm in diameter are used and function well. Defibrillation success may be higher with electrodes of 12-cm diameter compared with those of 8-cm diameter.[34,52]

Standard AEDs are suitable for use in children over the age of 8 years. In children between 1 and 8 years, use paediatric pads with an attenuator to reduce delivered energy, or a paediatric mode, if they are available; if not, use the unmodified machine, taking care to ensure that the adult pads do not overlap. Use of AEDs is not recommended in children less than 1 year.

Coupling agents

If using manual paddles, gel pads are preferable to electrode pastes and gels because the latter can spread between the two paddles, creating the potential for a spark. Do not use bare electrodes without a coupling material, because this causes high transthoracic impedance and may increase the severity of any cutaneous burns. Do not use medical gels or pastes of poor electrical conductivity (e.g., ultrasound gel). Electrode pads are preferred to electrode gel because they avoid the risk of smearing gel between the two paddles and the subsequent risk of arcing and ineffective defibrillation.

Pads versus paddles

Self-adhesive defibrillation pads are safe and effective and are preferable to standard defibrillation paddles.[52] Consideration should be given to use of self-adhesive pads in peri-arrest situations and in clinical situations where patient access is difficult. They have a similar transthoracic impedance[51] (and therefore efficacy)[53,54] to manual paddles, and enable the operator to defibrillate the patient from a safe distance rather than leaning over the patient (as occurs with paddles). When used for initial monitoring of a rhythm, both pads and paddles enable quicker delivery of the first shock compared with standard ECG electrodes, but pads are quicker than paddles.[55]

When gel pads are used with paddles, the electrolyte gel becomes polarised and thus is a poor conductor after defibrillation. This can cause spurious asystole that may persist for 3—4 min when used to monitor the rhythm; a phenomenon not reported with self-adhesive pads.[56,57] When using a gel pad/paddle combination, confirm a diagnosis of asystole with independent ECG electrodes rather than the paddles.

Fibrillation waveform analysis

It is possible to predict, with varying reliability, the success of defibrillation from the fibrillation waveform.[58—77] If optimal defibrillation waveforms and the optimal timing of shock delivery can be determined in prospective studies, it should be possible to prevent the delivery of unsuccessful high-energy shocks and minimise myocardial injury. This technology is under active development and investigation.

CPR versus defibrillation as the initial treatment

Although the previous guidelines have recommended immediate defibrillation for all shockable rhythms, recent evidence has suggested that a period of CPR before defibrillation may be beneficial after prolonged collapse. In clinical studies where response times exceeded 4—5 min, a period of 1.5—3 min of CPR by paramedics or EMS physicians before shock delivery improved ROSC, survival to hospital discharge[78,79] and 1-year survival[79] for adults with out-of-hospital VF or VT, compared

with immediate defibrillation. In contrast, a single randomised study in adults with out-of-hospital VF or VT failed to show improvements in ROSC or survival following 1.5 min of paramedic CPR.[80] In animal studies of VF lasting at least 5 min, CPR before defibrillation improved haemodynamics and survival.[81—83] It may not be possible to extrapolate the outcomes achieved by paramedic-provided CPR, which includes intubation and delivery of 100% oxygen,[79] to those that may be achieved by laypeople providing relative poor-quality CPR with mouth-to-mouth ventilation.

It is reasonable for EMS personnel to give a period of about 2 min of CPR (i.e., about five cycles at 30:2) before defibrillation in patients with prolonged collapse (>5 min). The duration of collapse is frequently difficult to estimate accurately, and it may be simplest if EMS personnel are instructed to provide this period of CPR before attempted defibrillation in any cardiac arrest they have not witnessed. Given the relatively weak evidence available, individual EMS directors should determine whether to implement a CPR-before-defibrillation strategy; inevitably, protocols will vary depending on the local circumstances.

Laypeople and first responders using AEDS should deliver the shock as soon as possible.

There is no evidence to support or refute CPR before defibrillation for in-hospital cardiac arrest. We recommend shock delivery as soon as possible following in-hospital cardiac arrest (see Section 4b and c).

The importance of early uninterrupted external chest compression is emphasised throughout these guidelines. In practice, it is often difficult to ascertain the exact time of collapse and, in any case, CPR should be started as soon as possible. The rescuer providing chest compressions should interrupt chest compressions only for rhythm analysis and shock delivery, and should be prepared to resume chest compressions as soon as a shock is delivered. When two rescuers are present, the rescuer operating the AED should apply the electrodes while CPR is in progress. Interrupt CPR only when it is necessary to assess the rhythm and deliver a shock. The AED operator should be prepared to deliver a shock as soon as analysis is complete and the shock is advised, ensuring all rescuers are not in contact with the victim. The single rescuer should practice coordination of CPR with efficient AED operation.

One-shock versus three-shock sequence

There are no published human or animal studies comparing a single-shock protocol with a three-stacked-shock protocol for treatment of VF cardiac arrest. Animal studies show that relatively short interruptions in external chest compression to deliver rescue breaths[84,85] or perform rhythm analysis[86] are associated with post-resuscitation myocardial dysfunction and reduced survival. Interruptions in external chest compression also reduce the chances of converting VF to another rhythm.[87] Analysis of CPR performance during out-of-hospital[16,88] and in-hospital[17] cardiac arrest has shown that significant interruptions are common, with external chest compressions comprising no more than 51%[16] to 76%[17] of total CPR time.

In the context of a three-shock protocol being recommended in the 2000 guidelines, interruptions in CPR to enable rhythm analysis by AEDs were significant. Delays of up to 37s between delivery of shocks and recommencing chest compressions have been reported.[89] With first shock efficacy of biphasic waveforms exceeding 90%,[90–93] failure to cardiovert VF successfully is more likely to suggest the need for a period of CPR rather than a further shock. Thus, immediately after giving a single shock, and without reassessing the rhythm or feeling for a pulse, resume CPR (30 compressions:2 ventilations) for 2 min before delivering another shock (if indicated) (see Section 4c). Even if the defibrillation attempt is successful in restoring a perfusing rhythm, it is very rare for a pulse to be palpable immediately after defibrillation, and the delay in trying to palpate a pulse will further compromise the myocardium if a perfusing rhythm has not been restored.[89] In one study of AEDs in out-of-hospital VF cardiac arrest, a pulse was detected in only 2.5% (12/481) of patients with the initial post shock pulse check, though a pulse was detected sometime after the initial shock sequence (and before a second shock sequence) in 24.5% (118/481) of patients.[93] If a perfusing rhythm has been restored, giving chest compressions does not increase the chance of VF recurring.[94] In the presence of post-shock asystole chest compressions may induce VF.[94]

This single shock strategy is applicable to both monophasic and biphasic defibrillators.

Waveforms and energy levels

Defibrillation requires the delivery of sufficient electrical energy to defibrillate a critical mass of myocardium, abolish the wavefronts of VF and enable restoration of spontaneous synchronised electrical activity in the form of an organised rhythm. The optimal energy for defibrillation is that which achieves defibrillation while causing the minimum of myocardial damage.[33] Selection of an appropriate energy level also reduces the number

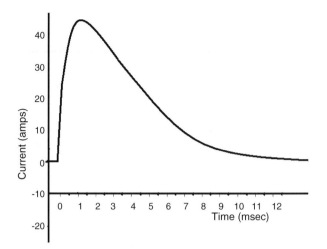

Figure 3.1 Monophasic damped sinusoidal waveform (MDS).

of repetitive shocks, which in turn limits myocardial damage.[95]

After a cautious introduction a decade ago, defibrillators delivering a shock with a biphasic waveform are now preferred. Monophasic defibrillators are no longer manufactured, although many remain in use. Monophasic defibrillators deliver current that is unipolar (i.e., one direction of current flow). There are two main types of monophasic waveform. The commonest waveform is the monophasic damped sinusoidal (MDS) waveform (Figure 3.1) which gradually returns to zero current flow. The monophasic truncated exponential (MTE) waveform is electronically terminated before current flow reaches zero (Figure 3.2). Biphasic defibrillators, in contrast, deliver current that flows in a positive direction for a specified duration before reversing and flowing in a negative direction for the remaining milliseconds of the electrical discharge. There are two main types of biphasic waveform: the biphasic truncated exponential (BTE) (Figure 3.3) and rectilinear biphasic (RLB) (Figure 3.4). Biphasic defibrillators compensate for the wide variations in transthoracic impedance by electronically

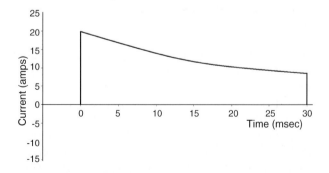

Figure 3.2 Monophasic truncated exponential waveform (MTE).

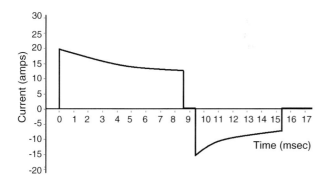

Figure 3.3 Biphasic truncated exponential waveform (BTE).

adjusting the waveform magnitude and duration. The optimal ratio of first-phase to second-phase duration and leading-edge amplitude has not been established. Whether different waveforms have differing efficacy for VF of differing durations is also unknown.

All manual defibrillators and AEDs that allow manual override of energy levels should be labelled to indicate their waveform (monophasic or biphasic) and recommended energy levels for attempted defibrillation of VF/VT. First-shock efficacy for long-duration VF/VT is greater with biphasic than monophasic waveforms,[96–98] and therefore use of the former is recommended whenever possible. Optimal energy levels for both monophasic and biphasic waveforms are unknown. The recommendations for energy levels are based on a consensus following careful review of the current literature.

Although energy levels are selected for defibrillation, it is the transmyocardial current flow that achieves defibrillation. Current correlates well with the successful defibrillation and cardioversion.[99]

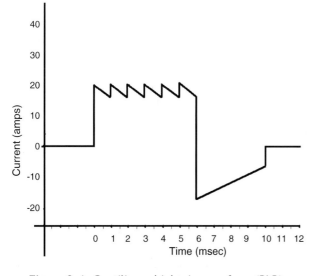

Figure 3.4 Rectilinear biphasic waveform (RLB).

The optimal current for defibrillation using a monophasic waveform is in the range of 30—40 A. Indirect evidence from measurements during cardioversion for atrial fibrillation suggest that the current during defibrillation using biphasic waveforms is in the range of 15—20 A.[100] Future technology may enable defibrillators to discharge according to transthoracic current: a strategy that may lead to greater consistency in shock success. Peak current amplitude, average current and phase duration all need to be studied to determine optimal values, and manufacturers are encouraged to explore further this move from energy-based to current-based defibrillation.

First shock

First-shock efficacy for long-duration cardiac arrest using monophasic defibrillation has been reported as 54%—63% for a 200-J monophasic truncated exponential (MTE) waveform[97,101] and 77%—91% using a 200-J monophasic damped sinusoidal (MDS) waveform.[96–98,101] Because of the lower efficacy of this waveform, the recommended initial energy level for the first shock using a monophasic defibrillator is 360 J. Although higher energy levels risk a greater degree of myocardial injury, the benefits of earlier conversion to a perfusing rhythm are paramount. Atrioventricular block is more common with higher monophasic energy levels, but is generally transient and has been shown not to affect survival to hospital discharge.[102] Only 1 of 27 animal studies demonstrated harm caused by attempted defibrillation using high-energy shocks.[103]

There is no evidence that one biphasic waveform or device is more effective than another. First-shock efficacy of the BTE waveform using 150—200 J has been reported as 86%—98%.[96,97,101,104,105] First-shock efficacy of the RLB waveform using 120 J is up to 85% (data not published in the paper but supplied by personnel communication).[98] The initial biphasic shock should be no lower than 120 J for RLB waveforms and 150 J for BTE waveforms. Ideally, the initial biphasic shock energy should be at least 150 J for all waveforms.

Manufacturers should display the effective waveform dose range on the face of the biphasic device. If the provider is unaware of the effective dose range of the device, use a dose of 200 J for the first shock. This 200 J default energy has been chosen because it falls within the reported range of selected doses that are effective for first and subsequent biphasic shocks and can be provided by every biphasic manual defibrillator available today. It is a consensus default dose and not a recommended ideal dose. If biphasic devices are clearly labelled and providers are familiar with the devices they use in clinical care, there will be no need for the default 200 J dose. Ongoing research is necessary to firmly establish the most appropriate initial settings for both monophasic and biphasic defibrillators.

Second and subsequent shocks

With monophasic defibrillators, if the initial shock has been unsuccessful at 360 J, second and subsequent shocks should all be delivered at 360 J. With biphasic defibrillators there is no evidence to support either a fixed or escalating energy protocol. Both strategies are acceptable; however, if the first shock is not successful and the defibrillator is capable of delivering shocks of higher energy, it is rational to increase the energy for subsequent shocks. If the provider is unaware of the effective dose range of the biphasic device and has used the default 200 J dose for the first shock, use either an equal or higher dose for second or subsequent shocks, depending on the capabilities of the device.

If a shockable rhythm (recurrent ventricular fibrillation) recurs after successful defibrillation (with or without ROSC), give the next shock with the energy level that had previously been successful.

Other related defibrillation topics

Defibrillation of children

Cardiac arrest is less common in children. Aetiology is generally related to hypoxia and trauma.[106–108] VF is relatively rare compared with adult cardiac arrest, occurring in 7%–15% of paediatric and adolescent arrests.[108–112] Common causes of VF in children include trauma, congenital heart disease, long QT interval, drug overdose and hypothermia. Rapid defibrillation of these patients may improve outcome.[112,113]

The optimal energy level, waveform and shock sequence are unknown but, as with adults, biphasic shocks appear to be at least as effective as, and less harmful than, monophasic shocks.[114–116] The upper limit for safe defibrillation is unknown, but doses in excess of the previously recommended maximum of 4 J kg^{-1} (as high as 9 J kg^{-1}) have defibrillated children effectively without significant adverse effects.[20,117,118] The recommended energy level for manual monophasic defibrillation is 4 J kg^{-1} for the initial shock and for subsequent shocks. The same energy level is recommended for manual biphasic defibrillation.[119] As with adults, if a shockable rhythm recurs, use the energy level for defibrillation that had previously been successful.

Blind defibrillation

Delivery of shocks without a monitor or an ECG rhythm diagnosis is referred to as ''blind'' defibrillation. Blind defibrillation is unnecessary. Handheld paddles with ''quick-look'' monitoring capabilities on modern manually operated defibrillators are widely available. AEDs use reliable and proven decision algorithms to identify VF.

Spurious asystole and occult ventricular fibrillation

Rarely, coarse VF can be present in some leads, with very small undulations seen in the orthogonal leads, which is called occult VF. A flat line that may resemble asystole is displayed; examine the rhythm in two leads to obtain the correct diagnosis. Of more importance, one study noted that spurious asystole, a flat line produced by technical errors (e.g., no power, leads unconnected, gain set to low, incorrect lead selection, or polarisation of electrolyte gel (see above)), was far more frequent than occult VF.[120]

There is no evidence that attempting to defibrillate true asystole is beneficial. Studies in children[121] and adults[122] have failed to show benefit from defibrillation of asystole. On the contrary, repeated shocks will cause myocardial injury.

Precordial thump

There are no prospective studies that evaluate use of precordial (chest) thump. The rationale for giving a thump is that the mechanical energy of the thump is converted to electrical energy, which may be sufficient to achieve cardioversion.[123] The electrical threshold of successful defibrillation increases rapidly after the onset of the arrhythmia, and the amount of electrical energy generated falls below this threshold within seconds. A precordial thump is most likely to be successful in converting VT to sinus rhythm. Successful treatment of VF by precordial thump is much less likely: in all the reported successful cases, the precordial thump was given within the first 10 s of VF.[123] Although three case series[124–126] reported that VF or pulseless VT was converted to a perfusing rhythm by a precordial thump, there are occasional reports of thump causing deterioration in cardiac rhythm, such as rate acceleration of VT, conversion of VT into VF, complete heart block or asystole.[125,127–132]

Consider giving a single precordial thump when cardiac arrest is confirmed rapidly after a witnessed, sudden collapse and a defibrillator is not immediately to hand. These circumstances are most likely to occur when the patient is monitored. Precordial thump should be undertaken immediately after confirmation of cardiac arrest and only by healthcare professionals trained in the technique. Using the ulnar edge of a tightly clenched fist, a sharp impact is delivered to the lower half of the sternum from a height of about 20 cm, followed by immediate retraction of the fist, which creates an impulse-like stimulus.

Cardioversion

If electrical cardioversion is used to convert atrial or ventricular tachyarrhythmias, the shock must be synchronised to occur with the R wave of the electrocardiogram rather than with the T wave: VF can be induced if a shock is delivered during the relative refractory portion of the cardiac cycle.[133] Synchronisation can be difficult in VT because of the wide-complex and variable forms of ventricular arrhythmia. If synchronisation fails, give unsynchronised shocks to the unstable patient in VT to avoid prolonged delay in restoring sinus rhythm. Ventricular fibrillation or pulseless VT requires unsynchronised shocks. Conscious patients must be anaesthetised or sedated before attempting synchronised cardioversion.

Atrial fibrillation

Biphasic waveforms are more effective than monophasic waveforms for cardioversion of AF[100,134,135]; when available, use a biphasic defibrillator in preference to a monophasic defibrillator.

Monophasic waveforms

A study of electrical cardioversion for atrial fibrillation indicated that 360-J MDS shocks were more effective than 100-J or 200-J MDS shocks.[136] Although a first shock of 360-J reduces overall energy requirements for cardioversion, 360 J may cause greater myocardial damage than occurs with lower monophasic energy levels, and this must be taken into consideration. Commence cardioversion of atrial fibrillation using an initial energy level of 200 J, increasing in a stepwise manner as necessary.

Biphasic waveforms

More data are needed before specific recommendations can be made for optimal biphasic energy levels. First-shock efficacy of a 70-J biphasic waveform has been shown to be significantly greater than that with a 100-monophasic waveform.[100,134,135] A

randomised study comparing escalating monophasic energy levels to 360 J and biphasic energy levels to 200 J found no difference in efficacy between the two waveforms.[137] An initial shock of 120—150 J, escalating if necessary, is a reasonable strategy based on current data.

Atrial flutter and paroxysmal supraventricular tachycardia

Atrial flutter and paroxysmal SVT generally require less energy than atrial fibrillation for cardioversion.[138] Give an initial shock of 100-J monophasic or 70—120 J biphasic waveform. Give subsequent shocks using stepwise increases in energy.[99]

Ventricular tachycardia

The energy required for cardioversion of VT depends on the morphological characteristics and rate of the arrhythmia.[139] Ventricular tachycardia with a pulse responds well to cardioversion using initial monophasic energies of 200 J. Use biphasic energy levels of 120—150 J for the initial shock. Give stepwise increases if the first shock fails to achieve sinus rhythm.[139]

Pacing

Consider pacing in patients with symptomatic bradycardia refractory to anticholinergic drugs or other second-line therapy (see Section 4f). Immediate pacing is indicated, especially when the block is at or below the His—Purkinje level. If transthoracic pacing is ineffective, consider transvenous pacing. Whenever a diagnosis of asystole is made, check the ECG carefully for the presence of P waves, because this may respond to cardiac pacing. Do not attempt pacing for asystole; it does not increase short-term or long-term survival in or out of hospital.[140—148]

References

1. American Heart Association in collaboration with International Liaison Committee on Resuscitation. Guidelines 2000 for Cardiopulmonary Resuscitation and Emergency Cardiovascular Care, Part 6: Advanced Cardiovascular Life Support: Section 2: Defibrillation. Circulation 2000;102(Suppl.):I90—4.
2. Larsen MP, Eisenberg MS, Cummins RO, Hallstrom AP. Predicting survival from out-of-hospital cardiac arrest: a graphic model. Ann Emerg Med 1993;22:1652—8.
3. Valenzuela TD, Roe DJ, Cretin S, Spaite DW, Larsen MP. Estimating effectiveness of cardiac arrest interventions: a logistic regression survival model. Circulation 1997;96:3308—13.

4. Waalewijn RA, de Vos R, Tijssen JGP, Koster RW. Survival models for out-of-hospital cardiopulmonary resuscitation from the perspectives of the bystander, the first responder, and the paramedic. Resuscitation 2001;51:113—22.

5. Myerburg RJ, Fenster J, Velez M, et al. Impact of community-wide police car deployment of automated external defibrillators on survival from out-of-hospital cardiac arrest. Circulation 2002;106:1058—64.

6. Capucci A, Aschieri D, Piepoli MF, Bardy GH, Iconomu E, Arvedi M. Tripling survival from sudden cardiac arrest via early defibrillation without traditional education in cardiopulmonary resuscitation. Circulation 2002;106:1065—70.

7. van Alem AP, Vrenken RH, de Vos R, Tijssen JG, Koster RW. Use of automated external defibrillator by first responders in out of hospital cardiac arrest: prospective controlled trial. BMJ 2003;327:1312.

8. Valenzuela TD, Bjerke HS, Clark LL, et al. Rapid defibrillation by nontraditional responders: the Casino Project. Acad Emerg Med 1998;5:414—5.

9. Swor RA, Jackson RE, Cynar M, et al. Bystander CPR, ventricular fibrillation, and survival in witnessed, unmonitored out-of-hospital cardiac arrest. Ann Emerg Med 1995;25:780—4.

10. Holmberg M, Holmberg S, Herlitz J. Effect of bystander cardiopulmonary resuscitation in out-of-hospital cardiac arrest patients in Sweden. Resuscitation 2000;47:59—70.

11. Monsieurs KG, Handley AJ, Bossaert LL. European Resuscitation Council Guidelines 2000 for Automated External Defibrillation. A statement from the Basic Life Support and Automated External Defibrillation Working Group (1) and approved by the Executive Committee of the European Resuscitation Council. Resuscitation 2001;48:207—9.

12. Cummins RO, Eisenberg M, Bergner L, Murray JA. Sensitivity accuracy, and safety of an automatic external defibrillator. Lancet 1984;2:318—20.

13. Davis EA, Mosesso Jr VN. Performance of police first responders in utilizing automated external defibrillation on victims of sudden cardiac arrest. Prehosp Emerg Care 1998;2:101—7.

14. White RD, Vukov LF, Bugliosi TF. Early defibrillation by police: initial experience with measurement of critical time intervals and patient outcome. Ann Emerg Med 1994;23:1009—13.

15. White RD, Hankins DG, Bugliosi TF. Seven years' experience with early defibrillation by police and paramedics in an emergency medical services system. Resuscitation 1998;39:145—51.

16. Wik L, Kramer-Johansen J, Myklebust H, et al. Quality of cardiopulmonary resuscitation during out-of-hospital cardiac arrest. JAMA 2005;293:299—304.

17. Abella BS, Alvarado JP, Myklebust H, et al. Quality of cardiopulmonary resuscitation during in-hospital cardiac arrest. JAMA 2005;293:305—10.

18. Kerber RE, Becker LB, Bourland JD, et al. Automatic external defibrillators for public access defibrillation: recommendations for specifying and reporting arrhythmia analysis algorithm performance, incorporating new waveforms, and enhancing safety. A statement for health professionals from the American Heart Association Task Force on Automatic External Defibrillation, Subcommittee on AED Safety and Efficacy. Circulation 1997;95:1677—82.

19. Dickey W, Dalzell GW, Anderson JM, Adgey AA. The accuracy of decision-making of a semi-automatic defibrillator during cardiac arrest. Eur Heart J 1992;13:608—15.

20. Atkinson E, Mikysa B, Conway JA, et al. Specificity and sensitivity of automated external defibrillator rhythm analysis in infants and children. Ann Emerg Med 2003;42:185—96.

21. Cecchin F, Jorgenson DB, Berul CI, et al. Is arrhythmia detection by automatic external defibrillator accurate for children? Sensitivity and specificity of an automatic external defibrillator algorithm in 696 pediatric arrhythmias. Circulation 2001;103:2483—8.

22. Zafari AM, Zarter SK, Heggen V, et al. A program encouraging early defibrillation results in improved in-hospital resuscitation efficacy. J Am Coll Cardiol 2004;44:846—52.

23. Destro A, Marzaloni M, Sermasi S, Rossi F. Automatic external defibrillators in the hospital as well? Resuscitation 1996;31:39—43.

24. Domanovits H, Meron G, Sterz F, et al. Successful automatic external defibrillator operation by people trained only in basic life support in a simulated cardiac arrest situation. Resuscitation 1998;39:47—50.

25. Cusnir H, Tongia R, Sheka KP, et al. In hospital cardiac arrest: a role for automatic defibrillation. Resuscitation 2004;63:183—8.

26. Kaye W, Mancini ME, Richards N. Organizing and implementing a hospital-wide first-responder automated external defibrillation program: strengthening the in-hospital chain of survival. Resuscitation 1995;30:151—6.

27. Miller PH. Potential fire hazard in defibrillation. JAMA 1972;221:192.

28. Hummel IIIrd RS, Ornato JP, Weinberg SM, Clarke AM. Spark-generating properties of electrode gels used during defibrillation. A potential fire hazard. JAMA 1988;260:3021—4.

29. Fires from defibrillation during oxygen administration. Health Devices 1994;23:307—9.

30. Lefever J, Smith A. Risk of fire when using defibrillation in an oxygen enriched atmosphere. Medical Devices Agency Safety Notices 1995;3:1—3.

31. Ward ME. Risk of fires when using defibrillators in an oxygen enriched atmosphere. Resuscitation 1996;31:173.

32. Theodorou AA, Gutierrez JA, Berg RA. Fire attributable to a defibrillation attempt in a neonate. Pediatrics 2003;112:677—9.

33. Kerber RE, Kouba C, Martins J, et al. Advance prediction of transthoracic impedance in human defibrillation and cardioversion: importance of impedance in determining the success of low-energy shocks. Circulation 1984;70:303—8.

34. Kerber RE, Grayzel J, Hoyt R, Marcus M, Kennedy J. Transthoracic resistance in human defibrillation. Influence of body weight, chest size, serial shocks, paddle size and paddle contact pressure. Circulation 1981;63:676—82.

35. Sado DM, Deakin CD, Petley GW, Clewlow F. Comparison of the effects of removal of chest hair with not doing so before external defibrillation on transthoracic impedance. Am J Cardiol 2004;93:98—100.

36. Deakin CD, Sado DM, Petley GW, Clewlow F. Differential contribution of skin impedance and thoracic volume to transthoracic impedance during external defibrillation. Resuscitation 2004;60:171—4.

37. Deakin C, Sado D, Petley G, Clewlow F. Determining the optimal paddle force for external defibrillation. Am J Cardiol 2002;90:812—3.

38. Deakin C, Bennetts S, Petley G, Clewlow F. What is the optimal paddle force for paediatric defibrillation? Resuscitation 2002;55:59.

39. Panacek EA, Munger MA, Rutherford WF, Gardner SF. Report of nitropatch explosions complicating defibrillation. Am J Emerg Med 1992;10:128—9.

40. Wrenn K. The hazards of defibrillation through nitroglycerin patches. Ann Emerg Med 1990;19:1327—8.

41. Pagan-Carlo LA, Spencer KT, Robertson CE, Dengler A, Birkett C, Kerber RE. Transthoracic defibrillation: importance of avoiding electrode placement directly on the female breast. J Am Coll Cardiol 1996;27:449—52.

42. Deakin CD, Sado DM, Petley GW, Clewlow F. Is the orientation of the apical defibrillation paddle of importance during manual external defibrillation? Resuscitation 2003;56:15—8.

43. Kirchhof P, Borggrefe M, Breithardt G. Effect of electrode position on the outcome of cardioversion. Card Electrophysiol Rev 2003;7:292—6.

44. Kirchhof P, Eckardt L, Loh P, et al. Anterior-posterior versus anterior-lateral electrode positions for external cardioversion of atrial fibrillation: a randomised trial. Lancet 2002;360:1275—9.

45. Botto GL, Politi A, Bonini W, Broffoni T, Bonatti R. External cardioversion of atrial fibrillation: role of paddle position on technical efficacy and energy requirements. Heart 1999;82:726—30.

46. Alp NJ, Rahman S, Bell JA, Shahi M. Randomised comparison of antero-lateral versus antero-posterior paddle positions for DC cardioversion of persistent atrial fibrillation. Int J Cardiol 2000;75:211—6.

47. Mathew TP, Moore A, McIntyre M, et al. Randomised comparison of electrode positions for cardioversion of atrial fibrillation. Heart 1999;81:576—9.

48. Walsh SJ, McCarty D, McClelland AJ, et al. Impedance compensated biphasic waveforms for transthoracic cardioversion of atrial fibrillation: a multi-centre comparison of antero-apical and antero-posterior pad positions. Eur Heart J 2005.

49. Deakin CD, McLaren RM, Petley GW, Clewlow F, Dalrymple-Hay MJ. Effects of positive end-expiratory pressure on transthoracic impedance—implications for defibrillation. Resuscitation 1998;37:9—12.

50. American National Standard: Automatic External Defibrillators and Remote Controlled Defibrillators (DF39). Arlington, Virgina: Association for the Advancement of Medical Instrumentation; 1993.

51. Deakin CD, McLaren RM, Petley GW, Clewlow F, Dalrymple-Hay MJ. A comparison of transthoracic impedance using standard defibrillation paddles and self-adhesive defibrillation pads. Resuscitation 1998;39:43—6.

52. Stults KR, Brown DD, Cooley F, Kerber RE. Self-adhesive monitor/defibrillation pads improve prehospital defibrillation success. Ann Emerg Med 1987;16:872—7.

53. Kerber RE, Martins JB, Kelly KJ, et al. Self-adhesive preapplied electrode pads for defibrillation and cardioversion. J Am Coll Cardiol 1984;3:815—20.

54. Kerber RE, Martins JB, Ferguson DW, et al. Experimental evaluation and initial clinical application of new self-adhesive defibrillation electrodes. Int J Cardiol 1985;8:57—66.

55. Perkins GD, Roberts C, Gao F. Delays in defibrillation: influence of different monitoring techniques. Br J Anaesth 2002;89:405—8.

56. Bradbury N, Hyde D, Nolan J. Reliability of ECG monitoring with a gel pad/paddle combination after defibrillation. Resuscitation 2000;44:203—6.

57. Chamberlain D. Gel pads should not be used for monitoring ECG after defibrillation. Resuscitation 2000;43:159—60.

58. Callaway CW, Sherman LD, Mosesso Jr VN, Dietrich TJ, Holt E, Clarkson MC. Scaling exponent predicts defibrillation success for out-of-hospital ventricular fibrillation cardiac arrest. Circulation 2001;103:1656—61.

59. Eftestol T, Sunde K, Aase SO, Husoy JH, Steen PA. Predicting outcome of defibrillation by spectral characterization

and nonparametric classification of ventricular fibrillation in patients with out-of-hospital cardiac arrest. Circulation 2000;102:1523—9.

60. Eftestol T, Wik L, Sunde K, Steen PA. Effects of cardiopulmonary resuscitation on predictors of ventricular fibrillation defibrillation success during out-of-hospital cardiac arrest. Circulation 2004;110:10—5.

61. Weaver WD, Cobb LA, Dennis D, Ray R, Hallstrom AP, Copass MK. Amplitude of ventricular fibrillation waveform and outcome after cardiac arrest. Ann Intern Med 1985;102:53—5.

62. Brown CG, Dzwonczyk R. Signal analysis of the human electrocardiogram during ventricular fibrillation: frequency and amplitude parameters as predictors of successful countershock. Ann Emerg Med 1996;27:184—8.

63. Callaham M, Braun O, Valentine W, Clark DM, Zegans C. Prehospital cardiac arrest treated by urban first-responders: profile of patient response and prediction of outcome by ventricular fibrillation waveform. Ann Emerg Med 1993;22:1664—77.

64. Strohmenger HU, Lindner KH, Brown CG. Analysis of the ventricular fibrillation ECG signal amplitude and frequency parameters as predictors of countershock success in humans. Chest 1997;111:584—9.

65. Strohmenger HU, Eftestol T, Sunde K, et al. The predictive value of ventricular fibrillation electrocardiogram signal frequency and amplitude variables in patients with out-of-hospital cardiac arrest. Anesth Analg 2001;93:1428—33.

66. Podbregar M, Kovacic M, Podbregar-Mars A, Brezocnik M. Predicting defibrillation success by 'genetic' programming in patients with out-of-hospital cardiac arrest. Resuscitation 2003;57:153—9.

67. Menegazzi JJ, Callaway CW, Sherman LD, et al. Ventricular fibrillation scaling exponent can guide timing of defibrillation and other therapies. Circulation 2004;109:926—31.

68. Povoas HP, Weil MH, Tang W, Bisera J, Klouche K, Barbatsis A. Predicting the success of defibrillation by electrocardiographic analysis. Resuscitation 2002;53:77—82.

69. Noc M, Weil MH, Tang W, Sun S, Pernat A, Bisera J. Electrocardiographic prediction of the success of cardiac resuscitation. Crit Care Med 1999;27:708—14.

70. Strohmenger HU, Lindner KH, Keller A, Lindner IM, Pfenninger EG. Spectral analysis of ventricular fibrillation and closed-chest cardiopulmonary resuscitation. Resuscitation 1996;33:155—61.

71. Noc M, Weil MH, Gazmuri RJ, Sun S, Biscera J, Tang W. Ventricular fibrillation voltage as a monitor of the effectiveness of cardiopulmonary resuscitation. J Lab Clin Med 1994;124:421—6.

72. Lightfoot CB, Nremt P, Callaway CW, et al. Dynamic nature of electrocardiographic waveform predicts rescue shock outcome in porcine ventricular fibrillation. Ann Emerg Med 2003;42:230—41.

73. Marn-Pernat A, Weil MH, Tang W, Pernat A, Bisera J. Optimizing timing of ventricular defibrillation. Crit Care Med 2001;29:2360—5.

74. Hamprecht FA, Achleitner U, Krismer AC, et al. Fibrillation power, an alternative method of ECG spectral analysis for prediction of countershock success in a porcine model of ventricular fibrillation. Resuscitation 2001;50:287—96.

75. Amann A, Achleitner U, Antretter H, et al. Analysing ventricular fibrillation ECG-signals and predicting defibrillation success during cardiopulmonary resuscitation employing N(alpha)-histograms. Resuscitation 2001;50:77—85.

76. Brown CG, Griffith RF, Van Ligten P, et al. Median frequency—a new parameter for predicting defibrillation success rate. Ann Emerg Med 1991;20:787—9.

77. Amann A, Rheinberger K, Achleitner U, et al. The prediction of defibrillation outcome using a new combination of mean frequency and amplitude in porcine models of cardiac arrest. Anesth Analg 2002;95:716—22.

78. Cobb LA, Fahrenbruch CE, Walsh TR, et al. Influence of cardiopulmonary resuscitation prior to defibrillation in patients with out-of-hospital ventricular fibrillation. JAMA 1999;281:1182—8.

79. Wik L, Hansen TB, Fylling F, et al. Delaying defibrillation to give basic cardiopulmonary resuscitation to patients with out-of-hospital ventricular fibrillation: a randomized trial. JAMA 2003;289:1389—95.

80. Jacobs IG, Finn JC, Oxer HF, Jelinek GA. CPR before defibrillation in out-of-hospital cardiac arrest: a randomized trial. Emerg Med Australas 2005;17:39—45.

81. Berg RA, Hilwig RW, Kern KB, Ewy GA. Precountershock cardiopulmonary resuscitation improves ventricular fibrillation median frequency and myocardial readiness for successful defibrillation from prolonged ventricular fibrillation: a randomized, controlled swine study. Ann Emerg Med 2002;40:563—70.

82. Berg RA, Hilwig RW, Ewy GA, Kern KB. Precountershock cardiopulmonary resuscitation improves initial response to defibrillation from prolonged ventricular fibrillation: a randomized, controlled swine study. Crit Care Med 2004;32:1352—7.

83. Kolarova J, Ayoub IM, Yi Z, Gazmuri RJ. Optimal timing for electrical defibrillation after prolonged untreated ventricular fibrillation. Crit Care Med 2003;31:2022—8.

84. Berg RA, Sanders AB, Kern KB, et al. Adverse hemodynamic effects of interrupting chest compressions for rescue breathing during cardiopulmonary resuscitation for ventricular fibrillation cardiac arrest. Circulation 2001;104:2465—70.

85. Kern KB, Hilwig RW, Berg RA, Sanders AB, Ewy GA. Importance of continuous chest compressions during cardiopulmonary resuscitation: improved outcome during a simulated single lay-rescuer scenario. Circulation 2002;105:645—9.

86. Yu T, Weil MH, Tang W, et al. Adverse outcomes of interrupted precordial compression during automated defibrillation. Circulation 2002;106:368—72.

87. Eftestol T, Sunde K, Steen PA. Effects of interrupting precordial compressions on the calculated probability of defibrillation success during out-of-hospital cardiac arrest. Circulation 2002;105:2270—3.

88. Valenzuela TD, Kern KB, Clark LL, et al. Interruptions of chest compressions during emergency medical systems resuscitation. Circulation 2005;112:1259—65.

89. van Alem AP, Sanou BT, Koster RW. Interruption of cardiopulmonary resuscitation with the use of the automated external defibrillator in out-of-hospital cardiac arrest. Ann Emerg Med 2003;42:449—57.

90. Bain AC, Swerdlow CD, Love CJ, et al. Multicenter study of principles-based waveforms for external defibrillation. Ann Emerg Med 2001;37:5—12.

91. Poole JE, White RD, Kanz KG, et al. Low-energy impedance-compensating biphasic waveforms terminate ventricular fibrillation at high rates in victims of out-of-hospital cardiac arrest. LIFE Investigators. J Cardiovasc Electrophysiol 1997;8:1373—85.

92. Schneider T, Martens PR, Paschen H, et al. Multicenter, randomized, controlled trial of 150-J biphasic shocks compared with 200- to 360-J monophasic shocks in the resuscitation of out-of-hospital cardiac arrest victims. Optimized Response to Cardiac Arrest (ORCA) Investigators. Circulation 2000;102:1780—7.

93. Rea TD, Shah S, Kudenchuk PJ, Copass MK, Cobb LA. Automated external defibrillators: to what extent does the algorithm delay CPR? Ann Emerg Med 2005;46:132—41.

94. Hess EP, White RD. Ventricular fibrillation is not provoked by chest compression during post-shock organized rhythms in out-of-hospital cardiac arrest. Resuscitation 2005;66:7—11.

95. Joglar JA, Kessler DJ, Welch PJ, et al. Effects of repeated electrical defibrillations on cardiac troponin I levels. Am J Cardiol 1999;83:270—2. A6.

96. van Alem AP, Chapman FW, Lank P, Hart AA, Koster RW. A prospective, randomised and blinded comparison of first shock success of monophasic and biphasic waveforms in out-of-hospital cardiac arrest. Resuscitation 2003;58:17—24.

97. Carpenter J, Rea TD, Murray JA, Kudenchuk PJ, Eisenberg MS. Defibrillation waveform and post-shock rhythm in out-of-hospital ventricular fibrillation cardiac arrest. Resuscitation 2003;59:189—96.

98. Morrison LJ, Dorian P, Long J, et al. Out-of-hospital cardiac arrest rectilinear biphasic to monophasic damped sine defibrillation waveforms with advanced life support intervention trial (ORBIT). Resuscitation 2005;66:149—57.

99. Kerber RE, Martins JB, Kienzle MG, et al. Energy, current, and success in defibrillation and cardioversion: clinical studies using an automated impedance-based method of energy adjustment. Circulation 1988;77:1038—46.

100. Koster RW, Dorian P, Chapman FW, Schmitt PW, O'Grady SG, Walker RG. A randomized trial comparing monophasic and biphasic waveform shocks for external cardioversion of atrial fibrillation. Am Heart J 2004;147:e20.

101. Martens PR, Russell JK, Wolcke B, et al. Optimal Response to Cardiac Arrest study: defibrillation waveform effects. Resuscitation 2001;49:233—43.

102. Weaver WD, Cobb LA, Copass MK, Hallstrom AP. Ventricular defibrillation: a comparative trial using 175-J and 320-J shocks. N Engl J Med 1982;307:1101—6.

103. Tang W, Weil MH, Sun S, et al. The effects of biphasic and conventional monophasic defibrillation on postresuscitation myocardial function. J Am Coll Cardiol 1999;34:815—22.

104. Gliner BE, Jorgenson DB, Poole JE, et al. Treatment of out-of-hospital cardiac arrest with a low-energy impedance-compensating biphasic waveform automatic external defibrillator. The LIFE Investigators. Biomed Instrum Technol 1998;32:631—44.

105. White RD, Blackwell TH, Russell JK, Snyder DE, Jorgenson DB. Transthoracic impedance does not affect defibrillation, resuscitation or survival in patients with out-of-hospital cardiac arrest treated with a non-escalating biphasic waveform defibrillator. Resuscitation 2005;64:63—9.

106. Kuisma M, Suominen P, Korpela R. Paediatric out-of-hospital cardiac arrests: epidemiology and outcome. Resuscitation 1995;30:141—50.

107. Sirbaugh PE, Pepe PE, Shook JE, et al. A prospective, population-based study of the demographics, epidemiology, management, and outcome of out-of-hospital pediatric cardiopulmonary arrest. Ann Emerg Med 1999;33:174—84.

108. Hickey RW, Cohen DM, Strausbaugh S, Dietrich AM. Pediatric patients requiring CPR in the prehospital setting. Ann Emerg Med 1995;25:495—501.

109. Appleton GO, Cummins RO, Larson MP, Graves JR. CPR and the single rescuer: at what age should you "call first" rather than "call fast"? Ann Emerg Med 1995;25:492—4.

110. Ronco R, King W, Donley DK, Tilden SJ. Outcome and cost at a children's hospital following resuscitation for out-of-

hospital cardiopulmonary arrest. Arch Pediatr Adolesc Med 1995;149:210—4.

111. Losek JD, Hennes H, Glaeser P, Hendley G, Nelson DB. Prehospital care of the pulseless, nonbreathing pediatric patient. Am J Emerg Med 1987;5:370—4.

112. Mogayzel C, Quan L, Graves JR, Tiedeman D, Fahrenbruch C, Herndon P. Out-of-hospital ventricular fibrillation in children and adolescents: causes and outcomes. Ann Emerg Med 1995;25:484—91.

113. Safranek DJ, Eisenberg MS, Larsen MP. The epidemiology of cardiac arrest in young adults. Ann Emerg Med 1992;21:1102—6.

114. Berg RA, Chapman FW, Berg MD, et al. Attenuated adult biphasic shocks compared with weight-based monophasic shocks in a swine model of prolonged pediatric ventricular fibrillation. Resuscitation 2004;61:189—97.

115. Tang W, Weil MH, Jorgenson D, et al. Fixed-energy biphasic waveform defibrillation in a pediatric model of cardiac arrest and resuscitation. Crit Care Med 2002;30:2736—41.

116. Clark CB, Zhang Y, Davies LR, Karlsson G, Kerber RE. Pediatric transthoracic defibrillation: biphasic versus monophasic waveforms in an experimental model. Resuscitation 2001;51:159—63.

117. Gurnett CA, Atkins DL. Successful use of a biphasic waveform automated external defibrillator in a high-risk child. Am J Cardiol 2000;86:1051—3.

118. Atkins DL, Jorgenson DB. Attenuated pediatric electrode pads for automated external defibrillator use in children. Resuscitation 2005;66:31—7.

119. Gutgesell HP, Tacker WA, Geddes LA, Davis S, Lie JT, McNamara DG. Energy dose for ventricular defibrillation of children. Pediatrics 1976;58:898—901.

120. Cummins RO, Austin Jr D. The frequency of 'occult' ventricular fibrillation masquerading as a flat line in prehospital cardiac arrest. Ann Emerg Med 1988;17:813—7.

121. Losek JD, Hennes H, Glaeser PW, Smith DS, Hendley G. Prehospital countershock treatment of pediatric asystole. Am J Emerg Med 1989;7:571—5.

122. Martin DR, Gavin T, Bianco J, et al. Initial countershock in the treatment of asystole. Resuscitation 1993;26:63—8.

123. Kohl P, King AM, Boulin C. Antiarrhythmic effects of acute mechanical stiumulation. In: Kohl P, Sachs F, Franz MR, editors. Cardiac mechano-electric feedback and arrhythmias: form pipette to patient. Philadelphia: Elsevier Saunders; 2005. p. 304—14.

124. Befeler B. Mechanical stimulation of the heart; its therapeutic value in tachyarrhythmias. Chest 1978;73:832—8.

125. Volkmann HKA, Kühnert H, Paliege R, Dannberg G, Siegert K. Terminierung von Kammertachykardien durch mechanische Herzstimulation mit Präkordialschlägen. (''Termination of Ventricular Tachycardias by Mechanical Cardiac Pacing by Means of Precordial Thumps''). Zeitschrift für Kardiologie 1990;79:717—24.

126. Caldwell G, Millar G, Quinn E. Simple mechanical methods for cardioversion: Defence of the precordial thump and cough version. Br Med J 1985;291:627—30.

127. Morgera T, Baldi N, Chersevani D, Medugno G, Camerini F. Chest thump and ventricular tachycardia. Pacing Clin Electrophysiol 1979;2:69—75.

128. Rahner E, Zeh E. Die Regularisierung von Kammertachykardien durch präkordialen Faustschlag. (''The Regularization of Ventricular Tachycardias by Precordial Thumping''). Medizinsche Welt 1978;29:1659—63.

129. Gertsch M, Hottinger S, Hess T. Serial chest thumps for the treatment of ventricular tachycardia in patients with coronary artery disease. Clin Cardiol 1992;15:181—8.

130. Krijne R. Rate acceleration of ventricular tachycardia after a precordial chest thump. Am J Cardiol 1984;53:964—5.

131. Sclarovsky S, Kracoff OH, Agmon J. Acceleration of ventricular tachycardia induced by a chest thump. Chest 1981;80:596—9.

132. Yakaitis RW, Redding JS. Precordial thumping during cardiac resuscitation. Crit Care Med 1973;1:22—6.

133. Lown B. Electrical reversion of cardiac arrhythmias. Br Heart J 1967;29:469—89.

134. Mittal S, Ayati S, Stein KM, et al. Transthoracic cardioversion of atrial fibrillation: comparison of rectilinear biphasic versus damped sine wave monophasic shocks. Circulation 2000;101:1282—7.

135. Page RL, Kerber RE, Russell JK, et al. Biphasic versus monophasic shock waveform for conversion of atrial fibrillation: the results of an international randomized, double-blind multicenter trial. J Am Coll Cardiol 2002;39:1956—63.

136. Joglar JA, Hamdan MH, Ramaswamy K, et al. Initial energy for elective external cardioversion of persistent atrial fibrillation. Am J Cardiol 2000;86:348—50.

137. Alatawi F, Gurevitz O, White R. Prospective, randomized comparison of two biphasic waveforms for the efficacy and safety of transthoracic biphasic cardioversion of atrial fibrillation. Heart Rhythm 2005;2:382—7.

138. Pinski SL, Sgarbossa EB, Ching E, Trohman RG. A comparison of 50-J versus 100-J shocks for direct-current cardioversion of atrial flutter. Am Heart J 1999;137:439—42.

139. Kerber RE, Kienzle MG, Olshansky B, et al. Ventricular tachycardia rate and morphology determine energy and current requirements for transthoracic cardioversion. Circulation 1992;85:158—63.

140. Hedges JR, Syverud SA, Dalsey WC, Feero S, Easter R, Shultz B. Prehospital trial of emergency transcutaneous cardiac pacing. Circulation 1987;76:1337—43.

141. Barthell E, Troiano P, Olson D, Stueven HA, Hendley G. Prehospital external cardiac pacing: a prospective, controlled clinical trial. Ann Emerg Med 1988;17:1221—6.

142. Cummins RO, Graves JR, Larsen MP, et al. Out-of-hospital transcutaneous pacing by emergency medical technicians in patients with asystolic cardiac arrest. N Engl J Med 1993;328:1377—82.

143. Ornato JP, Peberdy MA. The mystery of bradyasystole during cardiac arrest. Ann Emerg Med 1996;27:576—87.

144. Niemann JT, Adomian GE, Garner D, Rosborough JP. Endocardial and transcutaneous cardiac pacing, calcium chloride, and epinephrine in postcountershock asystole and bradycardias. Crit Care Med 1985;13:699—704.

145. Quan L, Graves JR, Kinder DR, Horan S, Cummins RO. Transcutaneous cardiac pacing in the treatment of out-of-hospital pediatric cardiac arrests. Ann Emerg Med 1992;21:905—9.

146. Dalsey WC, Syverud SA, Hedges JR. Emergency department use of transcutaneous pacing for cardiac arrests. Crit Care Med 1985;13:399—401.

147. Knowlton AA, Falk RH. External cardiac pacing during in-hospital cardiac arrest. Am J Cardiol 1986;57:1295—8.

148. Ornato JP, Carveth WL, Windle JR. Pacemaker insertion for prehospital bradyasystolic cardiac arrest. Ann Emerg Med 1984;13:101—3.

Resuscitation (2005) **67S1**, S39—S86

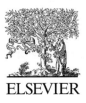

ELSEVIER

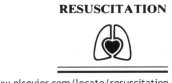

www.elsevier.com/locate/resuscitation

European Resuscitation Council Guidelines for Resuscitation 2005
Section 4. Adult advanced life support

Jerry P. Nolan, Charles D. Deakin, Jasmeet Soar,
Bernd W. Böttiger, Gary Smith

4a. Prevention of in-hospital cardiac arrest

The problem

This new section of the guidelines stresses the importance of preventing in-hospital cardiac arrest. Fewer than 20% of patients suffering an in-hospital cardiac arrest will survive to go home.[1,2] Most survivors have a witnessed and monitored VF arrest, primary myocardial ischaemia as the cause, and receive immediate defibrillation.

Cardiac arrest in patients in unmonitored ward areas is not usually a sudden unpredictable event, nor is it usually caused by primary cardiac disease. These patients often have slow and progressive physiological deterioration, involving hypoxia and hypotension, that is unnoticed by staff, or is recognised but poorly treated.[3,4] The underlying cardiac arrest rhythm in this group is usually non-shockable and survival to hospital discharge is very poor.[1,5]

The records of patients who have a cardiac arrest or unanticipated intensive care unit (ICU) admission often contain evidence of unrecognised, or untreated, breathing and circulation problems.[3,4,6—8] The ACADEMIA study showed

E-mail address: jerry.nolan@ukgateway.net (J.P. Nolan).

antecedents in 79% of cardiac arrests, 55% of deaths and 54% of unanticipated ICU admissions.[4] Early and effective treatment of seriously ill patients might prevent some cardiac arrests, deaths and unanticipated ICU admissions. A third of patients who have a false cardiac arrest call die subsequently.[9]

Nature of the deficiencies in acute care

These often involve simple aspects of care including: the failure to treat abnormalities of the patient's airway, breathing and circulation, incorrect use of oxygen therapy, failure to monitor patients, failure to involve experienced senior staff, poor communication, lack of teamwork and insufficient use of treatment limitation plans.[3,7]

Several studies show that medical and nursing staff lack knowledge and skills in acute care. For example, trainee doctors may lack knowledge about oxygen therapy,[10] fluid and electrolyte balance,[11] analgesia,[12] issues of consent,[13] pulse oximetry[14] and drug doses.[15] Medical students may be unable to recognise abnormal breathing patterns.[16] Medical school training provides poor preparation for doctors' early careers, and fails to teach them the essential aspects of applied physiology and acute care.[17] There is also little to suggest that the acute care training and knowledge of

0300-9572/$ — see front matter © 2005 European Resuscitation Council. All Rights Reserved. Published by Elsevier Ireland Ltd.
doi:10.1016/j.resuscitation.2005.10.009

senior medical staff is better.[18,19] Staff often lack confidence when dealing with acute care problems, and rarely use a systematic approach to the assessment of critically ill patients.[20]

Recognising the critically ill patient

In general, the clinical signs of acute illness are similar whatever the underlying process, as they reflect failing respiratory, cardiovascular and neurological systems. Abnormal physiology is common on general wards,[21] yet the measurement and recording of important physiological observations of sick patients occurs less frequently than is desirable.[3,4,8] This is surprising, as respiratory rate abnormalities may predict cardiorespiratory arrest.[22] To assist in the early detection of critical illness, many hospitals now use early warning scores (EWS) or calling criteria.[23–25] Early warning scoring systems allocate points to routine vital signs measurements on the basis of their derangement from an arbitrarily agreed 'normal' range.[23–25] The weighted score of one or more vital sign observations, or the total EWS, may be used to suggest increasing the frequency of vital signs monitoring to nurses, or to call ward doctors or critical care outreach teams to the patient. Alternatively, systems incorporating 'calling criteria' are based on routine observations, which activate a response when one or more variables reach an extremely abnormal value.[23,26] There are no data to establish the superiority of one system over another, but it may be preferable to use an EWS system, which can track changes in physiology and warn of impending physiological collapse, rather than the ''calling criteria'' approach, which is triggered only when an extreme value of physiology has been reached.

There is a clinical rationale to the use of EWS or calling criteria systems to identify sick patients early. However, their sensitivity, specificity and accuracy in predicting clinical outcomes has yet to be validated convincingly.[27,28] Several studies have identified abnormalities of heart rate, blood pressure, respiratory rate and conscious level as markers of impending critical events.[22,23,29] The suggestion that their incidence has predictive value must be questioned, as not all important vital signs are, or can be, recorded continuously in general ward areas. Several studies show that charting of vital signs is poor, with gaps in data recording.[3,4,8,30] Although the use of physiological systems can increase the frequency of vital signs monitoring,[31] they will be useful for outcome prediction only if widespread monitoring of hospitalised patients becomes available. Even when medical staff are alerted to a patient's abnormal physiology, there is often delay in attending the patient or referring to higher levels of care.[3,4,7] Whereas the use of a warning score based on physiological abnormalities is attractive, it is possible that a more subjective approach, based on staff experience and expertise, may also be effective.[32]

Response to critical illness

The traditional response to cardiac arrest is a reactive one in which hospital staff ('the cardiac arrest team') attend the patient after the cardiac arrest has occurred. Cardiac arrest teams appear to improve survival after cardiac arrest in circumstances where no team has previously existed.[33] However, the role of the cardiac arrest team has been questioned. In one study, only patients who had return of spontaneous circulation before the cardiac arrest team arrived were discharged from hospital alive.[34] When combined with the poor survival rate after in-hospital cardiac arrest, this emphasises the importance of early recognition and treatment of critically ill patients to prevent cardiac arrest. The name 'cardiac arrest team' implies that the team will be called only after cardiac arrest has occurred.

In some hospitals the cardiac arrest team has been replaced by a medical emergency team (MET) that responds, not only to patients in cardiac arrest, but also to those with acute physiological deterioration.[26] The MET usually comprises medical and nursing staff from intensive care and general medicine. and responds to specific calling criteria. Any member of the healthcare team can initiate a MET call. Early involvement of the MET may reduce cardiac arrests, deaths and unanticipated ICU admissions.[35,36] The MET may also be useful in detecting medical error, improving treatment limitation decisions and reducing postoperative ward deaths.[37,38] MET interventions often involve simple tasks such as starting oxygen therapy and intravenous fluids.[39] A circadian pattern of MET activation has been reported, which may suggest that systems for identifying and responding to medical emergencies may not be uniform throughout the 24-h period.[40] Studying the effect of the MET on patient outcomes is difficult. Many of the study findings to date can be criticised because of poor study design. A recent, well-designed, cluster-randomised controlled trial of the MET system demonstrated that the introduction of a MET increased the calling incidence for the team. However, it failed to show a reduction in the incidence of cardiac arrest, unexpected death or unplanned ICU admission.[41]

In the UK, a system of pre-emptive ward care, based predominantly on individual or teams of nurses known as critical care outreach, has developed.[42] Outreach services exist in many forms, ranging from a single nurse to a 24-h, 7 days per week multiprofessional team. An outreach team or system may reduce ward deaths, postoperative adverse events, ICU admissions and readmissions, and increase survival.[43–45]

Other attempts to improve the general ward care of patients and prevent physiological deterioration and cardiac arrest include new admission processes, early physiological monitoring and clinical intervention in the emergency department (ED), and the appointment of new grades of emergency physicians. Many of these models attempt to support the primary admitting team with the skills of 'resuscitation' specialists.[46] Medical and surgical assessment units act as a single location for all acute admissions until their required level of care is evaluated. Patients are monitored and observed for periods of up to 72 h, and there is usually rapid access to senior medical staff, diagnostics and urgent treatment.[47] The single location provides a central focus for on-call medical, nursing and physiotherapy staff, in contrast to the traditional system in which staff and patients are dispersed throughout the hospital.

Many acutely ill patients present to hospital via the ED and are obviously in need of immediate ICU-type interventions. Early goal-directed therapy in the ED reverses physiological derangement and appears to improve patient survival.[48]

Appropriate placement of patients

Ideally, the sickest patients should be admitted to an area that can provide the greatest supervision and the highest level of organ support and nursing care. This often occurs, but some patients are placed incorrectly.[49] International organisations have offered definitions of levels of care and produced admission and discharge criteria for high dependency units (HDUs) and ICUs.[50,51]

Staffing levels

Hospital staffing tends to be at its lowest during the night and at weekends. This may influence patient monitoring, treatment and outcomes. Admission to a general medical ward after 17:00 h[52] or to hospital at weekends[53] is associated with increased mortality. Patients who are discharged from ICUs to general wards at night have an increased risk of in-hospital death compared with those discharged during the day and those discharged to HDUs.[54] One study shows that higher nurse staffing is associated with reduction in cardiac arrest rates, as well as rates of pneumonia, shock and death.[55]

Resuscitation decisions

Consider 'do not attempt resuscitation' (DNAR) when the patient:

- does not wish to have CPR
- will not survive cardiac arrest even if CPR is attempted

Hospital staff often fail to consider whether resuscitation attempts are appropriate and resuscitation attempts in futile cases are common.[37] Even when there is clear evidence that cardiac arrest or death is likely, ward staff rarely make decisions about the patient's resuscitation status.[4] Many European countries have no formal policy for recording DNAR decisions and the practice of consulting patients about the decision is variable.[56] Improved knowledge, training and DNAR decision-making should improve patient care and prevent futile CPR attempts (see Section 8).

Guidelines for prevention of in-hospital cardiac arrest

The following strategies may prevent avoidable in-hospital cardiac arrests.

1. Provide care for patients who are critically ill or at risk of clinical deterioration in appropriate areas, with the level of care provided matched to the level of patient sickness.
2. Critically ill patients need regular observations: match the frequency and type of observations to the severity of illness or the likelihood of clinical deterioration and cardiopulmonary arrest. Often only simple vital sign observations (pulse, blood pressure, respiratory rate) are needed.
3. Use an EWS system to identify patients who are critically ill and or at risk of clinical deterioration and cardiopulmonary arrest.
4. Use a patient charting system that enables the regular measurement and recording of EWS.
5. Have a clear and specific policy that requires a clinical response to EWS systems. This should include advice on the further clinical management of the patient and the specific responsibilities of medical and nursing staff.
6. The hospital should have a clearly identified response to critical illness. This may include a designated outreach service or resuscitation team (e.g. MET) capable of responding to acute clinical crises identified by clinical triggers or

other indicators. This service must be available 24 h per day.

7. Train all clinical staff in the recognition, monitoring and management of the critically ill patient. Include advice on clinical management while awaiting the arrival of more experienced staff.

8. Identify patients for whom cardiopulmonary arrest is an anticipated terminal event and in whom CPR is inappropriate, and patients who do not wish to be treated with CPR. Hospitals should have a DNAR policy, based on national guidance, which is understood by all clinical staff.

9. Ensure accurate audit of cardiac arrest, 'false arrest', unexpected deaths and unanticipated ICU admissions using common datasets. Audit also the antecedents and clinical response to these events.

4b. In-hospital resuscitation

After in-hospital cardiac arrest, the division between basic life support and advanced life support is arbitrary; in practice, the resuscitation process is a continuum and is based on common sense. The public expect that clinical staff can undertake cardiopulmonary resuscitation (CPR). For all in-hospital cardiac arrests, ensure that:

- cardiorespiratory arrest is recognised immediately
- help is summoned using a standard telephone number
- CPR is started immediately using airway adjuncts, e.g. a pocket mask and, if indicated, defibrillation attempted within 3 min

The exact sequence of actions after in-hospital cardiac arrest will depend on many factors, including:

- location (clinical/non-clinical area; monitored/unmonitored area)
- training of the first responders
- number of responders
- equipment available
- hospital response system to cardiac arrest and medical emergencies, (e.g. MET) cardiac arrest team

Location

Patients who have monitored arrests are usually diagnosed rapidly. Ward patients may have had a period of deterioration and an unwitnessed arrest.[3,4,6–8] Ideally, all patients who are at high risk of cardiac arrest should be cared for in a monitored area where facilities for immediate resuscitation are available.

Training of first responders

All healthcare professionals should be able to recognise cardiac arrest, call for help and start CPR. Staff should do what they have been trained to do. For example, staff in critical care and emergency medicine will have more advanced resuscitation skills than staff who are not involved regularly in resuscitation in their normal clinical role. Hospital staff who attend a cardiac arrest may have different levels of skill to manage the airway, breathing and circulation. Rescuers must undertake the skills in which they are trained and competent.

Number of responders

The single responder must ensure that help is coming. If other staff are nearby, several actions can be undertaken simultaneously.

Equipment available

All clinical areas should have immediate access to resuscitation equipment and drugs to facilitate rapid resuscitation of the patient in cardiopulmonary arrest. Ideally, the equipment used for CPR (including defibrillators) and the layout of equipment and drugs should be standardised throughout the hospital.[57]

Resuscitation team

The resuscitation team may take the form of a traditional cardiac arrest team, which is called only when cardiac arrest is recognised. Alternatively, hospitals may have strategies to recognise patients at risk of cardiac arrest and summon a team (e.g., MET) before cardiac arrest occurs.[35,36,39,41,58] The term 'resuscitation team' reflects the range of response teams. In hospital cardiac arrests are rarely sudden or unexpected. A strategy of recognising patients at risk of cardiac arrest may enable some of these arrests to be prevented, or may prevent futile resuscitation attempts in those who are unlikely to benefit from CPR.

Immediate actions for a collapsed patient in a hospital

An algorithm for the initial management of in-hospital cardiac arrest is shown in Figure 4.1.

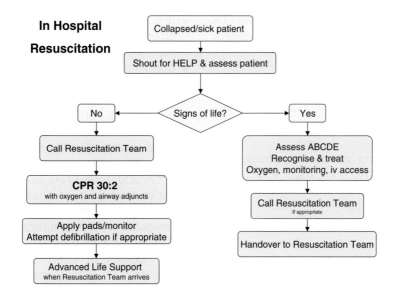

Figure 4.1 Algorithm for the treatment of in-hospital cardiac arrest.

- Ensure personal safety.
- Check the victim for a response.
- When healthcare professionals see a patient collapse or find a patient apparently unconscious in a clinical area, they should first shout for help, then assess if the patient is responsive. Gently shake the shoulders and ask loudly: ''Are you all right?''
- If other members of staff are nearby, it will be possible to undertake actions simultaneously.

The responsive patient

Urgent medical assessment is required. Depending on the local protocols, this may take the form of a resuscitation team (e.g., MET). While awaiting this team, give the patient oxygen, attach monitoring and insert an intravenous cannula.

The unresponsive patient

The exact sequence will depend on the training of staff and experience in assessment of breathing and circulation. Trained healthcare staff cannot assess the breathing and pulse sufficiently reliably to confirm cardiac arrest.[16,59,60] Agonal breathing (occasional gasps, slow, laboured or noisy breathing) is common in the early stages of cardiac arrest and is a sign of cardiac arrest and should not be confused as a sign of life/circulation.

- Shout for help (if not already)

Turn the victim on to his back and then open the airway:

- Open Airway and check breathing:

  - Open the airway using a head tilt chin lift
  - Look in the mouth. If a foreign body or debris is visible attempt to remove with forceps or suction as appropriate
  - If you suspect that there may have been an injury to the neck, try to open the airway using a jaw thrust. Remember that maintaining an airway and adequate ventilation is the overriding priority in managing a patient with a suspected spinal injury. If this is unsuccessful, use just enough head tilt to clear the airway. Use manual in-line stabilisation to minimise head movement if sufficient rescuers are available.

Keeping the airway open, look, listen, and feel for normal breathing (an occasional gasp, slow, laboured or noisy breathing is not normal):

- Look for chest movement
- Listen at the victim's mouth for breath sounds
- Feel for air on your cheek

Look, listen, and feel for no more than 10 s to determine if the victim is breathing normally

- Check for signs of a circulation:
  - It may be difficult to be certain that there is no pulse. If the patient has no signs of life (lack of movement, normal breathing, or coughing), start CPR until more experience help arrives or the patient shows signs of life.
  - Those experienced in clinical assessment should assess the carotid pulse whilst simultaneously looking for signs of life for not more than 10 s.
  - If the patient appears to have no signs of life, or if there is doubt, start CPR immediately. Delays

in diagnosis of cardiac arrest and starting CPR will adversely effect survival must be avoided.

If there is a pulse or signs of life, urgent medical assessment is required. Depending on the local protocols, this may take the form of a resuscitation team. While awaiting this team, give the patient oxygen, attach monitoring, and insert an intravenous cannula.

If there is no breathing, but there is a pulse (respiratory arrest), ventilate the patient's lungs and check for a circulation every 10 breaths.

Starting in-hospital CPR

- One person starts CPR as others call the resuscitation team and collect the resuscitation equipment and a defibrillator. If only one member of staff is present, this will mean leaving the patient.
- Give 30 chest compressions followed by 2 ventilations.
- Undertaking chest compressions properly is tiring; try to change the person doing chest compressions every 2 min.
- Maintain the airway and ventilate the lungs with the most appropriate equipment immediately to hand. A pocket mask, which may be supplemented with an oral airway, is usually readily available. Alternatively, use a laryngeal mask airway (LMA) and self-inflating bag, or bag-mask, according to local policy. Tracheal intubation should be attempted only by those who are trained, competent and experienced in this skill.
- Use an inspiratory time of 1 s and give enough volume to produce a normal chest rise. Add supplemental oxygen as soon as possible.
- Once the patient's trachea has been intubated, continue chest compressions uninterrupted (except for defibrillation or pulse checks when indicated), at a rate of $100\,min^{-1}$, and ventilate the lungs at approximately 10 breaths min^{-1}. Avoid hyperventilation.
- If there is no airway and ventilation equipment available, give mouth-to-mouth ventilation. If there are clinical reasons to avoid mouth-to-mouth contact, or you are unwilling or unable to do this, do chest compressions until help or airway equipment arrives.
- When the defibrillator arrives, apply the paddles to the patient and analyse the rhythm. If self-adhesive defibrillation pads are available, apply these without interrupting chest compressions. Pause briefly to assess the heart rhythm. If indicated, attempt either manual or automated external defibrillation (AED).

- Recommence chest compressions immediately after the defibrillation attempt. Minimise interruptions to chest compressions.
- Continue resuscitation until the resuscitation team arrives or the patient shows signs of life. Follow the voice prompts if using an AED. If using a manual defibrillator, follow the universal algorithm for advanced life support (Section 4c).
- Once resuscitation is underway, and if there are sufficient staff present, prepare intravenous cannulae and drugs likely to be used by the resuscitation team (e.g. adrenaline).
- Identify one person to be responsible for handover to the resuscitation team leader. Locate the patient's records.
- The quality of chest compressions during in-hospital CPR is frequently sub-optimal.[61,62] The team leader should monitor the quality of CPR and change CPR providers if the quality of CPR is poor. The person providing chest compressions should be changed every 2 min.

The monitored and witnessed cardiac arrest

If a patient has a monitored and witnessed cardiac arrest, act as follows.

- Confirm cardiac arrest and shout for help.
- Consider a precordial thump if the rhythm is VF/VT and a defibrillator is not immediately available.
- If the initial rhythm is VF/VT and a defibrillator is immediately available, give a shock first. The use of adhesive electrode pads or a 'quick-look' paddles technique will enable rapid assessment of heart rhythm compared with attaching ECG electrodes.[63]

Training for healthcare professionals

The Immediate Life Support course trains healthcare professionals in the skills required to start resuscitation, including defibrillation, and to be members of a cardiac arrest team (see Section 9).[64] The Advanced Life Support (ALS) course teaches the skills required for leading a resuscitation team.[65,66]

4c. ALS treatment algorithm

Introduction

Heart rhythms associated with cardiac arrest are divided into two groups: shockable rhythms (ventricular fibrillation/pulseless ventricular tachycardia (VF/VT)) and non-shockable rhythms (asystole

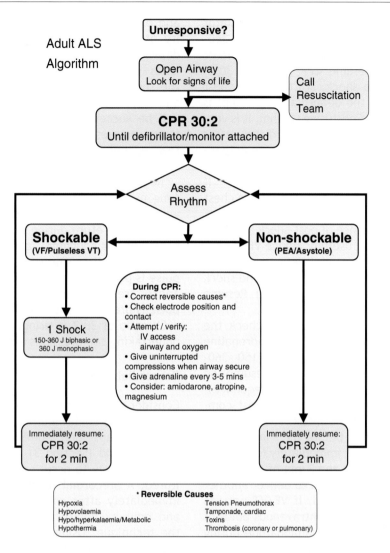

Adult ALS Algorithm

Figure 4.2 Advanced life support cardiac arrest algorithm.

and pulseless electrical activity (PEA)). The principal difference in the management of these two groups of arrhythmias is the need for attempted defibrillation in those patients with VF/VT. Subsequent actions, including chest compressions, airway management and ventilation, venous access, administration of adrenaline and the identification and correction of reversible factors, are common to both groups.

Although the ALS cardiac arrest algorithm (Figure 4.2) is applicable to all cardiac arrests, additional interventions may be indicated for cardiac arrest caused by special circumstances (Section 7).

The interventions that unquestionably contribute to improved survival after cardiac arrest are early defibrillation for VF/VT and prompt and effective bystander basic life support (BLS). Advanced airway intervention and the delivery of drugs have not been shown to increase survival to hospital

discharge after cardiac arrest, although they are still included among ALS interventions. Thus, during advanced life support, attention must be focused on early defibrillation and high-quality, uninterrupted BLS.

Shockable rhythms (ventricular fibrillation/pulseless ventricular tachycardia)

In adults, the commonest rhythm at the time of cardiac arrest is VF, which may be preceded by a period of VT or even supraventricular tachycardia (SVT).[67] Having confirmed cardiac arrest, summon help (including the request for a defibrillator) and start CPR, beginning with external chest compression, with a compression:ventilation (CV) ratio of 30:2. As soon as the defibrillator arrives, diagnose the rhythm by applying paddles or self-adhesive pads to the chest.

If VF/VT is confirmed, charge the defibrillator and give one shock (150—200-J biphasic or 360-J monophasic). Without reassessing the rhythm or feeling for a pulse, resume CPR (CV ratio 30:2) immediately after the shock, starting with chest compressions. Even if the defibrillation attempt is successful in restoring a perfusing rhythm, it is very rare for a pulse to be palpable immediately after defibrillation,[68] and the delay in trying to palpate a pulse will further compromise the myocardium if a perfusing rhythm has not been restored.[69] If a perfusing rhythm has been restored, giving chest compressions does not increase the chance of VF recurring.[70] In the presence of post-shock asystole, chest compressions may usefully induce VF.[70] Continue CPR for 2 min, then pause briefly to check the monitor: if there is still VF/VT, give a second shock (150—360-J biphasic or 360-J monophasic). Resume CPR immediately after the second shock.

Pause briefly after 2 min of CPR to check the monitor: if there is still VF/VT, give adrenaline followed immediately by a third shock (150—360-J biphasic or 360-J monophasic) and resumption of CPR (drug-shock-CPR-rhythm check sequence). Minimise the delay between stopping chest compressions and delivery of the shock. The adenaline that is given immediately before the shock will be circulated by the CPR that immediately follows the shock. After drug delivery and 2 min of CPR, analyse the rhythm and be prepared to deliver another shock immediately if indicated. If VF/VT persists after the third shock, give an intravenous bolus of amiodarone 300 mg. Inject the amiodarone during the brief rhythm analysis before delivery of the fourth shock.

When the rhythm is checked 2 min after giving a shock, if a nonshockable rhythm is present and the rhythm is organised (complexes appear regular or narrow), try to palpate a pulse. Rhythm checks must be brief, and pulse checks undertaken only if an organised rhythm is observed. If an organised rhythm is seen during a 2 min period of CPR, do not interrupt chest compressions to palpate a pulse unless the patient shows signs of life suggesting ROSC. If there is any doubt about the presence of a pulse in the presence of an organised rhythm, resume CPR. If the patient has ROSC, begin postresuscitation care. If the patient's rhythm changes to asystole or PEA, see non-shockable rhythms below.

During treatment of VF/VT, healthcare providers must practice efficient coordination between CPR and shock delivery. When VF is present for more than a few minutes, the myocardium is depleted of oxygen and metabolic substrates. A brief period of chest compressions will deliver oxygen and energy substrates and increase the probability of restoring a perfusing rhythm after shock delivery.[71] Analyses of VF waveform characteristics predictive of shock success indicate that the shorter the time between chest compression and shock delivery, the more likely the shock will be successful.[71,72] Reduction in the interval from compression to shock delivery by even a few seconds can increase the probability of shock success.[73]

Regardless of the arrest rhythm, give adrenaline 1 mg every 3—5 min until ROSC is achieved; this will be once every two loops of the algorithm. If signs of life return during CPR (movement, normal breathing, or coughing), check the monitor: if an organised rhythm is present, check for a pulse. If a pulse is palpable, continue post-resuscitation care and/or treatment of peri-arrest arrhythmia. If no pulse is present, continue CPR. Providing CPR with a CV ratio of 30:2 is tiring; change the individual undertaking compressions every 2 min.

Precordial thump

Consider giving a single precordial thump when cardiac arrest is confirmed rapidly after a witnessed, sudden collapse and a defibrillator is not immediately to hand (Section 3).[74] These circumstances are most likely to occur when the patient is monitored. A precordial thump should be undertaken immediately after confirmation of cardiac arrest and only by healthcare professionals trained in the technique. Using the ulnar edge of a tightly clenched fist, deliver a sharp impact to the lower half of the sternum from a height of about 20 cm, then retract the fist immediately to create an impulse-like stimulus. A precordial thump is most likely to be successful in converting VT to sinus rhythm. Successful treatment of VF by precordial thump is much less likely: in all the reported successful cases, the precordial thump was given within the first 10 s of VF.[75] There are very rare reports of a precordial thump converting a perfusing to a non-perfusing rhythm.[76]

Airway and ventilation

During the treatment of persistent VF, ensure good-quality chest compressions between defibrillation attempts. Consider reversible causes (4 H's and 4 T's) and, if identified, correct them. Check the electrode/defibrillating paddle positions and contacts, and the adequacy of the coupling medium, e.g. gel pads. Tracheal intubation provides the most reliable airway, but should be attempted only if the healthcare provider is properly trained and has adequate ongoing experience with the technique. Personnel skilled in advanced airway management should attempt laryngoscopy without stopping chest compressions; a brief pause in chest compressions may be required as the tube is passed through the vocal cords. Alternatively, to avoid any interruptions in chest compressions, the intubation attempt may be deferred until return of spontaneous circulation. No intubation attempt should take longer than 30 s: if intubation has not been achieved after this time, recommence bag-mask ventilation. After intubation, confirm correct tube position and secure it adequately. Once the patient's trachea has been intubated, continue chest compressions, at a rate of 100 min^{-1}, without pausing during ventilation. Ventilate the lungs at 10 breaths min^{-1}; do not hyperventilate the patient. A pause in the chest compressions allows the coronary perfusion pressure to fall substantially. On resuming compressions there is some delay before the original coronary perfusion pressure is restored, thus chest compressions that are not interrupted for ventilation result in a substantially higher mean coronary perfusion pressure.

In the absence of personnel skilled in tracheal intubation, acceptable alternatives are the Combitube, laryngeal mask airway (LMA), ProSeal LMA, or Laryngeal Tube (Section 4d). Once one of these airways has been inserted, attempt to deliver continuous chest compressions, uninterrupted during ventilation. If excessive gas leakage causes inadequate ventilation of the patient's lungs, chest compressions will have to be interrupted to enable ventilation (using a CV ratio of 30:2).

During continuous chest compressions, ventilate the lungs at 10 breaths min^{-1}.

Intravenous access and drugs

Peripheral versus central venous drug delivery. Establish intravenous access if this has not already been achieved. Although peak drug concentrations are higher and circulation times are shorter when drugs are injected into a central venous catheter compared with a peripheral cannula,[77] insertion of a central venous catheter requires interruption of CPR and is associated with several complications. Peripheral venous cannulation is quicker, easier to perform and safer. Drugs injected peripherally must be followed by a flush of at least 20 ml of fluid and elevation of the extremity for 10–20 s to facilitate drug delivery to the central circulation.

Intraosseous route. If intravenous access is difficult or impossible, consider the intraosseous route. Although normally considered as an alternative route for vascular access in children, it can also be effective in adults.[78] Intraosseous injection of drugs achieves adequate plasma concentrations in a time comparable with injection through a central venous catheter. The intraosseous route also enables withdrawal of marrow for venous blood gas analysis and measurement of electrolytes and haemoglobin concentration.

Tracheal route. If neither intravenous nor intraosseous access can be established, some drugs can be given by the tracheal route. However, unpredictable plasma concentrations are achieved when drugs are given via a tracheal tube, and the optimal tracheal dose of most drugs is unknown. During CPR, the equipotent dose of adrenaline given via the trachea is three to ten times higher than the intravenous dose.[79,80] Some animal studies suggest that the lower adrenaline concentrations achieved when the drug is given via the trachea may produce transient beta-adrenergic effects, which will cause hypotension and lower coronary artery perfusion pressure.[81–84] If given via the trachea, the dose of adrenaline is 3 mg diluted to at least 10 ml with sterile water. Dilution with water instead of 0.9% saline may achieve better drug absorption.[85] The solutions in prefilled syringes are acceptable for this purpose.

Adrenaline. Despite the widespread use of adrenaline during resuscitation, and several studies involving vasopressin, there is no placebo-controlled study that shows that the routine use of any vasopressor at any stage during human cardiac arrest increases survival to hospital discharge. Current evidence is insufficient to support or refute the routine use of any particular drug or sequence of drugs. Despite the lack of human data, the use of adrenaline is still recommended, based largely on animal data. The alpha-adrenergic actions of adrenaline cause vasoconstriction, which increases myocardial and cerebral perfusion pressure. The higher coronary blood flow increases the frequency of the VF waveform and should improve the chance of restoring a circulation when defibrillation is attempted.[86–88] The optimal duration of CPR and number of shocks that should be given before giving drugs is unknown. On the basis of expert consensus, if VF/VT persists after two shocks, give adrenaline and repeat every 3–5 min during cardiac arrest. Do not interrupt CPR to give drugs.

Anti-arrhythmic drugs. There is no evidence that giving any anti-arrhythmic drug routinely during human cardiac arrest increases survival to hospital discharge. In comparison with placebo[89] and lidocaine,[90] the use of amiodarone in shock-refractory VF improves the short-term outcome of survival to hospital admission. In these studies, the anti-arrhythmic therapy was given if VF/VT persisted after at least three shocks; however, these were delivered using the conventional three-stacked shocks strategy. There are no data on the use of amiodarone for shock-refractory VF/VT when single shocks are used. On the basis of expert consensus, if VF/VT persists after three shocks, give 300 mg amiodarone by bolus injection. A further dose of 150 mg may be given for recurrent or refractory VF/VT, followed by an infusion of 900 mg over 24. Lidocaine 1 mg kg^{-1} may be used as an alternative if amiodarone is not available, but do not give lidocaine if amiodarone has been given already.

Magnesium. Although the routine use of magnesium in cardiac arrest does not increase survival,[91-95] give magnesium (8 mmol = 4 ml 50% magnesium sulphate or 2 g) for refractory VF if there is any suspicion of hypomagnesaemia (e.g., patients on potassium-losing diuretics).

Bicarbonate. Administering sodium bicarbonate routinely during cardiac arrest and CPR (especially in out-of-hospital cardiac arrests) or after return of spontaneous circulation is not recommended. Give sodium bicarbonate (50 mmol) if cardiac arrest is associated with hyperkalaemia or tricyclic antidepressant overdose; repeat the dose according to the clinical condition and result of repeated blood gas analysis. Some experts give bicarbonate if the arterial pH is less than 7.1, but this is controversial. During cardiac arrest, arterial blood gas values do not reflect the acid—base state of the tissues[96]; the tissue pH will be lower than that in arterial blood. Mixed venous blood values give a more accurate estimate of the pH in the tissues,[96] but it is rare for a pulmonary artery catheter to be in situ at the time of cardiac arrest. If a central venous catheter is in situ, central venous blood gas analysis will provide a closer estimate of tissue acid/base state than that provided by arterial blood.

Persistent ventricular fibrillation

In VF persists, consider changing the position of the paddles (Section 3). Review all potentially reversible causes (see below) and treat any that are identified.

The duration of any individual resuscitation attempt is a matter of clinical judgement, taking into consideration the circumstances and the perceived prospect of a successful outcome. If it was considered appropriate to start resuscitation, it is usually considered worthwhile continuing as long as the patient remains in VF/VT.

Non-shockable rhythms (PEA and asystole)

Pulseless electrical activity (PEA) is defined as cardiac electrical activity in the absence of any palpable pulses. These patients often have some mechanical myocardial contractions, but these are too weak to produce a detectable pulse or blood pressure. PEA is often caused by reversible conditions, and can be treated if those conditions are identified and corrected (see below). Survival following cardiac arrest with asystole or PEA is unlikely unless a reversible cause can be found and treated effectively.

If the initial monitored rhythm is PEA or asystole, start CPR 30:2 and give adrenaline 1 mg as soon as intravascular access is achieved. If asystole is displayed, check without stopping CPR that the leads are attached correctly. Asystole is a condition that could be exacerbated or precipitated by excessive vagal tone and, theoretically, this could be reversed by a vagolytic drug; therefore, despite the lack of evidence that routine atropine for asystolic cardiac arrest increases survival, give atropine 3 mg (the dose that will provide maximum vagal blockade) if there is asystole or the rhythm is slow PEA (rate <60 min^{-1}). Secure the airway as soon as possible, to enable chest compressions to be delivered without pausing during ventilation. After 2 min of CPR, recheck the rhythm. If no rhythm is present (asystole), or if there is no change in the ECG appearance, resume CPR immediately. If an organised rhythm is present, attempt to palpate a pulse. If no pulse is present (or if there is any doubt about the presence of a pulse), continue CPR. If a pulse is present, begin post-resuscitation care. If signs of life return during CPR, check the rhythm and attempt to palpate a pulse.

Whenever a diagnosis of asystole is made, check the ECG carefully for the presence of P waves, because this may respond to cardiac pacing. There is no benefit in attempting to pace true asystole.

If there is doubt about whether the rhythm is asystole or fine VF, do not attempt defibrillation; instead, continue chest compressions and ventilation. Fine VF that is difficult to distinguish from asystole will not be shocked successfully into a perfusing rhythm. Continuing good-quality CPR may improve the amplitude and frequency of the VF and improve the chance of successful defibrillation to a perfusing rhythm. Delivering repeated shocks in an attempt to defibrillate what is thought to be fine VF will increase myocardial injury, both directly from the electricity and indirectly from the interruptions in coronary blood flow.

During the treatment of asystole or PEA, if the rhythm changes to VF, follow the left side of the algorithm. Otherwise, continue CPR and give adrenaline every 3—5 min (every other loop of the algorithm).

Potentially reversible causes

Potential causes or aggravating factors for which specific treatment exists must be considered during any cardiac arrest. For ease of memory, these are divided into two groups of four based upon their initial letter: either H or T. More details on many of these conditions are covered in Section 7.

The four Hs

Minimise the risk of hypoxia by ensuring that the patient's lungs are ventilated adequately with 100% oxygen. Make sure there is adequate chest rise and bilateral breath sounds. Using the techniques described in Section 4d, check carefully that the tracheal tube is not misplaced in a bronchus or the oesophagus.

Pulseless electrical activity caused by hypovolaemia is due usually to severe haemorrhage. This may be precipitated by trauma (Section 7i), gastrointestinal bleeding or rupture of an aortic aneurysm. Intravascular volume should be restored rapidly with fluid, coupled with urgent surgery to stop the haemorrhage.

Hyperkalaemia, hypokalaemia, hypocalcaemia, acidaemia and other metabolic disorders are detected by biochemical tests or suggested by the patient's medical history, e.g. renal failure (Section 7a). A 12-lead ECG may be diagnostic. Intravenous calcium chloride is indicated in the presence of hyperkalaemia, hypocalcaemia and calcium channel-blocker overdose.

Suspect hypothermia in any drowning incident (Sections 7c and d); use a low-reading thermometer.

The four Ts

A tension pneumothorax may be the primary cause of PEA and may follow attempts at central venous catheter insertion. The diagnosis is made clinically. Decompress rapidly by needle thoracocentesis, and then insert a chest drain.

Cardiac tamponade is difficult to diagnose because the typical signs of distended neck veins and hypotension are usually obscured by the arrest itself. Cardiac arrest after penetrating chest trauma is highly suggestive of tamponade and is an indication for needle pericardiocentesis or resuscitative thoracotomy (see Section 7i).

In the absence of a specific history, the accidental or deliberate ingestion of therapeutic or toxic substances may be revealed only by laboratory investigations (Section 7b). Where available, the appropriate antidotes should be used, but most often treatment is supportive.

The commonest cause of thromboembolic or mechanical circulatory obstruction is massive pulmonary embolus. If cardiac arrest is thought to be caused by pulmonary embolism, consider giving a thrombolytic drug immediately (Section 4e).[97]

4d. Airway management and ventilation

Introduction

Patients requiring resuscitation often have an obstructed airway, usually secondary to loss of consciousness, but occasionally it may be the primary cause of cardiorespiratory arrest. Prompt assessment, with control of the airway and ventilation of the lungs, is essential. This will help to prevent secondary hypoxic damage to the brain and other vital organs. Without adequate oxygenation it may be impossible to restore a spontaneous cardiac output. These principles may not apply to the witnessed primary cardiac arrest in the vicinity of a defibrillator; in this case, the priority is immediate attempted defibrillation.

Airway obstruction

Causes of airway obstruction

Obstruction of the airway may be partial or complete. It may occur at any level, from the nose and mouth down to the trachea (Figure 4.3). In the unconscious patient, the commonest site of airway obstruction is at the level of the pharynx. Until recently this obstruction had been attributed to posterior displacement of the tongue caused by decreased muscle tone; with the tongue ultimately touching the posterior pharyngeal wall. The precise cause of airway obstruction in the unconscious state has been identified by studying patients under general anaesthesia.[98,99] These studies of anaesthetised patients have shown that the site of airway obstruction is at the soft palate and epiglottis and not the tongue. Obstruction may be caused also by vomit or blood (regurgitation of gastric contents or trauma), or by foreign bodies. Laryngeal obstruction may be caused by oedema from burns, inflammation or anaphylaxis. Upper airway stimulation may cause laryngeal spasm. Obstruction of the airway below the larynx is less com-

Causes of airway obstruction

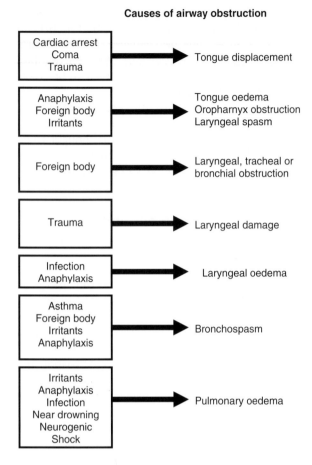

Figure 4.3 Causes of airway obstruction.

mon, but may arise from excessive bronchial secretions, mucosal oedema, bronchospasm, pulmonary oedema or aspiration of gastric contents.

Recognition of airway obstruction

Airway obstruction can be subtle and is often missed by healthcare professionals, let alone by lay people. The 'look, listen and feel' approach is a simple, systematic method of detecting airway obstruction.

- Look for chest and abdominal movements.
- Listen and feel for airflow at the mouth and nose.

In partial airway obstruction, air entry is diminished and usually noisy. Inspiratory stridor is caused by obstruction at the laryngeal level or above. Expiratory wheeze implies obstruction of the lower airways, which tend to collapse and obstruct during expiration. Other characteristic sounds include the following:

- Gurgling is caused by liquid or semisolid foreign material in the main airways.
- Snoring arises when the pharynx is partially occluded by the soft palate or epiglottis.
- Crowing is the sound of laryngeal spasm.

In a patient who is making respiratory efforts, complete airway obstruction causes paradoxical chest and abdominal movement, often described as 'see-saw breathing'. As the patient attempts to breathe in, the chest is drawn in and the abdomen expands; the opposite occurs during expiration. This is in contrast to the normal breathing pattern of synchronous movement upwards and outwards of the abdomen (pushed down by the diaphragm) with the lifting of the chest wall. During airway obstruction, other accessory muscles of respiration are used, with the neck and the shoulder muscles contracting to assist movement of the thoracic cage. Full examination of the neck, chest and abdomen is required to differentiate the paradoxical movements that may mimic normal respiration. The examination must include listening for the absence of breath sounds in order to diagnose complete airway obstruction reliably; any noisy breathing indicates partial airway obstruction. During apnoea, when spontaneous breathing movements are absent, complete airway obstruction is recognised by failure to inflate the lungs during attempted positive pressure ventilation. Unless airway patency can be re-established to enable adequate lung ventilation within a period of a very few minutes, neurological and other vital organ injury may occur, leading to cardiac arrest.

Basic airway management

Once any degree of obstruction is recognised, immediate measures must be taken to create and maintain a clear airway. There are three manoeuvres that may improve the patency of an airway obstructed by the tongue or other upper airway structures: head tilt, chin lift, and jaw thrust.

Head tilt and chin lift

The rescuer's hand is placed on the patient's forehead and the head gently tilted back; the fingertips of the other hand are placed under the point of the patient's chin, which is gently lifted to stretch the anterior neck structures (Figure 4.4).[100–105]

Jaw thrust

Jaw thrust is an alternative manoeuvre for bringing the mandible forward and relieving obstruction by the soft palate and epiglottis. The rescuer's index and other fingers are placed behind the angle of the mandible, and pressure is applied upwards and forwards. Using the thumbs, the mouth is opened slightly by downward displacement of the chin (Figure 4.5).

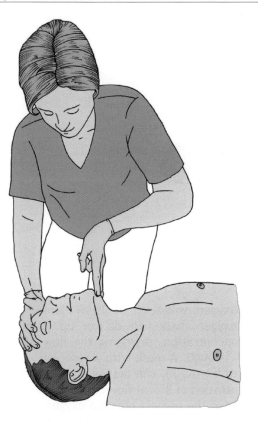

Figure 4.4 Head tilt and chin lift. © 2005 European Resuscitation Council.

These simple positional methods are successful in most cases where airway obstruction results from relaxation of the soft tissues. If a clear airway cannot be achieved, look for other causes of airway obstruction. Use a finger sweep to remove any solid foreign body seen in the mouth. Remove broken or displaced dentures, but leave well-fitting dentures as they help to maintain the contours of the mouth, facilitating a good seal for ventilation.

Airway management in patients with suspected cervical spine injury

If spinal injury is suspected (e.g., if the victim has fallen, been struck on the head or neck, or has been rescued after diving into shallow water), maintain the head, neck, chest and lumbar region in the neutral position during resuscitation. Excessive head tilt could aggravate the injury and damage the cervical spinal cord[106–110]; however, this complication has not been documented and the relative risk is unknown. When there is a risk of cervical spine injury, establish a clear upper airway by using jaw thrust or chin lift in combination with manual in-line stabilisation (MILS) of the head and neck by an assistant.[111,112] If life-threatening airway obstruction persists despite effective application of jaw thrust or chin lift, add head tilt a small amount at a time until the airway is open; establishing a patent airway takes priority over concerns about a potential cervical spine injury.

Adjuncts to basic airway techniques

Simple airway adjuncts are often helpful, and sometimes essential, to maintain an open airway, particularly when resuscitation is prolonged. The position of the head and neck must be maintained to keep the airway aligned. Oropharyngeal and nasopharyngeal airways overcome backward displacement of the soft palate and tongue in an unconscious patient, but head tilt and jaw thrust may also be required.

Oropharyngeal airways. Oropharyngeal airways are available in sizes suitable for the newborn to large adults. An estimate of the size required is obtained by selecting an airway with a length corresponding to the vertical distance between

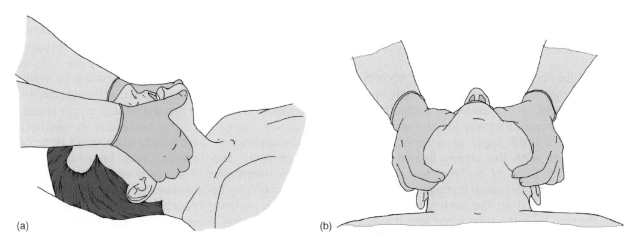

(a)   (b)

Figure 4.5 Jaw thrust. © 2005 European Resuscitation Council.

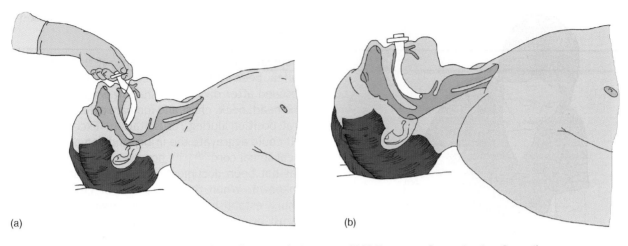

(a)   (b)

Figure 4.6 Insertion of oropharyngeal airway. © 2005 European Resuscitation Council.

the patient's incisors and the angle of the jaw (Figure 4.6). The most common sizes are 2, 3 and 4 for small, medium and large adults, respectively.

If the glossopharyngeal and laryngeal reflexes are present, vomiting or laryngospasm may be caused by inserting an oropharyngeal airway; thus, insertion should be attempted only in comatose patients. The oropharyngeal airway can become obstructed at three possible sites:[113] part of the tongue can occlude the end of the airway; the airway can lodge in the vallecula; and the airway can be obstructed by the epiglottis.

Nasopharyngeal airways. In patients who are not deeply unconscious, a nasopharyngeal airway is tolerated better than an oropharyngeal airway. The nasopharyngeal airway may be life saving in patients with clenched jaws, trismus or maxillofacial injuries, when insertion of an oral airway is impossible. Inadvertent insertion of a nasopharyngeal airway through a fracture of the skull base and into the cranial vault is possible, but extremely rare.[114,115] In the presence of a known or suspected basal skull fracture an oral airway is preferred but, if this is not possible and the airway is obstructed, gentle insertion of a nasopharyngeal airway may be life saving (i.e., the benefits may far outweigh the risks).

The tubes are sized in millimetres according to their internal diameter, and the length increases with diameter. The traditional methods of sizing a nasopharyngeal airway (measurement against the patient's little finger or anterior nares) do not correlate with the airway anatomy and are unreliable.[116] Sizes of 6—7 mm are suitable for adults. Insertion can cause damage to the mucosal lining of the nasal airway, with bleeding in up to 30% of cases.[117] If the tube is too long it may stimulate the laryngeal or glossopharyngeal reflexes to produce laryngospasm or vomiting.

Oxygen

Give oxygen whenever it is available. A standard oxygen mask will deliver up to 50% oxygen concentration, providing the flow of oxygen is high enough. A mask with a reservoir bag (non-rebreathing mask), can deliver an inspired oxygen concentration of 85% at flows of 10—15 l min^{-1}. Initially, give the highest possible oxygen concentration, which can then be titrated to the oxygen saturation by pulse oximeter (SpO$_2$) or arterial blood gases.

Suction

Use a wide-bore rigid sucker (Yankauer) to remove liquid (blood, saliva and gastric contents) from the upper airway. Use the sucker cautiously if the patient has an intact gag reflex; the sucker can provoke vomiting.

Ventilation

Provide artificial ventilation as soon as possible for any patient in whom spontaneous ventilation is inadequate or absent. Expired air ventilation (rescue breathing) is effective, but the rescuer's expired oxygen concentration is only 16—17%, so it must be replaced as soon as possible by ventilation with oxygen-enriched air. Although mouth-to-mouth ventilation has the benefit of not requiring any equipment, the technique is aesthetically unpleasant, particularly when vomit or blood is present, and rescuers may be reluctant to place themselves in intimate contact with a victim who may be unknown to them.[118—121] There are only isolated reports of individuals acquiring infections after providing CPR, e.g. tuberculosis[122] and severe acute respiratory distress syndrome (SARS).[123] Transmission of human immunodefi-

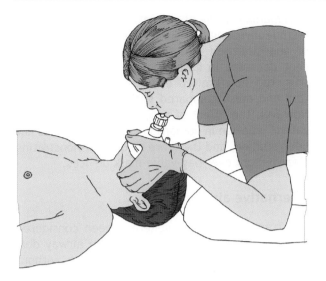

Figure 4.7 Mouth-to-mask ventilation. © 2005 European Resuscitation Council.

ciency virus (HIV) during provision of CPR has never been reported. Simple adjuncts are available to enable direct person-to-person contact to be avoided; some of these devices may reduce the risk of cross-infection between patient and rescuer, although they are unlikely to offer significant protection from SARS.[123] The pocket resuscitation mask is used widely. It is similar to an anaesthetic facemask, and enables mouth-to-mask ventilation. It has a unidirectional valve, which directs the patient's expired air away from the rescuer. The mask is transparent so that vomit or blood from the patient can be seen. Some masks have a connector for the addition of oxygen. When using masks without a connector, supplemental oxygen can be given by placing the tubing underneath one side and ensuring an adequate seal. Use a two-hand technique to maximise the seal with the patient's face (Figure 4.7).

High airway pressures can be generated if the tidal volumes or inspiratory flows are excessive, predisposing to gastric inflation and subsequent risk of regurgitation and pulmonary aspiration. The possibility of gastric inflation is increased by

- malalignment of the head and neck, and an obstructed airway
- an incompetent oesophageal sphincter (present in all patients with cardiac arrest)
- a high inflation pressure

Conversely, if inspiratory flow is too low, inspiratory time will be prolonged and the time available to give chest compressions is reduced. Deliver each breath over approximately 1 s and transfer a volume that corresponds to normal chest movement; this represents a compromise between giving

an adequate volume, minimising the risk of gastric inflation, and allowing adequate time for chest compressions. During CPR with an unprotected airway, give two ventilations after each sequence of 30 chest compressions.

Self-inflating bag

The self-inflating bag can be connected to a facemask, tracheal tube or alternative airway device such as the LMA or Combitube. Without supplemental oxygen, the self-inflating bag ventilates the patient's lungs with ambient air (21% oxygen). This can be increased to about 45% by attaching oxygen directly to the bag. If a reservoir system is attached and the oxygen flow is increased to approximately 10 l min^{-1}, an inspired oxygen concentration of approximately 85% can be achieved.

Although the bag-mask device enables ventilation with high concentrations of oxygen, its use by a single person requires considerable skill. When used with a face mask, it is often difficult to achieve a gas-tight seal between the mask and the patient's face, and to maintain a patent airway with one hand while squeezing the bag with the other.[124] Any significant leak will cause hypoventilation and, if the airway is not patent, gas may be forced into the stomach.[125,126] This will reduce ventilation further and greatly increase the risk of regurgitation and aspiration.[127] Cricoid pressure can reduce this risk but requires the presence of a trained assistant. Poorly applied cricoid pressure may make it more difficult to ventilate the patient's lungs.[128]

The two-person technique for bag-mask ventilation is preferable (Figure 4.8). One person holds the facemask in place using a jaw thrust with both

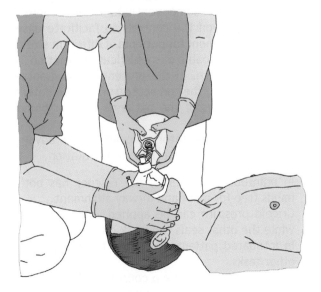

Figure 4.8 The two-person technique for bag-mask ventilation. © 2005 European Resuscitation Council.

hands, and an assistant squeezes the bag. In this way, a better seal can be achieved and the patient's lungs can be ventilated more effectively and safely.

Once a tracheal tube, Combitube or supraglottic airway device has been inserted, ventilate the lungs at a rate of 10 breaths min^{-1} and continue chest compressions without pausing during ventilations. The seal of the LMA around the larynx is unlikely to be good enough to prevent at least some gas leaking when inspiration coincides with chest compressions. Moderate gas leakage is acceptable, particularly as most of this gas will pass up through the patient's mouth; if excessive gas leakage results in inadequate ventilation of the patient's lungs, chest compressions will have to be interrupted to enable ventilation, using a compression—ventilation ratio of 30:2.

Automatic ventilators

Very few studies address specific aspects of ventilation during advanced life support. There are some data indicating that the ventilation rates delivered by healthcare personnel during cardiac arrest are excessive.[61,129] Automatic ventilators or resuscitators provide a constant flow of gas to the patient during inspiration; the volume delivered is dependent on the inspiratory time (a longer time provides a greater tidal volume). Because pressure in the airway rises during inspiration, these devices are often pressure limited to protect the lungs against barotrauma. An automatic ventilator can be used with either a facemask or other airway device (e.g., tracheal tube, LMA).

An automatic resuscitator should be set initially to deliver a tidal volume of 6—7 ml kg^{-1} at 10 breaths min^{-1}. Some ventilators have coordinated markings on the controls to facilitate easy and rapid adjustment for patients of different sizes, and others are capable of sophisticated variation in respiratory pattern. In the presence of a spontaneous circulation, the correct setting will be determined by analysis of the patient's arterial blood gases.

Automatic resuscitators provide many advantages over alternative methods of ventilation.

- In unintubated patients, the rescuer has both hands free for mask and airway alignment.
- Cricoid pressure can be applied with one hand while the other seals the mask on the face.
- In intubated patients they free the rescuer for other tasks.
- Once set, they provide a constant tidal volume, respiratory rate and minute ventilation; thus, they may help to avoid excessive ventilation.

A manikin study of simulated cardiac arrest and a study involving fire-fighters ventilating the lungs of anaesthetised patients both showed a significant decrease in gastric inflation with manually-triggered flow-limited oxygen-powered resuscitators and mask compared with a bag-mask.[130,131] However, the effect of automatic resuscitators on gastric inflation in humans in cardiac arrest has not been studied, and there are no data demonstrating clear benefit over bag-valve-mask devices.

Alternative airway devices

The tracheal tube has generally been considered the optimal method of managing the airway during cardiac arrest. There is evidence that, without adequate training and experience, the incidence of complications, such as unrecognised oesophageal intubation (6—14% in some studies)[132—135] and dislodgement, is unacceptably high.[136] Prolonged attempts at tracheal intubation are harmful; the cessation of chest compressions during this time will compromise coronary and cerebral perfusion. Several alternative airway devices have been considered for airway management during CPR. The Combitube, the LMA, and the Laryngeal Tube (LT) are the only alternative devices to be studied during CPR, but none of these studies have been powered adequately to enable survival to be studied as a primary endpoint; instead, most researchers have studied insertion and ventilation success rates. There are no data supporting the routine use of any specific approach to airway management during cardiac arrest. The best technique is dependent on the precise circumstances of the cardiac arrest and the competence of the rescuer.

Laryngeal mask airway (LMA)

The laryngeal mask airway comprises a wide-bore tube with an elliptical inflated cuff designed to seal around the laryngeal opening (Figure 4.9). It is easier to insert than a tracheal tube.[137—143] The LMA has been studied during CPR, but none of these studies has compared it directly with the tracheal tube. During CPR, successful ventilation is achieved with the LMA in 72—98% of cases.[144—150]

Ventilation using the LMA is more efficient and easier than with a bag-mask.[124] When an LMA can be inserted without delay it is preferable to avoid bag-mask ventilation altogether. When used for intermittent positive pressure ventilation, provided high inflation pressures (>20 cm H_2O) are avoided, gastric inflation can be minimised. In comparison with bag-mask ventilation, use of a self-inflating bag and

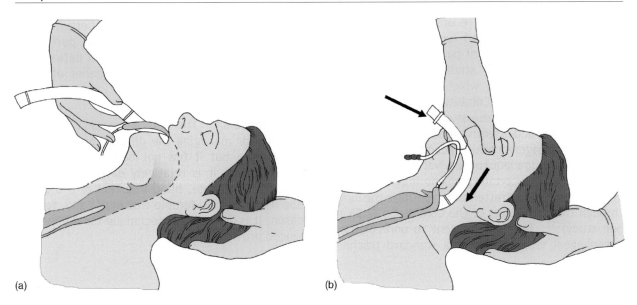

Figure 4.9   Insertion of a laryngeal mask airway. © 2005 European Resuscitation Council.

LMA during cardiac arrest reduces the incidence of regurgitation.[127]

In comparison with tracheal intubation, the perceived disadvantages of the LMA are the increased risk of aspiration and inability to provide adequate ventilation in patients with low lung and/or chest-wall compliance. There are no data demonstrating whether or not it is possible to provide adequate ventilation via an LMA without interruption of chest compressions. The ability to ventilate the lungs adequately while continuing to compress the chest

may be one of the main benefits of a tracheal tube. There are remarkably few cases of pulmonary aspiration reported in the studies of the LMA during CPR.

The Combitube

The Combitube is a double-lumen tube introduced blindly over the tongue, and provides a route for ventilation whether the tube has passed into the oesophagus (Figure 4.10a) or the tra-

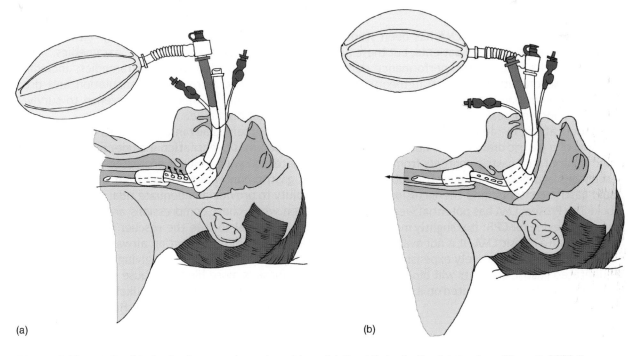

Figure 4.10   (a) Combitube in the oesophageal position. (b) Combitube in the tracheal position. © 2005 European Resuscitation Council.

chea (Figure 4.10b). There are many studies of the Combitube in CPR and successful ventilation was achieved in 79—98% of patients.[146,151—157] All except one[151] of these studies involved out-of-hospital cardiac arrest, which reflects the infrequency with which the Combitube is used in hospitals. On the basis of these studies, the Combitube appears as safe and effective as tracheal intubation for airway management during cardiac arrest; however, there are inadequate survival data to be able to comment with certainty on the impact on outcome. It is possible to attempt to ventilate the lungs through the wrong port of the Combitube (2.2% in one study)[152]: This is equivalent to unrecognised oesophageal intubation with a standard tracheal tube.

Other airway devices

Laryngeal Tube. The LT is a relatively new airway device; its function in anaesthetised patients has been reported in several studies. The performance of the LT is favourable in comparison with the classic LMA and LMA,[158,159] and successful insertion rates have been reported even in studies of paramedics.[160] There are sporadic case reports relating to use of the laryngeal tube during CPR.[161,162] In a recent study, the LT was placed in 30 patients in cardiac arrest out of hospital by minimally trained nurses.[163] LT insertion was successful within two attempts in 90% of patients, and ventilation was adequate in 80% of cases. No regurgitation occurred in any patient.

ProSeal LMA. The ProSeal LMA has been studied extensively in anaesthetised patients, but there are no studies of its function and performance during CPR. It has several attributes that, in theory, make it more suitable than the classic LMA for use during CPR: improved seal with the larynx enabling ventilation at higher airway pressures,[164,165] the inclusion of a gastric drain tube enabling venting of liquid regurgitated gastric contents from the upper oesophagus and passage of a gastric tube to drain liquid gastric contents, and the inclusion of a bite block. The Proseal LMA has potential weaknesses as an airway device for CPR: it is slightly more difficult to insert than a classic LMA, it is not available in disposable form and is relatively expensive, and solid regurgitated gastric contents will block the gastric drainage tube. Data are awaited on its performance during CPR.

Airway management device. In anaesthetised patients, the airway management device (AMD) performed poorly in one study,[166] but a modified version appeared to function slightly better.[167] The pharyngeal airway express (PAX) also performed poorly in one study of anaesthetised patients.[168] There are no data on the use of either of these devices during CPR.

Intubating LMA. The intubating LMA (ILMA) is valuable for managing the difficult airway during anaesthesia, but it has not been studied during CPR. Although it is relatively easy to insert the ILMA,[169,170] reliable, blind insertion of a tracheal tube requires considerable training[171] and, for this reason, it is not an ideal technique for the inexperienced provider.

Tracheal intubation

There is insufficient evidence to support or refute the use of any specific technique to maintain an airway and provide ventilation in adults with cardiopulmonary arrest. Despite this, tracheal intubation is perceived as the optimal method of providing and maintaining a clear and secure airway. It should be used only when trained personnel are available to carry out the procedure with a high level of skill and confidence. The only randomised controlled trial comparing tracheal intubation with bag-mask ventilation was undertaken in children requiring airway management out-of-hospital.[172] In this investigation there was no difference in survival to discharge, but it is unclear how applicable this paediatric study is to adult resuscitation. Two reports compared outcomes from out-of-hospital cardiac arrest in adults when treated by either emergency medical technicians or paramedics.[173,174] The skills provided by the paramedics, including intubation and intravenous cannulation and drug administration,[174] made no difference to survival to hospital discharge.

The perceived advantages of tracheal intubation over bag-mask ventilation include: maintenance of a patent airway, which is protected from aspiration of gastric contents or blood from the oropharynx; ability to provide an adequate tidal volume reliably even when chest compressions are uninterrupted; the potential to free the rescuer's hands for other tasks; the ability to suction airway secretions; and the provision of a route for giving drugs. Use of the bag-mask is more likely to cause gastric distension which, theoretically, is more likely to cause regurgitation with risk of aspiration. However, there are no reliable data to indicate that the incidence of aspiration is any more in cardiac arrest patients ventilated with bag-mask versus those that are ventilated via tracheal tube.

The perceived disadvantages of tracheal intubation over bag-mask ventilation include: the risk of an unrecognised misplaced tracheal tube, which in patients with out-of-hospital cardiac arrest in some studies ranges from 6%[132–134] to 14%[135]; a prolonged period without chest compressions while intubation is attempted; and a comparatively high failure rate. Intubation success rates correlate with the intubation experience attained by individual paramedics.[175] Rates for failure to intubate are as high as 50% in prehospital systems with a low patient volume and providers who do not perform intubation frequently.[134] The cost of training prehospital staff to undertake intubation should also be considered. Healthcare personnel who undertake prehospital intubation should do so only within a structured, monitored programme, which should include comprehensive competency-based training and regular opportunities to refresh skills.

In some cases, laryngoscopy and attempted intubation may prove impossible or cause life-threatening deterioration in the patient's condition. Such circumstances include acute epiglottal conditions, pharyngeal pathology, head injury (where straining may occur further rise in intracranial pressure) or cervical spine injury. In these circumstances, specialist skills such as the use of anaesthetic drugs or fibreoptic laryngoscopy may be required. These techniques require a high level of skill and training.

Rescuers must weigh the risks and benefits of intubation against the need to provide effective chest compressions. The intubation attempt will require interruption of chest compressions but, once an advanced airway is in place, ventilation will not require interruption of chest compressions. Personnel skilled in advanced airway management should be able to undertake laryngoscopy without stopping chest compressions; a brief pause in chest compressions will be required only as the tube is passed through the vocal cords. Alternatively, to avoid any interruptions in chest compressions, the intubation attempt may be deferred until return of spontaneous circulation. No intubation attempt should take longer than 30 s; if intubation has not been achieved after this time, recommence bag-mask ventilation. After intubation, tube placement must be confirmed and the tube secured adequately.

Confirmation of correct placement of the tracheal tube

Unrecognised oesophageal intubation is the most serious complication of attempted tracheal intubation. Routine use of primary and secondary techniques to confirm correct placement of the tracheal tube should reduce this risk. Primary assessment includes observation of chest expansion bilaterally, auscultation over the lung fields bilaterally in the axillae (breath sounds should be equal and adequate) and over the epigastrium (breath sounds should not be heard). Clinical signs of correct tube placement (condensation in the tube, chest rise, breath sounds on auscultation of lungs, and inability to hear gas entering the stomach) are not completely reliable. Secondary confirmation of tracheal tube placement by an exhaled carbon dioxide or oesophageal detection device should reduce the risk of unrecognised oesophageal intubation. If there is doubt about correct tube placement, use the laryngoscope and look directly to see if the tube passes through the vocal cords.

None of the secondary confirmation techniques will differentiate between a tube placed in a main bronchus and one placed correctly in the trachea. There are inadequate data to identify the optimal method of confirming tube placement during cardiac arrest, and all devices should be considered as adjuncts to other confirmatory techniques.[176] There are no data quantifying their ability to monitor tube position after initial placement.

The oesophageal detector device creates a suction force at the tracheal end of the tracheal tube, either by pulling back the plunger on a large syringe or releasing a compressed flexible bulb. Air is aspirated easily from the lower airways through a tracheal tube placed in the cartilage-supported rigid trachea. When the tube is in the oesophagus, air cannot be aspirated because the oesophagus collapses when aspiration is attempted. The oesophageal detector device is generally reliable in patients with both a perfusing and a non-perfusing rhythm, but it may be misleading in patients with morbid obesity, late pregnancy or severe asthma or when there are copious tracheal secretions; in these conditions the trachea may collapse when aspiration is attempted.[133,177–180]

Carbon dioxide detector devices measure the concentration of exhaled carbon dioxide from the lungs. The persistence of exhaled carbon dioxide after six ventilations indicates placement of the tracheal tube in the trachea or a main bronchus.[181] Confirmation of correct placement above the carina will require auscultation of the chest bilaterally in the mid-axillary lines. In patients with a spontaneous circulation, a lack of exhaled carbon dioxide indicates that the tube is in the oesophagus. During cardiac arrest, pulmonary blood flow may be so low that there is insufficient exhaled carbon dioxide, so the detector does not identify a correctly placed tracheal tube. When exhaled carbon dioxide is detected in cardiac arrest, it indicates reliably that the tube is in the trachea or main bronchus but, when it is absent, tracheal tube placement is best confirmed with an oesophageal detector device. A variety of electronic as well as simple, inexpensive, colorimetric carbon dioxide detectors are available for both in-hospital and out-of-hospital use.

Cricoid pressure

During bag-mask ventilation and attempted intubation, cricoid pressure applied by a trained assistant should prevent passive regurgitation of gastric contents and the consequent risk of pulmonary aspiration. If the technique is applied imprecisely or with excessive force, ventilation and intubation can be made more difficult.[128] If ventilation of the patient's lungs is not possible, reduce the pressure applied to the cricoid cartilage or remove it completely. If the patient vomits, release the cricoid immediately.

Securing the tracheal tube

Accidental dislodgement of a tracheal tube can occur at any time, but may be more likely during resuscitation and during transport. The most effective method for securing the tracheal tube has yet to be determined; use either conventional tapes or ties, or purpose-made tracheal tube holders.

Cricothyroidotomy

Occasionally, it will be impossible to ventilate an apnoeic patient with a bag-mask, or to pass a tracheal tube or alternative airway device. This may occur in patients with extensive facial trauma or laryngeal obstruction due to oedema or foreign material. In these circumstances, delivery of oxygen through a needle or surgical cricothyroidotomy may be life-saving. A tracheostomy is contraindicated in an emergency, as it is time consuming, hazardous and requires considerable surgical skill and equipment.

Surgical cricothyroidotomy provides a definitive airway that can be used to ventilate the patient's lungs until semi-elective intubation or tracheostomy is performed. Needle cricothyroidotomy is a much more temporary procedure providing only short-term oxygenation. It requires a wide-bore, non-kinking cannula, a high-pressure oxygen source, runs the risk of barotrauma and can be particularly ineffective in patients with chest trauma. It is also prone to failure because of kinking of the cannula, and is unsuitable for patient transfer.

4e. Assisting the circulation

Drugs and fluids for cardiac arrest

This topic is divided into: drugs used during the management of a cardiac arrest; anti-arrhythmic drugs used in the peri-arrest period; other drugs used in the peri-arrest period; fluids; and routes for drug delivery. Every effort has been made to provide accurate information on the drugs in these guidelines, but literature from the relevant pharmaceutical companies will provide the most up-to-date data.

Drugs used during the treatment of cardiac arrest

Only a few drugs are indicated during the immediate management of a cardiac arrest, and there is limited scientific evidence supporting their use. Drugs should be considered only after initial shocks have been delivered (if indicated) and chest compressions and ventilation have been started.

There are three groups of drugs relevant to the management of cardiac arrest that were reviewed during the 2005 Consensus Conference: vasopressors, anti-arrhythmics and other drugs. Routes of drug delivery other than the optimal intravenous route were also reviewed and are discussed.

Vasopressors

There are currently no placebo-controlled studies showing that the routine use of any vasopressor at any stage during human cardiac arrest increases survival to hospital discharge. The primary goal of cardiopulmonary resuscitation is to re-establish blood flow to vital organs until the restoration of spontaneous circulation. Despite the lack of data from cardiac arrest in humans, vasopressors continue to be recommended as a means of increasing cerebral and coronary perfusion during CPR.

Adrenaline (epinephrine) versus vasopressin. Adrenaline has been the primary sympathomimetic agent for the management of cardiac arrest for 40 years.[182] Its primary efficacy is due to its alpha-adrenergic, vasoconstrictive effects causing systemic vasoconstriction, which increases coronary and cerebral perfusion pressures. The beta-adrenergic actions of adrenaline (inotropic, chronotropic) may increase coronary and cerebral blood flow, but concomitant increases in myocardial oxygen consumption, ectopic ventricular arrhythmias (particularly when the myocardium is acidotic) and transient hypoxaemia due to pulmonary arteriovenous shunting may offset these benefits.

The potentially deleterious beta-effects of adrenaline have led to exploration of alternative vasopressors. Vasopressin is a naturally occurring antidiuretic hormone. In very high doses it is a powerful vasoconstrictor that acts by stimulation of smooth muscle V1 receptors. The importance of vasopressin in cardiac arrest was first recognised in studies of out-of-hospital cardiac arrest patients, where vasopressin levels were found to be higher in successfully resuscitated patients.[183,184] Although clinical[185,186] and animal[187-189] studies demonstrated improved haemodynamic variables when using vasopressin as an alternative to adrenaline during resuscitation from cardiac arrest, some,[186] but not all, demonstrated improved survival.[190,191]

The first clinical use of vasopressin during cardiac arrest was reported in 1996 and appeared promising. In a study of cardiac arrest patients refractory to standard therapy with adrenaline, vasopressin restored a spontaneous circulation in all eight patients, three of whom were discharged neurologically intact.[186] The following year, the same group published a small randomised trial of out-of-hospital ventricular fibrillation, in which the rates of successful resuscitation and survival for 24 h were significantly higher in patients treated with vasopressin than in those treated with adrenaline.[192] Following these two studies, the American Heart Association (AHA) recommended that vasopressin could be used as an alternative to adrenaline for the treatment of adult shock-refractory VF.[182] The success of these small studies led to two large randomised studies comparing vasopressin with adrenaline for in-hospital[193] and out-of-hospital[194] cardiac arrest. Both studies randomised patients to receive vasopressin or adrenaline initially, and used adrenaline as a rescue treatment in patients refractory to the initial drug. Both studies were unable to demonstrate an overall increase in the rates of ROSC or survival for vasopressin 40 U,[193] with the dose repeated in one study,[194] when compared with adrenaline (1 mg, repeated), as the initial vasopressor. In the large out-of-hospital cardiac arrest study,[194] post-hoc analysis suggested that the subset of patients with asystole had significant improvement in survival to discharge, but survival neurologically intact was no different.

A recent meta-analysis of five randomised trials[195] showed no statistically significant difference between vasopressin and adrenaline for ROSC, death within 24 h or death before hospital discharge. The subgroup analysis based on initial cardiac rhythm did not show any statistically significant difference in the rate of death before hospital discharge.[195]

Participants at the 2005 Consensus Conference debated in depth the treatment recommendations that should follow from this evidence. Despite the absence of placebo-controlled trials, adrenaline has been the standard vasopressor in cardiac arrest. It was agreed that there is currently insufficient evidence to support or refute the use of vasopressin as an alternative to, or in combination with, adrenaline in any cardiac arrest rhythm. Current practice still supports adrenaline as the primary vasopressor for the treatment of cardiac arrest of all rhythms.

Adrenaline
Indications

- Adrenaline is the first drug used in cardiac arrest of any aetiology: it is included in the ALS algorithm for use every 3–5 min of CPR.
- Adrenaline is preferred in the treatment of anaphylaxis (Section 7g).
- Adrenaline is second-line treatment for cardiogenic shock.

Dose. During cardiac arrest, the initial intravenous dose of adrenaline is 1 mg. When intravascular (intravenous or intra-osseous) access is delayed or cannot be achieved, give 2–3 mg, diluted to 10 ml with sterile water, via the tracheal tube. Absorption via the tracheal route is highly variable.

There is no evidence supporting the use of higher doses of adrenaline for patients in refractory cardiac arrest. In some cases, an adrenaline infusion is required in the post-resuscitation period.

Following return of spontaneous circulation, excessive ($\geq$1 mg) doses of adrenaline may induce tachycardia, myocardial ischaemia, VT and VF. Once a perfusing rhythm is established, if further adrenaline is deemed necessary, titrate the dose carefully to achieve an appropriate blood pressure. Intravenous doses of 50–100 mcg are usually sufficient for most hypotensive patients. Use adrenaline cautiously in patients with cardiac arrest associated with cocaine or other sympathomimetic drugs.

Use. Adrenaline is available most commonly in two dilutions:

- 1 in 10,000 (10 ml of this solution contains 1 mg of adrenaline)
- 1 in 1000 (1 ml of this solution contains 1 mg of adrenaline)

Both these dilutions are used routinely in European countries.

Various other pressor drugs (e.g., noradrenaline)[196] have been used experimentally as an alternative to adrenaline for the treatment of cardiac arrest.

Anti-arrhythmics

As with vasopressors, the evidence that anti-arrhythmic drugs are of benefit in cardiac arrest is limited. No anti-arrhythmic drug given during human cardiac arrest has been shown to increase survival to hospital discharge, although amiodarone has been shown to increase survival to hospital admission.[89,90] Despite the lack of human long-term outcome data, the balance of evidence is in favour of the use anti-arrhythmic drugs for the management of arrhythmias in cardiac arrest.

Amiodarone. Amiodarone is a membrane-stabilising anti-arrhythmic drug that increases the duration of the action potential and refractory period in atrial and ventricular myocardium. Atrioventricular conduction is slowed, and a similar effect is seen with accessory pathways. Amiodarone has a mild negative inotropic action and causes peripheral vasodilation through non-competitive alpha-blocking effects. The hypotension that occurs with intravenous amiodarone is related to the rate of delivery and is due more to the solvent (Polysorbate 80), which causes histamine release, rather than the drug itself.[197] The use of an aqueous amiodarone preparation that is relatively free from these side effects is encouraged but is not yet widely available [198,199].

Following three initial shocks, amiodarone in shock-refractory VF improves the short-term outcome of survival to hospital admission compared with placebo[89] or lignocaine.[90] Amiodarone also appears to improve the response to defibrillation when given to humans or animals with VF or haemodynamically unstable ventricular tachycardia.[198–202] There is no evidence to indicate the time at which amiodarone should be given when using a single shock strategy. In the clinical studies to date, the amiodarone was given if VF/VT persisted after at least three shocks. For this reason, and in the absence of any other data, amiodarone 300 mg is recommended if VF/VT persists after three shocks.

Indications. Amiodarone is indicated in

- refractory VF/VT
- haemodynamically stable ventricular tachycardia (VT) and other resistant tachyarrhythmias (Section 4f)

Dose. Consider an initial intravenous dose of 300 mg amiodarone, diluted in 5% dextrose to a volume of 20 ml (or from a pre-filled syringe), if VF/VT persists after the third shock. Amiodarone can cause thrombophlebitis when injected into a peripheral vein; use a central venous catheter if one is in situ but, if not, use a large peripheral vein and a generous flush. Details about the use of amiodarone for the treatment of other arrhythmias are given in Section 4f.

Clinical aspects of use. Amiodarone may paradoxically be arrhythmogenic, especially if given concurrently with drugs that prolong the QT interval. However, it has a lower incidence of pro-arrhythmic effects than other anti-arrhythmic drugs under similar circumstances. The major acute adverse effects from amiodarone are hypotension and bradycardia, which can be prevented by slowing the rate of drug infusion, or can be treated with fluids and/or inotropic drugs. The side effects associated with prolonged oral use (abnormalities of thyroid function, corneal microdeposits, peripheral neuropathy, and pulmonary/hepatic infiltrates) are not relevant in the acute setting.

Lidocaine. Until the publication of the 2000 ILCOR guidelines, lidocaine was the antiarrhythmic drug of choice. Comparative studies with amiodarone[90] have displaced it from this position, and lidocaine is now recommended only when amiodarone is unavailable. Amiodarone should be available at all hospital arrests and to all out-of-hospital arrests attended by ambulance crew.

Lidocaine is a membrane-stabilising anti-arrhythmic drug that acts by increasing the myocyte refractory period. It decreases ventricular automaticity, and its local anaesthetic action suppresses ventricular ectopic activity. Lidocaine suppresses activity of depolarised, arrhythmogenic tissues while interfering minimally with the electrical activity of normal tissues. Therefore, it is effective in suppressing arrhythmias associated with depolarisation (e.g. ischaemia, digitalis toxicity) but is relatively ineffective against arrhythmias occurring in normally polarised cells (e.g., atrial fibrillation/flutter). Lidocaine raises the threshold for ventricular fibrillation.

Lidocaine toxicity causes paraesthesia, drowsiness, confusion and muscular twitching progressing to convulsions. It is considered generally that a safe dose of lidocaine must not exceed $3 \, mg \, kg^{-1}$ over the first hour. If there are signs of toxicity, stop the infusion immediately; treat seizures if they occur. Lidocaine depresses myocardial function, but to a much lesser extent than amiodarone. The myocardial depression is usually transient and can be treated with intravenous fluids or vasopressors.

Indications. Lidocaine is indicated in refractory VF/VT (when amiodarone is unavailable).

Dose. When amiodarone is unavailable, consider an initial dose of 100 mg (1—1.5 mg kg^{-1}) of lidocaine for VF/pulseless VT refractory to three shocks. Give an additional bolus of 50 mg if necessary. The total dose should not exceed 3 mg kg^{-1} during the first hour.

Clinical aspects of use. Lidocaine is metabolised by the liver, and its half-life is prolonged if the hepatic blood flow is reduced, e.g. in the presence of reduced cardiac output, liver disease or in the elderly. During cardiac arrest normal clearance mechanisms do not function, thus high plasma concentrations may be achieved after a single dose. After 24 h of continuous infusion, the plasma half-life increases significantly. Reduce the dose in these circumstances, and regularly review the indication for continued therapy. Lidocaine is less effective in the presence of hypokalaemia and hypomagnesaemia, which should be corrected immediately.

Magnesium sulphate. Magnesium is an important constituent of many enzyme systems, especially those involved with ATP generation in muscle. It plays a major role in neurochemical transmission, where it decreases acetylcholine release and reduces the sensitivity of the motor endplate. Magnesium also improves the contractile response of the stunned myocardium, and limits infarct size by a mechanism that has yet to be fully elucidated.[203] The normal plasma range of magnesium is 0.8—1.0 mmol l^{-1}.

Hypomagnesaemia is often associated with hypokalaemia, and may contribute to arrhythmias and cardiac arrest. Hypomagnesaemia increases myocardial digoxin uptake and decreases cellular Na$^+$/K$^+$-ATP-ase activity. Patients with hypomagnesaemia, hypokalaemia, or both may become cardiotoxic even with therapeutic digitalis levels. Magnesium deficiency is not uncommon in hospitalised patients and frequently coexists with other electrolyte disturbances, particularly hypokalaemia, hypophosphataemia, hyponatraemia and hypocalcaemia.

Although the benefits of giving magnesium in known hypomagnesaemic states are recognised, the benefit of giving magnesium routinely during cardiac arrest is unproven. Studies in adults in and out of hospital[91—95,204] have failed to demonstrate any increase in the rate of ROSC when magnesium is given routinely during CPR. There is some evidence that magnesium may be beneficial in refractory VF.[205]

Indications. Magnesium sulphate is indicated in

- shock-refractory VF in the presence of possible hypomagnesaemia
- ventricular tachyarrhythmias in the presence of possible hypomagnesaemia
- torsades de pointes
- digoxin toxicity

Dose. In shock-refractory VF, give an initial intravenous dose of 2 g (4 ml (8 mmol)) of 50% magnesium sulphate) peripherally over 1—2 min; it may be repeated after 10—15 min. Preparations of magnesium sulphate solutions differ among European countries.

Clinical aspects of use. Hypokalaemic patients are often hypomagnesaemic. If ventricular tachyarrhythmias arise, intravenous magnesium is a safe, effective treatment. The role of magnesium in acute myocardial infarction is still in doubt. Magnesium is excreted by the kidneys, but side effects associated with hypermagnesaemia are rare, even in renal failure. Magnesium inhibits smooth muscle contraction, causing vasodilation and a dose-related hypotension, which is usually transient and responds to intravenous fluids and vasopressors.

Other drugs

The evidence for the benefits of other drugs, including atropine, aminophylline and calcium, given routinely during human cardiac arrest, is limited. Recommendations for the use of these drugs are based on our understanding of their pharmacodynamic properties and the pathophysiology of cardiac arrest.

Atropine. Atropine antagonises the action of the parasympathetic neurotransmitter acetylcholine at muscarinic receptors. Therefore, it blocks the effect of the vagus nerve on both the sinoatrial (SA) node and the atrioventricular (AV) node, increasing sinus automaticity and facilitating AV node conduction.

Side effects of atropine are dose-related (blurred vision, dry mouth and urinary retention); they are not relevant during a cardiac arrest. Acute confusional states may occur after intravenous injection, particularly in elderly patients. After cardiac arrest, dilated pupils should not be attributed solely to atropine.

Atropine is indicated in:

- asystole
- pulseless electrical activity (PEA) with a rate <60 min^{-1}
- sinus, atrial, or nodal bradycardia when the haemodynamic condition of the patient is unstable

The recommended adult dose of atropine for asystole or PEA with a rate <60 min^{-1} is 3 mg intravenously in a single bolus. Its use in the treatment of bradycardia is covered in Section 4f. Several recent studies have failed to demonstrate any benefit from atropine in out-of-hospital or in-hospital cardiac arrests[174,206–210]; however, asystole carries a grave prognosis and there are anecdotal accounts of success after giving atropine. It is unlikely to be harmful in this situation.

Theophylline (aminophylline). Theophylline is a phosphodiesterase inhibitor that increases tissue concentrations of cAMP and releases adrenaline from the adrenal medulla. It has chronotropic and inotropic actions. The limited studies of aminophylline in bradyasystolic cardiac arrest have failed to demonstrate an increase in ROSC or survival to hospital discharge[211–214]; the same studies have not shown that harm is caused by aminophylline.

Aminophylline is indicated in:

- asystolic cardiac arrest
- peri-arrest bradycardia refractory to atropine

Theophylline is given as aminophylline, a mixture of theophylline with ethylenediamine, which is 20 times more soluble than theophylline alone. The recommended adult dose is 250–500 mg (5 mg kg^{-1}) given by slow intravenous injection.

Theophylline has a narrow therapeutic window with an optimal plasma concentration of 10–20 mg l^{-1} (55–110 mmol l^{-1}). Above this concentration, side effects such as arrhythmias and convulsions may occur, especially when given rapidly by intravenous injection.

Calcium. Calcium plays a vital role in the cellular mechanisms underlying myocardial contraction. There are very few data supporting any beneficial action for calcium after most cases of cardiac arrest. High plasma concentrations achieved after injection may be harmful to the ischaemic myocardium and may impair cerebral recovery. Give calcium during resuscitation only when indicated specifically, i.e. in pulseless electrical activity caused by

- hyperkalaemia
- hypocalcaemia
- overdose of calcium channel-blocking drugs

The initial dose of 10 ml 10% calcium chloride (6.8 mmol Ca^{2+}) may be repeated if necessary. Calcium can slow the heart rate and precipitate arrhythmias. In cardiac arrest, calcium may be given by rapid intravenous injection. In the presence of a spontaneous circulation give it slowly. Do not give calcium solutions and sodium bicarbonate simultaneously by the same route.

Buffers. Cardiac arrest results in combined respiratory and metabolic acidosis caused by cessation of pulmonary gas exchange and the development of anaerobic cellular metabolism, respectively. The best treatment of acidaemia in cardiac arrest is chest compression; some additional benefit is gained by ventilation. If the arterial blood pH is less than 7.1 (or base excess more negative than −10 mmol l^{-1}) during or following resuscitation from cardiac arrest, consider giving small doses of sodium bicarbonate (50 ml of an 8.4% solution). During cardiac arrest, arterial gas values may be misleading and bear little relationship to the tissue acid–base state[96]; analysis of central venous blood may provide a better estimation of tissue pH (see Section 4c). Bicarbonate causes generation of carbon dioxide, which diffuses rapidly into cells. This has the following effects.

- It exacerbates intracellular acidosis.
- It produces a negative inotropic effect on ischaemic myocardium.
- It presents a large, osmotically active, sodium load to an already compromised circulation and brain.
- It produces a shift to the left in the oxygen dissociation curve, further inhibiting release of oxygen to the tissues.

Mild acidaemia causes vasodilation and can increase cerebral blood flow. Therefore, full correction of the arterial blood pH may theoretically reduce cerebral blood flow at a particularly critical time. As the bicarbonate ion is excreted as carbon dioxide via the lungs, ventilation needs to be increased. For all these reasons, metabolic acidosis must be severe to justify giving sodium bicarbonate.

Several animal and clinical studies have examined the use of buffers during cardiac arrest. Clinical studies using Tribonate®[215] or sodium bicarbonate as buffers have failed to demonstrate any advantage.[216–220] Only one study has found clinical benefit, suggesting that EMS systems using sodium bicarbonate earlier and more frequently had significantly higher ROSC and hospital discharge rates and better long-term neurological outcome.[221] Animal studies have generally been inconclusive, but some have shown benefit in giving sodium bicarbonate to treat cardiovascular toxicity (hypotension, cardiac arrhythmias) caused by tricyclic antidepressants and other fast sodium channel blockers (Section 7b).[222] Giving sodium bicarbonate routinely during cardiac arrest and CPR (especially in out-of-hospital cardiac arrests) or after return of spontaneous circulation is not recommended. Consider sodium bicarbonate for life-threatening hyperkalaemia or cardiac arrest associated with hyperkalaemia, severe metabolic acidosis, or tricyclic overdose. Give 50 mmol (50 ml of an 8.4% solution) of sodium bicarbonate intravenously. Repeat the dose as necessary, but use acid/base analysis (either arterial or central venous) to guide therapy. Severe tissue damage may be caused by subcutaneous extravasation of concentrated sodium bicarbonate. The solution is incompatible with calcium salts as it causes the precipitation of calcium carbonate.

Thrombolysis during CPR. Adult cardiac arrest is usually caused by acute myocardial ischaemia following coronary artery occlusion by thrombus. There are several reports on the successful use of thrombolytics during cardiac arrest, particularly when the arrest was caused by pulmonary embolism. The use of thrombolytic drugs to break down coronary artery and pulmonary artery thrombus has been the subject of several studies. Thrombolytics have also been demonstrated in animal studies to have beneficial effects on cerebral blood flow during cardiopulmonary resuscitation,[223,224] and a clinical study has reported less anoxic encephalopathy after thrombolytic therapy during CPR.[225]

Several studies have examined the use of thrombolytic therapy given during non-traumatic cardiac arrest refractory to standard therapy. Two studies have shown an increase in ROSC with non-significant improvements in survival to hospital discharge,[97,226] and a further study demonstrated greater ICU survival.[225] A small series of case reports has also reported survival to discharge in three cases refractory to standard therapy with VF or PEA treated with thrombolytics[227]; conversely, one large clinical trial[228] failed to show any significant benefit for thrombolytics in cases of undifferentiated PEA out-of-hospital cardiac arrest unresponsive to initial interventions.

When given to cardiac arrest patients with suspected or proven pulmonary embolus, two studies have demonstrated possible benefits[229,230]; one found an improvement in 24-h survival.[229] Several clinical studies[97,226,229,231] and case series[227,230,232–234] have not demonstrated any increase in bleeding complications with thrombolysis during CPR in non-traumatic cardiac arrest.

There are insufficient clinical data to recommend the routine use of thrombolysis during non-traumatic cardiac arrest. Consider thrombolytic therapy when cardiac arrest is thought to be due to proven or suspected acute pulmonary embolus. Thrombolysis may be considered in adult cardiac arrest on a case by case basis following initial failure of standard resuscitation in patients in whom an acute thrombotic aetiology for the arrest is suspected. Ongoing CPR is not a contraindication to thrombolysis.

Following thrombolysis during CPR for acute pulmonary embolism, survival and good neurological outcome have been reported in cases requiring in excess of 60 min of CPR. If a thrombolytic drug is given in these circumstances, consider performing CPR for at least 60–90 min before termination of resuscitation attempts.[235,236]

Intravenous fluids

Hypovolaemia is a potentially reversible cause of cardiac arrest. Infuse fluids rapidly if hypovolaemia is suspected. In the initial stages of resuscitation there are no clear advantages to using colloid, so use saline or Hartmann's solution. Avoid dextrose, which is redistributed away from the intravascular space rapidly and causes hyperglycaemia, which may worsen neurological outcome after cardiac arrest.[237–244]

Whether fluids should be infused routinely during cardiac arrest is controversial. There are no published human studies of routine fluid use compared to no fluids during normovolaemic cardiac arrest. Four animal studies[245–248] of experimental ventricular fibrillation neither support nor refute the use of intravenous fluids routinely. In the absence of hypovolaemia, infusion of an excessive volume of fluid is likely to be harmful. Use intravenous fluid to flush peripherally injected drugs into the central circulation.

Alternative routes for drug delivery

Intraosseous route

If intravenous access cannot be established, intraosseous delivery of resuscitation drugs will achieve adequate plasma concentrations. Several studies indicate that intraosseous access is safe and effective for fluid resuscitation, drug delivery and laboratory evaluation.[78,249–255] Traditionally, the intraosseous route is used mainly for children, but it is also effective in adults.

Drugs given via the tracheal tube

Resuscitation drugs can also be given via the tracheal tube, but the plasma concentrations achieved using this route are variable and substantially lower than those achieved by the intravenous or intraosseous routes.

Doses of adrenaline 3–10 times higher than when given intravenously are required to achieve similar plasma concentrations.[79,80] During CPR, lung perfusion is only 10–30% of the normal value, resulting in a pulmonary adrenaline depot. When cardiac output is restored after a high dose of endobronchial adrenaline, prolonged reabsorption of adrenaline from the lungs into the pulmonary circulation may occur, causing arterial hypertension, malignant arrhythmias and recurrence of VF.[80] Lidocaine and atropine can also be given via a tracheal tube, but the plasma concentrations achieved are also variable.[256–258] If intravenous access is delayed or cannot be achieved, consider obtaining intraosseous access. Give drugs via the tracheal tube if intravascular (intravenous or intraosseous) access is delayed or cannot be achieved. There are no benefits from endobronchial injection compared with injection of the drug directly into the tracheal tube.[256] Dilution with water instead of 0.9% saline may achieve better drug absorption and cause less reduction in PaO_2.[85,259]

CPR techniques and devices

At best, standard manual CPR produces coronary and cerebral perfusion that is just 30% of normal.[260] Several CPR techniques and devices may improve haemodynamics or short-term survival when used by well-trained providers in selected cases. To date, no adjunct has consistently been shown to be superior to conventional manual CPR. CPR techniques include the following.

High-frequency chest compressions (HFCC)

High-frequency (>100 compressions min^{-1}) manual or mechanical chest compressions improve haemodynamics but have not been shown to improve long term outcome.[261–265]

Open-chest CPR

Open-chest CPR produces better coronary perfusion coronary pressure than standard CPR[266] and may be indicated for patients with cardiac arrest due to trauma (see Section 7i), in the early postoperative phase after cardiothoracic surgery[267,268] (see Section 7h) or when the chest or abdomen is already open (transdiaphragmatic approach), for example, in trauma surgery.

Interposed abdominal compression (IAC-CPR)

The IAC-CPR technique involves compression of the abdomen during the relaxation phase of chest compression.[269,270] This enhances venous return during CPR[271,272] and improves ROSC and short-term survival.[273,274] One study showed improved survival to hospital discharge with IAC-CPR compared with standard CPR for out-of-hospital cardiac arrest,[274] but another showed no survival advantage.[275] CPR devices include the following.

Active compression-decompression CPR (ACD-CPR)

ACD-CPR is achieved with a hand-held device equipped with a suction cup to lift the anterior chest actively during decompression. Decreasing intrathoracic pressure during the decompression phase increases venous return to the heart and increases cardiac output and subsequent coronary and cerebral perfusion pressures during the compression phase.[276–279] Results of ACD-CPR have been mixed. In some clinical studies ACD-CPR improved haemodynamics compared with standard CPR,[173,277,279,280] but in another study it did not.[281] In three randomised studies,[280,282,283] ACD-CPR improved long-term survival after out-of-hospital cardiac arrest; however, in five other randomised studies, ACD-CPR made no difference to outcome.[284–288] The efficacy of ACD-CPR may be highly dependent on the quality and duration of training.[289]

A meta-analysis of 10 trials of out-of-hospital cardiac arrest and two of in-hospital cardiac arrest showed no early or late survival benefit to ACD-CPR over conventional CPR.[290] Two post-mortem studies have shown more rib and sternal fractures after ACD-CPR compared with conventional CPR,[291,292] but another found no difference.[293]

Impedance threshold device (ITD)

The impedance threshold device (ITD) is a valve that limits air entry into the lungs during chest recoil between chest compressions; this decreases intrathoracic pressure and increases venous return to the heart. When used with a cuffed tracheal tube and active compression-decompression (ACD),[294–296] the ITD is thought to act synergistically to enhance venous return during active decompression. The ITD has also been used during conventional CPR with a tracheal tube or facemask.[297] If rescuers can maintain a tight facemask seal, the ITD may create the same negative intrathoracic pressure as when used with a tracheal tube.[297]

In two randomised studies of out-of-hospital cardiac arrest, ACD-CPR plus the ITD improved ROSC and 24-h survival compared with standard CPR alone.[296,298] When used during standard CPR, the ITD increased 24-h survival after PEA out-of-hospital cardiac arrest.[297]

Mechanical piston CPR

Mechanical piston devices depress the sternum by means of a compressed gas-powered plunger mounted on a backboard. In several studies in animals,[299,300] mechanical piston CPR improved end-tidal carbon dioxide, cardiac output, cerebral blood flow, MAP and short-term neurological outcome. Studies in humans also document improvement in end-tidal carbon dioxide and mean arterial pressure when using mechanical piston CPR compared with conventional CPR.[301–303]

Lund University cardiac arrest system (LUCAS) CPR

The Lund University cardiac arrest system (LUCAS) is a gas-driven sternal compression device that incorporates a suction cup for active decompression. There are no published randomised human studies comparing LUCAS-CPR with standard CPR. A study of pigs with VF showed that LUCAS-CPR improves haemodynamic and short-term survival compared with standard CPR.[304] The LUCAS was also used in 20 patients, but incomplete outcome data were reported.[304] In another pig study, in comparison with standard CPR, LUCAS-CPR increased cerebral blood flow and cardiac output.[305] The LUCAS enables delivery of continuous compressions during transport and defibrillation.

Mechanical piston CPR or LUCAS CPR may be particularly useful when prolonged CPR is required; this might include during transport to hospital or after cardiac arrest following hypothermia[306] or poisoning.

Load-distributing band CPR or vest CPR

The load distributing band (LDB) is a circumferential chest compression device comprising a pneumatically actuated constricting band and backboard. The use of LDB CPR improves haemodynamics.[307–309] A case—control study documented improvement in survival to the emergency department when LDB-CPR was delivered after out-of-hospital cardiac arrest.[310]

Phased thoracic—abdominal compression—decompression CPR (PTACD-CPR)

Phased thoracic—abdominal compression—decompression CPR combines the concepts of IAC-CPR and ACD-CPR. It comprises a hand-held device that alternates chest compression and abdominal decompression with chest decompression and abdominal compression. One randomised study of adults in cardiac arrest documented no improvement in survival from use of PTACD-CPR.[311]

Minimally invasive direct cardiac massage

Minimally invasive direct cardiac massage (MIDCM) is accomplished by insertion of a small plunger-like device through a 2—4-cm incision in the chest wall. In one clinical study the MIDCM generated improved blood pressure over standard CPR, but the device caused cardiac rupture in one postoperative cardiovascular surgical patient.[312] The plunger device is no longer manufactured.

4f. Peri-arrest arrhythmias

Introduction

A successful strategy to reduce the mortality and morbidity of cardiac arrest includes measures to prevent other potentially serious arrhythmias, and optimal treatment should they occur. Cardiac arrhythmias are well recognised complications of myocardial infarction. They may precede ventricular fibrillation or follow successful defibrillation. The treatment algorithms described in this section have been designed to enable the non-specialist ALS provider to treat the patient effectively and safely in an emergency; for this reason, they have been kept as simple as possible. If patients are not acutely ill there may be several other treatment options, including the use of drugs (oral or parenteral), that will be less familiar to the non-expert. In this situation there will be time to seek advice from cardiologists or other doctors with the appropriate expertise.

More comprehensive information on the management of arrhythmias can be found at www.escardio.org.

Principles of treatment

In all cases, give oxygen and insert an intravenous cannula while the arrhythmia is assessed. Whenever possible, record a 12-lead ECG; this will help determine the precise rhythm, either before treatment or retrospectively, if necessary with the help of an expert. Correct any electrolyte abnormalities (e.g., K^+, Mg^{2+}, Ca^{2+}) (Section 7a).

The assessment and treatment of all arrhythmias addresses two factors: the condition of the patient (stable versus unstable), and the nature of the arrhythmia.

Adverse signs

The presence or absence of adverse signs or symptoms will dictate the appropriate treatment for most arrhythmias. The following adverse factors indicate a patient who is unstable because of the arrhythmia.

1. Clinical evidence of low cardiac output. This is seen as pallor, sweating, cold and clammy extremities (increased sympathetic activity), impaired consciousness (reduced cerebral blood flow), and hypotension (e.g., systolic blood pressure <90 mmHg).
2. Excessive tachycardia. Coronary blood flow occurs predominantly during diastole. Very high heart rates (e.g., >150 min⁻¹) reduce diastole critically, decreasing coronary blood flow and causing myocardial ischaemia. Broad, complex tachycardias are tolerated less well by the heart than narrow, complex tachycardias.
3. Excessive bradycardia. This is defined as a heart rate of <40 beats min⁻¹, but rates of <60 beats min⁻¹ may not be tolerated by patients with poor cardiac reserve. Even a higher heart rate may be inappropriately slow for a patient with a low stroke-volume.
4. Heart failure. By reducing coronary artery blood flow, arrhythmias compromise myocardial performance. In acute situations this is manifested by pulmonary oedema (failure of the left ventricle) or raised jugular venous pressure, and hepatic engorgement (failure of the right ventricle).
5. Chest pain. The presence of chest pain implies that the arrhythmia (particularly a tachyarrhythmia) is causing myocardial ischaemia. This is especially important if there is underlying coronary artery disease or structural heart disease in which myocardial ischaemia is likely to lead to further life-threatening complications including cardiac arrest.

Treatment options

Having determined the rhythm and the presence or absence of adverse signs, there are broadly three options for immediate treatment:

1. anti-arrhythmic (and other) drugs
2. attempted electrical cardioversion
3. cardiac pacing

All anti-arrhythmic treatments—physical manoeuvres, drugs, or electrical treatment—can also be pro-arrhythmic, so that clinical deterioration may be caused by the treatment rather than lack of effect. Furthermore, the use of multiple anti-arrhythmic drugs or high doses of a single drug can cause myocardial depression and hypotension. This may cause a deterioration of the cardiac rhythm. Anti-arrhythmic drugs are slower in effect and less reliable than electrical cardioversion in converting a tachycardia to sinus rhythm; thus, drugs tend to be reserved for stable patients without adverse signs, and electrical cardioversion is usually the preferred treatment for the unstable patient displaying adverse signs.

Once the arrhythmia has been treated successfully, repeat the 12-lead ECG to enable detection of any underlying abnormalities that may require long-term therapy.

Bradycardia

A bradycardia is defined strictly as a heart rate of <60 beats min⁻¹. However, it is more helpful to classify a bradycardia as absolute (<40 beats min⁻¹) or relative, when the heart rate is inappropriately slow for the haemodynamic state of the patient.

The first step in the assessment of bradycardia is to determine if the patient is unstable (Figure 4.11). The following adverse signs may indicate instability:

- systolic blood pressure <90 mmHg
- heart rate <40 beats min⁻¹
- ventricular arrhythmias requiring suppression
- heart failure

If adverse signs are present, give atropine, 500 mcg, intravenously and, if necessary, repeat every 3—5 min to a total of 3 mg. Doses of atropine of less than 500 mcg paradoxically may cause further slowing of the heart rate.[313] In healthy volunteers a dose of 3 mg produces the maximum achievable increase in resting heart rate.[314] Use atropine cautiously in the presence of acute coronary ischaemia or myocardial infarction; increased heart rate may worsen ischaemia or increase the zone of infarction. If a satisfactory response is achieved with atropine, or the patient is stable, next determine the risk of asystole, which is indicated by:

- recent asystole

Bradycardia Algorithm

(includes rates inappropriately slow for haemodynamic state)

If appropriate, give oxygen, cannulate a vein, and record a 12-lead ECG

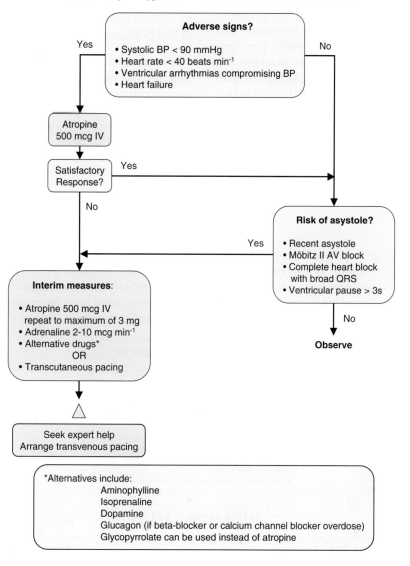

Figure 4.11 Bradycardia algorithm.

- Möbitz type II AV block
- complete (third-degree) heart block (especially with broad QRS or initial heart rate <40 beats min^{-1})
- ventricular standstill of more than 3 s

Atrioventricular (AV) blocks are divided into first, second, and third degrees and may be associated with multiple medications or electrolyte disturbances, as well as structural problems caused by acute myocardial infarction and myocarditis. A first-degree AV block is defined by a prolonged P—R interval (>0.20 s), and is usually benign. Second-degree AV block is divided into Möbitz types I and II. In Möbitz type I, the block is at the AV node, is often transient and may be asymptomatic. In Möbitz type II, the block is most often below the AV node at the bundle of His or at the bundle branches, and is often symptomatic, with the potential to progress to complete AV block. Third-degree heart block is defined by AV dissociation which may be permanent or transient, depending on the underlying cause.

Pacing is likely to be required if there is a risk of asystole, or if the patient is unstable and has failed to respond satisfactorily to atropine. Under these circumstances, the definitive treatment is transvenous pacing. One or more of the following interventions can be used to improve the patient's condition while waiting for the appropriate personnel and facilities:

- transcutaneous pacing
- adrenaline infusion in the range of 2—10 mcg min^{-1} titrated to response

Other drugs that can be given for symptomatic bradycardia include dopamine, isoprenaline and theophylline. Consider giving intravenous glucagon if beta-blockers or calcium channel blockers are a potential cause of the bradycardia. Do not give atropine to patients with cardiac transplants— paradoxically, it can cause a high-degree AV block or even sinus arrest.[315]

Complete heart block with a narrow QRS is not an absolute indication for pacing, because AV junctional ectopic pacemakers (with a narrow QRS) may provide a reasonable and stable heart rate.

Pacing

Transcutaneous pacing. Initiate transcutaneous pacing immediately if there is no response to atropine, if atropine is unlikely to be effective or if the patient is severely symptomatic, particularly if there is high-degree block (Möbitz Type II second- or third-degree block). Transcutaneous pacing can be painful and may fail to produce effective mechanical capture. Verify mechanical capture and reassess the patient's condition. Use analgesia and sedation to control pain, and attempt to identify the cause of the bradyarrhythmia.

Fist pacing. If atropine is ineffective and transcutaneous pacing is not immediately available, fist pacing can be attempted while waiting for pacing equipment[316–318]: give serial rhythmic blows with the closed fist over the left lower edge of the sternum to pace the heart at a physiological rate of 50—70 beats min^{-1}.

Tachycardias

Previous ERC guidelines have included three separate tachycardia algorithms: broad-complex tachycardia, narrow-complex tachycardia and atrial fibrillation. In the peri-arrest setting, many treatment principles are common to all the tachycardias; for this reason, they have been combined into a single tachycardia algorithm (Figure 4.12).

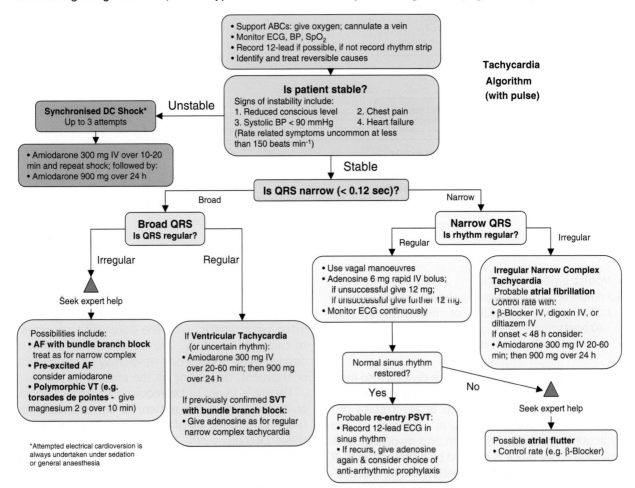

Figure 4.12 Tachycardia algorithm.

If the patient is unstable and deteriorating, with signs and symptoms caused by the tachycardia (e.g., impaired conscious level, chest pain, heart failure, hypotension or other signs of shock), attempt synchronised cardioversion immediately. In patients with otherwise normal hearts, serious signs and symptoms are uncommon if the ventricular rate is <150 beats min^{-1}. Patients with impaired cardiac function or significant comorbidity may be symptomatic and unstable at lower heart rates. If cardioversion fails to restore sinus rhythm and the patient remains unstable, give amiodarone 300 mg intravenously over 10—20 min and re-attempt electrical cardioversion. The loading dose of amiodarone can be followed by an infusion of 900 mg over 24 h. Serial DC shocks are not appropriate for recurrent (within hours or days) paroxysms (self-terminating episodes) of atrial fibrillation. This is relatively common in critically ill patients who may have ongoing precipitating factors causing the arrhythmia (e.g., metabolic disturbance, sepsis). Cardioversion does not prevent subsequent arrhythmias. If there are recurrent episodes, treat them with drugs.

Synchronised electrical cardioversion

If electrical cardioversion is used to convert atrial or ventricular tachyarrhythmias, the shock must be synchronised with the R wave of the ECG rather than with the T wave. By avoiding the relative refractory period in this way, the risk of inducing ventricular fibrillation is minimised. Conscious patients must be anaesthetised or sedated before synchronised cardioversion is attempted. For a broad-complex tachycardia and AF, start with 200-J monophasic or 120—150 J biphasic and increase in increments if this fails (see Section 3). Atrial flutter and paroxysmal SVT will often convert with lower energies: start with 100-J monophasic or 70—120-J biphasic.

If the patient with tachycardia is stable (no serious signs or symptoms caused by the tachycardia) and is not deteriorating, there is time to evaluate the rhythm using the 12-lead ECG and determine treatment options. The ALS provider may not have the expertise to diagnose the tachycardia precisely, but should be capable of differentiating between sinus tachycardia, narrow-complex SVT and broad-complex tachycardia. If the patient is stable there is normally time to consult an expert. If the patient becomes unstable, proceed immediately to synchronised electrical cardioversion. Management of patients with significant comorbid conditions and symptomatic tachycardia requires treatment of the comorbid conditions.

Broad-complex tachycardia

In broad-complex tachycardias the QRS complexes are >0.12 s and are usually ventricular in origin. Although broad-complex tachycardias may be caused by supraventricular rhythms with aberrant conduction, in the unstable patient in the peri-arrest context assume they are ventricular in origin. In the stable patient with broad-complex tachycardia, the next step is to determine if the rhythm is regular or irregular.

Regular broad complex tachycardia. A regular broad-complex tachycardia is likely to be ventricular tachycardia or SVT with bundle branch block. Stable ventricular tachycardia can be treated with amiodarone 300 mg intravenously over 20—60 min followed by an infusion of 900 mg over 24 h. If the broad-complex regular tachycardia is thought to be SVT with bundle branch block, give adenosine, using the strategy indicated for narrow-complex tachycardia (below).

Irregular broad complex tachycardia. Irregular broad complex tachycardia is most likely to be AF with bundle branch block, but careful examination of a 12-lead ECG (if necessary by an expert) may enable confident identification of the rhythm. Another possible cause is AF with ventricular pre-excitation (in patients with Wolff—Parkinson—White (WPW) syndrome). There is more variation in the appearance and width of the QRS complexes than in AF with bundle branch block. A third possible cause is polymorphic VT (e.g., torsade de pointes), but polymorphic VT is relatively unlikely to be present without adverse features.

Seek expert help with the assessment and treatment of irregular broad-complex tachyarrhythmia. If treating AF with bundle branch block, treat as for AF (see below). If pre-excited AF (or atrial flutter) is suspected, avoid adenosine, digoxin, verapamil and diltiazem. These drugs block the AV node and cause a relative increase in pre-excitation. Electrical cardioversion is usually the safest treatment option.

Treat torsades de pointes VT immediately by stopping all drugs known to prolong QT interval. Correct electrolyte abnormalities, especially hypokalaemia. Give magnesium sulphate, 2 g, intravenously over 10 min.[319,320] Obtain expert help, as other treatment (e.g., overdrive pacing) may be indicated to prevent relapse once the arrhythmia has been corrected. If adverse features develop (which is usual), arrange immediate synchronised cardioversion. If the patient becomes pulseless, attempt defibrillation immediately (cardiac arrest algorithm).

Narrow-complex tachycardia

Regular narrow-complex tachycardias include:

- sinus tachycardia
- AV nodal re-entry tachycardia (AVNRT, the commonest type of SVT)
- AV re-entry tachycardia (AVRT (due to WPW syndrome))
- atrial flutter with regular AV conduction (usually 2:1)

Irregular narrow-complex tachycardia is most commonly AF or sometimes atrial flutter with variable AV conduction ('variable block').

Regular narrow-complex tachycardia

Sinus tachycardia. Sinus tachycardia is a common physiological response to a stimulus such as exercise or anxiety. In a sick patient it may be seen in response to many stimuli, such as pain, fever, anaemia, blood loss and heart failure. Treatment is almost always directed at the underlying cause; trying to slow sinus tachycardia that has occurred in response to most of these situations will make the situation worse.

AVNRT and AVRT (paroxysmal SVT). AVNRT is the commonest type of paroxysmal SVT, often seen in people without any other form of heart disease and is relatively uncommon in a peri-arrest setting. It causes a regular narrow-complex tachycardia, often with no clearly visible atrial activity on the ECG, with heart rates usually well above the typical range of sinus rates at rest ($60-120$ beats min^{-1}). It is usually benign, unless there is additional co-incidental structural heart disease or coronary disease, but may cause symptoms that the patient finds frightening.

AV re-entry tachycardia (AVRT) is seen in patients with the WPW syndrome and is also usually benign unless there happens to be additional structural heart disease. The common type of AVRT is a regular narrow-complex tachycardia, also often having no visible atrial activity on the ECG.

Atrial flutter with regular AV conduction (often 2:1 block). Atrial flutter with regular AV conduction (often 2:1 block) produces a regular narrow-complex tachycardia in which it may be difficult to see atrial activity and identify flutter waves with confidence, so it may be indistinguishable initially from AVNRT and AVRT. When atrial flutter with 2:1 block or even 1:1 conduction is accompanied by bundle branch block, it produces a regular broad-complex tachycardia that will usually be very difficult to distinguish from VT; treatment of this rhythm as if it were VT will usually be effective,

or will slow the ventricular response enabling identification of the rhythm. Most typical atrial flutter has an atrial rate of about 300 beats min^{-1}, so atrial flutter with 2:1 block tends to produce a tachycardia of about 150 beats min^{-1}. Much faster rates (170 beats min^{-1} or more) are unlikely to be due to atrial flutter with 2:1 block.

Treatment of regular narrow complex tachycardia. If the patient is unstable with adverse features caused by the arrhythmia, attempt synchronised electrical cardioversion. It is reasonable to give adenosine to an unstable patient with a regular narrow-complex tachycardia while preparations are made for synchronised cardioversion; however, do not delay electrical cardioversion if the adenosine fails to restore sinus rhythm. In the absence of adverse features, proceed as follows.

- Start with vagal manoeuvres. Carotid sinus massage or the Valsalva manoeuvre will terminate up to a quarter of episodes of paroxysmal SVT. A Valsalva manoeuvre (forced expiration against a closed glottis) in the supine position may be the most effective technique. A practical way of achieving this without protracted explanation is to ask the patient to blow into a 20-ml syringe with enough force to push back the plunger. Avoid carotid massage if a carotid bruit is present; rupture of an atheromatous plaque could cause cerebral embolism and stroke. In the context of acute ischaemia or digitalis toxicity, sudden bradycardia may trigger VF. Record an ECG (preferably multi-lead) during each manoeuvre. If the rhythm is atrial flutter, slowing of the ventricular response will often occur and demonstrate flutter waves.
- If the arrhythmia persists and is not atrial flutter, use adenosine. Give 6 mg as a rapid intravenous bolus. Record an ECG (preferably multi-lead) during each injection. If the ventricular rate slows transiently but the arrhythmia then persists, look for atrial activity such as atrial flutter or other atrial tachycardia and treat accordingly. If there is no response to adenosine 6 mg, give a 12-mg bolus; if there is no response, give one further 12 mg-bolus.
- Successful termination of a tachyarrhythmia by vagal manoeuvres or adenosine indicates that it was almost certainly AVNRT or AVRT. Monitor the patients for further rhythm abnormalities. Treat recurrence either with further adenosine or with a longer-acting drug with AV nodal-blocking action (e.g., diltiazem or beta-blocker).
- Vagal manoeuvres or adenosine will terminate almost all AVNRT or AVRT within seconds. Failure to terminate a regular narrow-complex tachycar-

dia with adenosine suggests an atrial tachycardia such as atrial flutter.

- If adenosine is contraindicated or fails to terminate a regular narrow-complex tachycardia without demonstrating that it is atrial flutter, give a calcium channel blocker (e.g., verapamil 2.5—5 mg intravenously over 2 min).

Irregular narrow-complex tachycardia

An irregular narrow-complex tachycardia is most likely to be AF with an uncontrolled ventricular response or, less commonly, atrial flutter with variable AV block. Record a 12-lead ECG to identify the rhythm. If the patient is unstable with adverse features caused by the arrhythmia, attempt synchronised electrical cardioversion.

If there are no adverse features, treatment options include:

- rate control by drug therapy
- rhythm control using drugs to encourage chemical cardioversion
- rhythm control by electrical cardioversion
- treatment to prevent complications (e.g., anticoagulation)

Obtain expert help to determine the most appropriate treatment for the individual patient. The longer a patient remains in AF, the greater is the likelihood of atrial clot developing. In general, patients who have been in AF for more than 48 h should not be treated by cardioversion (electrical or chemical) until they have received full anticoagulation or absence of atrial clot has been shown by transoesophageal echocardiography. If the aim is to control heart rate, options include a beta-blocker,[321,322] digoxin, diltiazem,[323,324] magnesium[325,326] or combinations of these.

If the duration of AF is less than 48 h and rhythm control is considered appropriate, this may be attempted using amiodarone (300 mg intravenously over 20—60 min followed by 900 mg over 24 h). Ibutilide or flecainide can also be given for rhythm control, but expert advice should be obtained before using these drugs for this purpose. Electrical cardioversion remains an option in this setting and will restore sinus rhythm in more patients than chemical cardioversion.

Seek expert help if any patient with AF is known or found to have ventricular pre-excitation (WPW syndrome). Avoid using adenosine, diltiazem, verapamil or digoxin to patients with pre-excited AF or atrial flutter, as these drugs block the AV node and cause a relative increase in pre-excitation.

Antiarrhythmic drugs

Adenosine

Adenosine is a naturally occurring purine nucleotide. It slows transmission across the AV node but has little effect on other myocardial cells or conduction pathways. It is highly effective for terminating paroxysmal SVT with re-entrant circuits that include the AV node (AVNRT). In other narrow-complex tachycardias, adenosine will reveal the underlying atrial rhythms by slowing the ventricular response. It has an extremely short half-life of 10—15 s and, therefore, is given as a rapid bolus into a fast running intravenous infusion or followed by a saline flush. The smallest dose likely to be effective is 6 mg (which is outside some current licences for an initial dose) and, if unsuccessful this can be followed with up to two doses each of 12 mg every 1—2 min. Patients should be warned of transient unpleasant side effects, in particular nausea, flushing, and chest discomfort.[327] Adenosine is not available in some European countries, but adenosine triphosphate (ATP) is an alternative. In a few European countries neither preparation may be available; verapamil is probably the next best choice. Theophylline and related compounds block the effect of adenosine. Patients receiving dipyridamole or carbamazepine, or with denervated (transplanted) hearts, display a markedly exaggerated effect that may be hazardous. In these patients, or if injected into a central vein, reduce the initial dose of adenosine to 3 mg. In the presence of WPW syndrome, blockage of conduction across the AV node by adenosine may promote conduction across an accessory pathway. In the presence of supraventricular arrhythmias this may cause a dangerously rapid ventricular response. In the presence of WPW syndrome, rarely, adenosine may precipitate atrial fibrillation associated with a dangerously rapid ventricular response.

Amiodarone

Intravenous amiodarone has effects on sodium, potassium and calcium channels as well as alpha- and beta-adrenergic blocking properties. Indications for intravenous amiodarone include:

- control of haemodynamically stable VT, polymorphic VT and wide-complex tachycardia of uncertain origin
- paroxysmal SVT uncontrolled by adenosine, vagal manoeuvres or AV nodal blockade
- to control rapid ventricular rate due to accessory pathway conduction in pre-excited atrial arrhythmias

Give amiodarone, 300 mg intravenously, over 10—60 min depending on the circumstances and haemodynamic stability of the patient. This loading dose is followed by an infusion of 900 mg over 24 h. Additional infusions of 150 mg can be repeated as necessary for recurrent or resistant arrhythmias to a maximum manufacturer-recommended total daily dose of 2 g (this maximum licensed dose varies between countries). In patients known to have severely impaired heart function, intravenous amiodarone is preferable to other anti-arrhythmic drugs for atrial and ventricular arrhythmias. Major adverse effects from amiodarone are hypotension and bradycardia, which can be prevented by slowing the rate of drug infusion. The hypotension associated with amiodarone is caused by vasoactive solvents (Polysorbate 80 and benzyl alcohol). A new aqueous formulation of amiodarone does not contain these solvents and causes no more hypotension than lidocaine.[198] Whenever possible, intravenous amiodarone should be given via a central venous catheter; it causes thrombophlebitis when infused into a peripheral vein. In an emergency it should be injected into a large peripheral vein.

Calcium channel blockers: verapamil and diltiazem

Verapamil and diltiazem are calcium channel blocking drugs that slow conduction and increase refractoriness in the AV node. Intravenous diltiazem is not available in some countries. These actions may terminate re-entrant arrhythmias and control ventricular response rate in patients with a variety of atrial tachycardias. Indications include:

- stable regular narrow-complex tachycardias uncontrolled or unconverted by adenosine or vagal manoeuvres
- to control ventricular rate in patients with AF or atrial flutter and preserved ventricular function when the duration of the arrhythmia is less than 48 h

The initial dose of verapamil is 2.5—5 mg intravenously given over 2 min. In the absence of a therapeutic response or drug-induced adverse event, give repeated doses of 5—10 mg every 15—30 min to a maximum of 20 mg. Verapamil should be given only to patients with narrow-complex paroxysmal SVT or arrhythmias known with certainty to be of supraventricular origin.

Diltiazem at a dose of 250 mcg kg^{-1}, followed by a second dose of 350 mcg kg^{-1}, is as effective as verapamil. Verapamil and, to a lesser extent, diltiazem may decrease myocardial contractility and critically reduce cardiac output in patients with

severe LV dysfunction. For the reasons stated under adenosine (above), calcium channel blockers are considered harmful when given to patients with AF or atrial flutter associated with known pre-excitation (WPW) syndrome.

Beta-adrenergic blockers

Beta-blocking drugs (atenolol, metoprolol, labetalol (alpha- and beta-blocking effects), propranolol, esmolol) reduce the effects of circulating catecholamines and decrease heart rate and blood pressure. They also have cardioprotective effects for patients with acute coronary syndromes. Beta-blockers are indicated for the following tachycardias:

- narrow-complex regular tachycardias uncontrolled by vagal manoeuvres and adenosine in the patient with preserved ventricular function
- to control rate in AF and atrial flutter when ventricular function is preserved

The intravenous dose of atenolol (beta$_1$) is 5 mg given over 5 min, repeated if necessary after 10 min. Metoprolol (beta$_1$) is given in doses of 2—5 mg at 5-min intervals to a total of 15 mg. Propranolol (beta$_1$ and beta$_2$ effects), 100 mcg kg^{-1}, is given slowly in three equal doses at 2—3-min intervals.

Intravenous esmolol is a short-acting (half-life of 2—9 min) beta$_1$-selective beta-blocker. It is given as an intravenous loading dose of 500 mcg kg^{-1} over 1 min, followed by an infusion of 50—200 mcg kg^{-1} min^{-1}.

Side effects of beta-blockade include bradycardias, AV conduction delays and hypotension. Contraindications to the use of beta-adrenergic blocking agents include second- or third-degree heart block, hypotension, severe congestive heart failure and lung disease associated with bronchospasm.

Magnesium

Magnesium can be given for control of ventricular rate in atrial fibrillation.[326,328—330] Give magnesium sulphate 2 g (8 mmol) over 10 min. This can be repeated once if necessary.

4g. Post-resuscitation care

Introduction

ROSC is the just the first step toward the goal of complete recovery from cardiac arrest. Interventions in the post-resuscitation period are likely to influence the final outcome significantly,[237,331] yet there are relatively few data relating to this phase. Of 22,105 patients admitted to intensive care units in the UK after cardiac arrest, 9974 (45%) survived to leave intensive care and 6353 (30%) survived to hospital discharge (data from Intensive Care National Audit and Research Centre (ICNARC), London, December 1995 to October 2004). To return the patient to a state of normal cerebral function with no neurological deficit, a stable cardiac rhythm and normal haemodynamic function, further resuscitation tailored to each patient's individual needs is required. The post-resuscitation phase starts at the location where ROSC is achieved but, once stabilised, the patient is transferred to the most appropriate high-care area (e.g., intensive care unit, coronary care unit) for continued monitoring and treatment.

Airway and breathing

Patients who have had a brief period of cardiac arrest responding immediately to appropriate treatment may achieve an immediate return of normal cerebral function. These patients do not require tracheal intubation and ventilation but should be given oxygen via a facemask. Hypoxia and hypercarbia both increase the likelihood of a further cardiac arrest and may contribute to secondary brain injury. Consider tracheal intubation, sedation and controlled ventilation in any patient with obtunded cerebral function. Ensure the tracheal tube is positioned correctly well above the carina. Hypocarbia causes cerebral vasoconstriction and a decreased cerebral blood flow.[332] After cardiac arrest, hypocapnia induced by hyperventilation causes cerebral ischaemia.[333–336] There are no data to support the targeting of a specific arterial PCO_2 after resuscitation from cardiac arrest, but it is reasonable to adjust ventilation to achieve normocarbia and to monitor this using the end-tidal PCO_2 and arterial blood gas values. Adjust the inspired oxygen concentrations to achieve adequate arterial oxygen saturation.

Insert a gastric tube to decompress the stomach; gastric distension caused by mouth-to-mouth or bag-mask-valve ventilation will splint the diaphragm and impair ventilation. Avoid coughing; this will increase intracranial pressure and may cause transient hypoxaemia. Give adequate doses of sedative and, if absolutely necessary, give a neuromuscular blocking drug. Obtain a chest radiograph to check the position of the tracheal tube and central venous lines, etc., assess for pulmonary oedema and to detect complications from CPR such as a pneumothorax associated with rib fractures.

Circulation

If there is evidence of coronary occlusion, consider the need for immediate revascularisation by thrombolysis or percutaneous coronary intervention (see acute coronary syndromes).

Haemodynamic instability is common after cardiac arrest and manifests as hypotension, low cardiac index and arrhythmias.[337] This post-resuscitation myocardial dysfunction (or myocardial stunning) is usually transient and often reverses within 24–48 h.[338] The post-resuscitation period is associated with marked elevations in plasma cytokine concentrations, manifesting as a sepsis-like syndrome and multiple organ dysfunction.[339]

Infusion of fluids may be required to increase right heart filling pressures or, conversely, diuretics and vasodilators may be needed to treat left ventricular failure. In the ICU an arterial line for continuous blood pressure monitoring is essential, and the use of a non-invasive or invasive (pulmonary artery catheter) cardiac output monitor may be helpful. There are very few randomised trials evaluating the role of blood pressure on the outcome after cardiac arrest. One randomised study demonstrated no difference in the neurological outcome among patients randomised to a mean arterial blood pressure of >100 mmHg versus ≤100 mmHg 5 min after ROSC; however, good functional recovery was associated with a higher blood pressure during the first 2 h after ROSC.[340] In the absence of definitive data, target the mean arterial blood pressure to achieve an adequate urine output, taking into consideration the patient's normal blood pressure.

Immediately after a cardiac arrest there is typically a period of hyperkalaemia. Subsequent endogenous catecholamine release promotes intracellular transportation of potassium, causing hypokalaemia. Hypokalaemia may predispose to ventricular arrhythmias. Give potassium to maintain the serum potassium concentration between 4.0 and 4.5 mmol l^{-1}.

Disability (optimising neurological recovery)

Cerebral perfusion

Immediately after ROSC there is a period of cerebral hyperaemia.[341] After 15–30 min of reperfusion, however, global cerebral blood flow decreases and there is generalised hypoperfusion. Normal cerebral autoregulation is lost, leaving cerebral perfusion dependent on mean arterial pressure. Under these circumstances, hypotension will compromise cerebral blood flow severely and will compound any neurological injury. Thus, after ROSC, maintain mean arterial pressure at the patient's normal level.

Sedation

Although it has been common practice to sedate and ventilate patients for up to 24 h after ROSC, there are no data to support a defined period of ventilation, sedation and neuromuscular blockade after cardiac arrest. The duration of sedation and ventilation may be influenced by the use of therapeutic hypothermia (see below). There are no data to indicate whether or not the choice of sedation influences outcome, but short-acting drugs (e.g., propofol, alfentanil, remifentanil) will enable earlier neurological assessment. There is an increased incidence of pneumonia when sedation is prolonged beyond 48 h after prehospital or in-hospital cardiac arrest.[342]

Control of seizures

Seizures and/or myoclonus occur in 5—15% of adult patients who achieve ROSC, and in approximately 40% of those who remain comatose.[343] Seizures increase cerebral metabolism by up to four-fold. Prolonged seizure activity may cause cerebral injury, and should be controlled with benzodiazepines, phenytoin, propofol or a barbiturate. Each of these drugs can cause hypotension, and this must be treated appropriately. Seizures and myoclonus per se are not related significantly to outcome, but status epilepticus and, in particular, status myoclonus are associated with a poor outcome.[343,344]

Temperature control

Treatment of hyperpyrexia. A period of hyperthermia (hyperpyrexia) is common in the first 48 h after cardiac arrest.[345—347] The risk of a poor neurological outcome increases for each degree of body temperature $>37\,^{\circ}$C.[348] Antipyretics and/or physical cooling methods decrease infarct volumes in animal models of global ischaemia.[349,350] Treat any hyperthermia occurring in the first 72 h after cardiac arrest with antipyretics or active cooling.

Therapeutic hypothermia. Mild therapeutic hypothermia is thought to suppress many of the chemical reactions associated with reperfusion injury. These reactions include free-radical production, excitatory amino acid release, and calcium shifts, which can in turn lead to mitochondrial damage and apoptosis (programmed cell death).[351—353] Two randomised clinical trials showed improved outcome in adults remaining comatose after initial resuscitation from out-of-hospital VF cardiac arrest, who were cooled within minutes to hours after ROSC.[354,355] The subjects were cooled to $32—34\,^{\circ}$C for 12—24 h. One study documented improved metabolic endpoints (lactate and O_2 extraction) when comatose adult patients were cooled after ROSC from out-of-hospital cardiac arrest in which the initial rhythm was PEA/asystole.[356] A small study showed benefit after therapeutic hypothermia in comatose survivors of non-VF arrest.[357]

External and/or internal cooling techniques can be used to initiate cooling.[354—356,358—361] An infusion of $30\,mg\,kg^{-1}$ of $4\,^{\circ}$C-saline decreases core temperature by $1.5\,^{\circ}$C.[358,359,361,362] Intravascular cooling enables more precise control of core temperature than external methods, but it is unknown whether this improves outcome.[360,363—365]

Complications of mild therapeutic hypothermia include increased infection, cardiovascular instability, coagulopathy, hyperglycaemia and electrolyte abnormalities such as hypophosphataemia and hypomagnesaemia.[366,367]

Unconscious adult patients with spontaneous circulation after out-of-hospital VF cardiac arrest should be cooled to $32—34\,^{\circ}$C. Cooling should be started as soon as possible and continued for at least 12—24 h.[368—374] Induced hypothermia might also benefit unconscious adult patients with spontaneous circulation after out-of-hospital cardiac arrest from a non-shockable rhythm, or cardiac arrest in hospital. Treat shivering by ensuring adequate sedation and giving neuromuscular blocking drugs. Bolus doses of neuromuscular blockers are usually adequate, but infusions are necessary occasionally. Rewarm the patient slowly $(0.25—0.5\,^{\circ}C\,h^{-1})$ and avoid hyperthermia. The optimum target temperature, rate of cooling, duration of hypothermia and rate of rewarming have yet to be determined; further studies are essential.

Blood glucose control

There is a strong association between high blood glucose after resuscitation from cardiac arrest and poor neurological outcome.[237—244] Persistent hyperglycaemia after stroke is also associated with a worse neurological outcome.[375—378] Tight control of blood glucose ($4.4—6.1\,mmol\,l^{-1}$ or $80—110\,mg\,dl^{-1}$) using insulin reduces hospital mortality in critically ill adults,[379,380] but this has not been demonstrated in post-cardiac arrest patients specifically. The benefit is thought to result from the strict glycaemic control rather than the dose of insulin infused.[381] One rat study has shown that glucose plus insulin improves cerebral outcome after asphyxial cardiac arrest.[382] There are no randomised controlled human trials of glucose control after cardiac arrest. The optimal blood glucose target in critically ill patients has not been determined. Comatose patients are at particular risk from unrecognised hypoglycaemia, and the risk of this complication occurring increases as the target blood glucose concentration is lowered.

In common with all critically ill patients, patients admitted to a critical care environment after cardiac arrest should have their blood glucose monitored frequently and hyperglycaemia treated with an insulin infusion. The blood glucose concentration that triggers insulin therapy, and the target range of blood glucose concentrations, should be determined by local policy. There is a need for studies of glucose control after cardiac arrest.

Prognostication

Once a heart has been resuscitated to a stable rhythm and cardiac output, the organ that influences an individual's survival most significantly is the brain. Two thirds of those dying after admission to ICU following out-of-hospital cardiac arrest die from neurological injury.[383] A quarter of those dying after admission to ICU following in-hospital cardiac arrest die from neurological injury. A means of predicting neurological outcome that can be applied to individual patients immediately after ROSC is required. Such a test of prognosis must have 100% specificity.

Clinical tests

There are no neurological signs that can predict outcome in the first hours after ROSC. By 3 days after the onset of coma relating to cardiac arrest, 50% of patients with no chance of ultimate recovery have died. In the remaining patients, the absence of pupil light reflexes on day 3 and an absent motor response to pain on day 3 are both independently predictive of a poor outcome (death or vegetative state) with very high specificity.[384–386]

Biochemical tests

Measurement of serum neuron-specific enolase (NSE) and protein S-100b may be useful in determining the outcome of a cardiac arrest.[237,243,244,387–399] However, the 95% confidence interval (CI) in the trials undertaken to date is wide, and in many of the studies return to consciousness (without comment on level of function) was considered a ''good'' outcome. The

only meta-analysis to look at this topic estimated that to obtain 95% CI with 5% false-positive rate would require a study population of approximately 600 patients.[400] No study this large has been conducted, and these biochemical tests remain unreliable for predicting outcome in individual cases.

Electrophysiological tests

Median nerve somatosensory evoked potentials in normothermic patients, comatose for at least 72 h after cardiac arrest, predict poor outcome with 100% specificity.[384] Bilateral absence of the N20 component of the evoked potentials in comatose patients with coma of hypoxic-anoxic origin is uniformly fatal. When recorded at least 24–48 h after ROSC, the electroencephalogram (EEG), provides limited prognostic information.[401–413] A normal or grossly abnormal EEG predicts outcome reliably, but an EEG between these extremes is unreliable for prognostication.

References

1. Gwinnutt CL, Columb M, Harris R. Outcome after cardiac arrest in adults in UK hospitals: effect of the 1997 guidelines. Resuscitation 2000;47:125–35.
2. Peberdy MA, Kaye W, Ornato JP, et al. Cardiopulmonary resuscitation of adults in the hospital: a report of 14720 cardiac arrests from the National Registry of Cardiopulmonary Resuscitation. Resuscitation 2003;58:297–308.
3. Hodgetts TJ, Kenward G, Vlackonikolis I, et al. Incidence, location and reasons for avoidable in-hospital cardiac arrest in a district general hospital. Resuscitation 2002;54:115–23.
4. Kause J, Smith G, Prytherch D, Parr M, Flabouris A, Hillman K. A comparison of antecedents to cardiac arrests, deaths and emergency intensive care admissions in Australia and New Zealand, and the United Kingdom—the ACADEMIA study. Resuscitation 2004;62:275–82.
5. Herlitz J, Bang A, Aune S, Ekstrom L, Lundstrom G, Holmberg S. Characteristics and outcome among patients suffering in-hospital cardiac arrest in monitored and non-monitored areas. Resuscitation 2001;48:125–35.
6. Franklin C, Mathew J. Developing strategies to prevent inhospital cardiac arrest: analyzing responses of physicians and nurses in the hours before the event. Crit Care Med 1994;22:244–7.
7. McQuillan P, Pilkington S, Allan A, et al. Confidential inquiry into quality of care before admission to intensive care. BMJ 1998;316:1853–8.
8. National Confidential Enquiry into Patient Outcome and Death. An Acute Problem? London, National Confidential Enquiry into Patient Outcome and Death, 2005.
9. Cashman JN. In-hospital cardiac arrest: what happens to the false arrests? Resuscitation 2002;53:271–6.
10. Smith GB, Poplett N. Knowledge of aspects of acute care in trainee doctors. Postgrad Med J 2002;78:335–8.
11. Meek T. New house officers' knowledge of resuscitation, fluid balance and analgesia. Anaesthesia 2000;55:1128–9.

12. Gould TH, Upton PM, Collins P. A survey of the intended management of acute postoperative pain by newly quali-fied doctors in the south west region of England in August 1992. Anaesthesia 1994;49:807—10.

13. Jackson E, Warner J. How much do doctors know about consent and capacity? J R Soc Med 2002;95:601—3.

14. Kruger PS, Longden PJ. A study of a hospital staff's knowledge of pulse oximetry. Anaesth Intensive Care 1997;25:38—41.

15. Wheeler DW, Remoundos DD, Whittlestone KD, et al. Doctors' confusion over ratios and percentages in drug solutions: the case for standard labelling. J R Soc Med 2004;97:380—3.

16. Perkins GD, Stephenson B, Hulme J, Monsieurs KG. Birming-ham assessment of breathing study (BABS). Resuscitation 2005;64:109—13.

17. Goldacre MJ, Lambert T, Evans J, Turner G. Preregistra-tion house officers' views on whether their experience at medical school prepared them well for their jobs: national questionnaire survey. BMJ 2003;326:1011—2.

18. Thwaites BC, Shankar S, Niblett D, Saunders J. Can consul-tants resuscitate? J R Coll Physicians Lond 1992;26:265—7.

19. Saravanan P, Soar J. A survey of resuscitation training needs of senior anaesthetists. Resuscitation 2005;64:93—6.

20. Featherstone P, Smith GB, Linnell M, Easton S, Osgood VM. Impact of a one-day inter-professional course (ALERT™) on attitudes and confidence in managing critically ill adult patients. Resuscitation 2005;65:329—36.

21. Harrison GA, Jacques TC, Kilborn G, McLaws ML. The preva-lence of recordings of the signs of critical conditions and emergency responses in hospital wards—the SOCCER study. Resuscitation 2005;65:149—57.

22. Buist M, Bernard S, Nguyen TV, Moore G, Anderson J. Asso-ciation between clinically abnormal observations and sub-sequent in-hospital mortality: a prospective study. Resus-citation 2004;62:137—41.

23. Goldhill DR, Worthington L, Mulcahy A, Tarling M, Sumner A. The patient-at-risk team: identifying and managing seri-ously ill ward patients. Anaesthesia 1999;54:853—60.

24. Hodgetts TJ, Kenward G, Vlachonikolis IG, Payne S, Castle N. The identification of risk factors for cardiac arrest and formulation of activation criteria to alert a medical emer-gency team. Resuscitation 2002;54:125—31.

25. Subbe CP, Davies RG, Williams E, Rutherford P, Gemmell L. Effect of introducing the Modified Early Warning score on clinical outcomes, cardio-pulmonary arrests and intensive care utilisation in acute medical admissions. Anaesthesia 2003;58:797—802.

26. Lee A, Bishop G, Hillman KM, Daffurn K. The Medical Emer-gency Team. Anaesth Intensive Care 1995;23:183—6.

27. Cuthbertson BH. Outreach critical care—cash for no ques-tions? Br J Anaesth 2003;90:4—6.

28. Parr M. Critical care outreach: some answers, more ques-tions. Intensive Care Med 2004;30:1261—2.

29. Goldhill DR, McNarry AF. Physiological abnormalities in early warning scores are related to mortality in adult inpa-tients. Br J Anaesth 2004;92:882—4.

30. Subbe CP, Williams EM, Gemmell LW. Are medical emer-gency teams picking up enough patients with increased respiratory rate? Crit Care Med 2004;32:1983—4.

31. McBride J, Knight D, Piper J, Smith GB. Long-term effect of introducing an early warning score on respiratory rate charting on general wards. Resuscitation 2005;65:41—4.

32. Carberry M. Implementing the modified early warning sys-tem: our experiences. Nurs Crit Care 2002;7:220—6.

33. Sandroni C, Ferro G, Santangelo S, et al. In-hospital car-diac arrest: survival depends mainly on the effective-ness of the emergency response. Resuscitation 2004;62: 291—7.

34. Soar J, McKay U. A revised role for the hospital cardiac arrest team? Resuscitation 1998;38:145—9.

35. Bellomo R, Goldsmith D, Uchino S, et al. A prospective before-and-after trial of a medical emergency team. Med J Aust 2003;179:283—7.

36. Buist MD, Moore GE, Bernard SA, Waxman BP, Anderson JN, Nguyen TV. Effects of a medical emergency team on reduction of incidence of and mortality from unex-pected cardiac arrests in hospital: preliminary study. BMJ 2002;324:387—90.

37. Parr MJ, Hadfield JH, Flabouris A, Bishop G, Hillman K. The Medical Emergency Team: 12 month analysis of reasons for activation, immediate outcome and not-for-resuscitation orders. Resuscitation 2001;50:39—44.

38. Bellomo R, Goldsmith D, Uchino S, et al. Prospective con-trolled trial of effect of medical emergency team on post-operative morbidity and mortality rates. Crit Care Med 2004;32:916—21.

39. Kenward G, Castle N, Hodgetts T, Shaikh L. Evaluation of a medical emergency team one year after implementation. Resuscitation 2004;61:257—63.

40. Jones D, Bates S, Warrillow S, et al. Circadian pattern of activation of the medical emergency team in a teaching hospital. Crit Care 2005;9:R303—6.

41. The MERIT study investigators. Introduction of the medi-cal emergency team (MET) system: a cluster-randomised controlled trial. Lancet 2005;365:2091—7.

42. Critical care outreach 2003: progress in developing ser-vices. The National Outreach Report 2003. London, Depart-ment of Health and National Health Service Modernisation Agency; 2003.

43. Ball C, Kirkby M, Williams S. Effect of the critical care out-reach team on patient survival to discharge from hospital and readmission to critical care: non-randomised popula-tion based study. BMJ 2003;327:1014.

44. Priestley G, Watson W, Rashidian A, et al. Introducing Crit-ical Care Outreach: a ward-randomised trial of phased introduction in a general hospital. Intensive Care Med 2004;30:1398—404.

45. Story DA, Shelton AC, Poustie SJ, Colin-Thome NJ, McNi-col PL. The effect of critical care outreach on post-operative serious adverse events. Anaesthesia 2004;59: 762—6.

46. Szalados JE. Critical care teams managing floor patients: the continuing evolution of hospitals into intensive care units? Crit Care Med 2004;32:1071—2.

47. Cooke MW, Higgins J, Kidd P. Use of emergency observa-tion and assessment wards: a systematic literature review. Emerg Med J 2003;20:138—42.

48. Rivers E, Nguyen B, Havstad S, et al. Early goal-directed therapy in the treatment of severe sepsis and septic shock. N Engl J Med 2001;345:1368—77.

49. Leeson-Payne CG, Aitkenhead AR. A prospective study to assess the demand for a high dependency unit. Anaesthesia 1995;50:383—7.

50. Guidelines for the utilisation of intensive care units. Euro-pean Society of Intensive Care Medicine. Intensive Care Med 1994;20:163—4.

51. Haupt MT, Bekes CE, Brilli RJ, et al. Guidelines on critical care services and personnel: recommendations based on a system of categorization of three levels of care. Crit Care Med 2003;31:2677—83.

52. Hillson SD, Rich EC, Dowd B, Luxenberg MG. Call nights and patients care: effects on inpatients at one teaching hospital. J Gen Intern Med 1992;7:405—10.

53. Bell CM, Redelmeier DA. Mortality among patients admitted to hospitals on weekends as compared with weekdays. N Engl J Med 2001;345:663—8.

54. Beck DH, McQuillan P, Smith GB. Waiting for the break of dawn? The effects of discharge time, discharge TISS scores and discharge facility on hospital mortality after intensive care. Intensive Care Med 2002;28:1287—93.

55. Needleman J, Buerhaus P, Mattke S, Stewart M, Zelevinsky K. Nurse-staffing levels and the quality of care in hospitals. N Engl J Med 2002;346:1715—22.

56. Baskett PJ, Lim A. The varying ethical attitudes towards resuscitation in Europe. Resuscitation 2004;62:267—73.

57. Gabbott D, Smith G, Mitchell S, et al. Cardiopulmonary resuscitation standards for clinical practice and training in the UK. Resuscitation 2005;64:13—9.

58. Bristow PJ, Hillman KM, Chey T, et al. Rates of in-hospital arrests, deaths and intensive care admissions: the effect of a medical emergency team. Med J Aust 2000;173:236—40.

59. Eberle B, Dick WF, Schneider T, Wisser G, Doetsch S, Tzanova I. Checking the carotid pulse check: diagnostic accuracy of first responders in patients with and without a pulse. Resuscitation 1996;33:107—16.

60. Ruppert M, Reith MW, Widmann JH, et al. Checking for breathing: evaluation of the diagnostic capability of emergency medical services personnel, physicians, medical students, and medical laypersons. Ann Emerg Med 1999;34:720—9.

61. Abella BS, Alvarado JP, Myklebust H, et al. Quality of cardiopulmonary resuscitation during in-hospital cardiac arrest. JAMA 2005;293:305—10.

62. Abella BS, Sandbo N, Vassilatos P, et al. Chest compression rates during cardiopulmonary resuscitation are suboptimal: a prospective study during in-hospital cardiac arrest. Circulation 2005;111:428—34.

63. Perkins GD, Roberts C, Gao F. Delays in defibrillation: influence of different monitoring techniques. Br J Anaesth 2002;89:405—8.

64. Soar J, Perkins GD, Harris S, Nolan JP. The immediate life support course. Resuscitation 2003;57:21—6.

65. Nolan J. Advanced life support training. Resuscitation 2001;50:9—11.

66. Perkins G, Lockey A. The advanced life support provider course. BMJ 2002;325:S81.

67. Bayes de Luna A, Coumel P, Leclercq JF. Ambulatory sudden cardiac death: mechanisms of production of fatal arrhythmia on the basis of data from 157 cases. Am Heart J 1989;117:151—9.

68. Rea TD, Shah S, Kudenchuk PJ, Copass MK, Cobb LA. Automated external defibrillators: to what extent does the algorithm delay CPR? Ann Emerg Med 2005;46:132—41.

69. van Alem AP, Sanou BT, Koster RW. Interruption of cardiopulmonary resuscitation with the use of the automated external defibrillator in out-of-hospital cardiac arrest. Ann Emerg Med 2003;42:449—57.

70. Hess EP, White RD. Ventricular fibrillation is not provoked by chest compression during post-shock organized rhythms in out-of-hospital cardiac arrest. Resuscitation 2005;66:7—11.

71. Eftestol T, Wik L, Sunde K, Steen PA. Effects of cardiopulmonary resuscitation on predictors of ventricular fibrillation defibrillation success during out-of-hospital cardiac arrest. Circulation 2004;110:10—5.

72. Eftestol T, Sunde K, Aase SO, Husoy JH, Steen PA. Predicting outcome of defibrillation by spectral characterization and nonparametric classification of ventricular fibrillation in patients with out-of-hospital cardiac arrest. Circulation 2000;102:1523—9.

73. Eftestol T, Sunde K, Steen PA. Effects of interrupting precordial compressions on the calculated probability of defibrillation success during out-of-hospital cardiac arrest. Circulation 2002;105:2270—3.

74. Caldwell G, Millar G, Quinn E. Simple mechanical methods for cardioversion: defence of the precordial thump and cough version. Br Med J 1985;291:627—30.

75. Kohl P, King AM, Boulin C. Antiarrhythmic effects of acute mechanical stiumulation. In: Kohl P, Sachs F, Franz MR, editors. Cardiac mechano-electric feedback and arrhythmias: form pipette to patient. Philadelphia: Elsevier Saunders; 2005. p. 304—14.

76. Krijne R. Rate acceleration of ventricular tachycardia after a precordial chest thump. Am J Cardiol 1984;53:964—5.

77. Emerman CL, Pinchak AC, Hancock D, Hagen JF. Effect of injection site on circulation times during cardiac arrest. Crit Care Med 1988;16:1138—41.

78. Glaeser PW, Hellmich TR, Szewczuga D, Losek JD, Smith DS. Five-year experience in prehospital intraosseous infusions in children and adults. Ann Emerg Med 1993;22:1119—24.

79. Schuttler J, Bartsch A, Ebeling BJ, et al. Endobronchial administration of adrenaline in preclinical cardiopulmonary resuscitation. Anasth Intensivther Notfallmed 1987;22:63—8.

80. Hornchen U, Schuttler J, Stoeckel H, Eichelkraut W, Hahn N. Endobronchial instillation of epinephrine during cardiopulmonary resuscitation. Crit Care Med 1987;15:1037—9.

81. Vaknin Z, Manisterski Y, Ben-Abraham R, et al. Is endotracheal adrenaline deleterious because of the beta adrenergic effect? Anesth Analg 2001;92:1408—12.

82. Manisterski Y, Vaknin Z, Ben-Abraham R, et al. Endotracheal epinephrine: a call for larger doses. Anesth Analg 2002;95:1037—41 [table of contents].

83. Efrati O, Ben-Abraham R, Barak A, et al. Endobronchial adrenaline: should it be reconsidered? Dose response and haemodynamic effect in dogs. Resuscitation 2003;59:117—22.

84. Elizur A, Ben-Abraham R, Manisterski Y, et al. Tracheal epinephrine or norepinephrine preceded by beta blockade in a dog model. Can beta blockade bestow any benefits? Resuscitation 2003;59:271—6.

85. Naganobu K, Hasebe Y, Uchiyama Y, Hagio M, Ogawa H. A comparison of distilled water and normal saline as diluents for endobronchial administration of epinephrine in the dog. Anesth Analg 2000;91:317—21.

86. Eftestol T, Wik L, Sunde K, Steen PA. Effects of cardiopulmonary resuscitation on predictors of ventricular fibrillation defibrillation success during out-of-hospital cardiac arrest. Circulation 2004;110:10—5.

87. Berg RA, Hilwig RW, Kern KB, Ewy GA. Precountershock cardiopulmonary resuscitation improves ventricular fibrillation median frequency and myocardial readiness for successful defibrillation from prolonged ventricular fibrillation: a randomized, controlled swine study. Ann Emerg Med 2002;40:563—70.

88. Achleitner U, Wenzel V, Strohmenger HU, et al. The beneficial effect of basic life support on ventricular fibrillation mean frequency and coronary perfusion pressure. Resuscitation 2001;51:151—8.

89. Kudenchuk PJ, Cobb LA, Copass MK, et al. Amiodarone for resuscitation after out-of-hospital cardiac arrest due to ventricular fibrillation. N Engl J Med 1999;341:871—8.

90. Dorian P, Cass D, Schwartz B, Cooper R, Gelaznikas R, Barr A. Amiodarone as compared with lidocaine for shock-resistant ventricular fibrillation. N Engl J Med 2002;346:884—90.

91. Thel MC, Armstrong AL, McNulty SE, Califf RM, O'Connor CM. Randomised trial of magnesium in in-hospital cardiac arrest. Lancet 1997;350:1272—6.

92. Allegra J, Lavery R, Cody R, et al. Magnesium sulfate in the treatment of refractory ventricular fibrillation in the prehospital setting. Resuscitation 2001;49:245—9.

93. Fatovich D, Prentice D, Dobb G. Magnesium in in-hospital cardiac arrest. Lancet 1998;351:446.

94. Hassan TB, Jagger C, Barnett DB. A randomised trial to investigate the efficacy of magnesium sulphate for refractory ventricular fibrillation. Emerg Med J 2002;19:57—62.

95. Miller B, Craddock L, Hoffenberg S, et al. Pilot study of intravenous magnesium sulfate in refractory cardiac arrest: safety data and recommendations for future studies. Resuscitation 1995;30:3—14.

96. Weil MH, Rackow EC, Trevino R, Grundler W, Falk JL, Griffel MI. Difference in acid—base state between venous and arterial blood during cardiopulmonary resuscitation. N Engl J Med 1986;315:153—6.

97. Bottiger BW, Bode C, Kern S, et al. Efficacy and safety of thrombolytic therapy after initially unsuccessful cardiopulmonary resuscitation: a prospective clinical trial. Lancet 2001;357:1583—5.

98. Boidin MP. Airway patency in the unconscious patient. Br J Anaesth 1985;57:306—10.

99. Nandi PR, Charlesworth CH, Taylor SJ, Nunn JF, Dore CJ. Effect of general anaesthesia on the pharynx. Br J Anaesth 1991;66:157—62.

100. Guildner CW. Resuscitation: opening the airway. A comparative study of techniques for opening an airway obstructed by the tongue. JACEP 1976;5:588—90.

101. Safar P, Aguto-Escarraga L. Compliance in apneic anesthetized adults. Anesthesiology 1959;20:283—9.

102. Greene DG, Elam JO, Dobkin AB, Studley CL. Cinefluorographic study of hyperextension of the neck and upper airway patency. Jama 1961;176:570—3.

103. Morikawa S, Safar P, Decarlo J. Influence of the head-jaw position upon upper airway patency. Anesthesiology 1961;22:265—70.

104. Ruben HM, Elam JO, Ruben AM, Greene DG. Investigation of upper airway problems in resuscitation. 1. Studies of pharyngeal X-rays and performance by laymen. Anesthesiology 1961;22:271—9.

105. Elam JO, Greene DG, Schneider MA, et al. Head-tilt method of oral resuscitation. JAMA 1960;172:812—5.

106. Aprahamian C, Thompson BM, Finger WA, Darin JC. Experimental cervical spine injury model: evaluation of airway management and splinting techniques. Ann Emerg Med 1984;13:584—7.

107. Donaldson 3rd WF, Heil BV, Donaldson VP, Silvaggio VJ. The effect of airway maneuvers on the unstable C1-C2 segment. A cadaver study. Spine 1997;22:1215—8.

108. Donaldson 3rd WF, Towers JD, Doctor A, Brand A, Donaldson VP. A methodology to evaluate motion of the unstable spine during intubation techniques. Spine 1993;18:2020—3.

109. Hauswald M, Sklar DP, Tandberg D, Garcia JF. Cervical spine movement during airway management: cinefluoroscopic appraisal in human cadavers. Am J Emerg Med 1991;9:535—8.

110. Brimacombe J, Keller C, Kunzel KH, Gaber O, Boehler M, Puhringer F. Cervical spine motion during airway management: a cinefluoroscopic study of the posteriorly destabilized third cervical vertebrae in human cadavers. Anesth Analg 2000;91:1274—8.

111. Majernick TG, Bieniek R, Houston JB, Hughes HG. Cervical spine movement during orotracheal intubation. Ann Emerg Med 1986;15:417—20.

112. Lennarson PJ, Smith DW, Sawin PD, Todd MM, Sato Y, Traynelis VC. Cervical spinal motion during intubation: efficacy of stabilization maneuvers in the setting of complete segmental instability. J Neurosurg Spine 2001;94:265—70.

113. Marsh AM, Nunn JF, Taylor SJ, Charlesworth CH. Airway obstruction associated with the use of the Guedel airway. Br J Anaesth 1991;67:517—23.

114. Schade K, Borzotta A, Michaels A. Intracranial malposition of nasopharyngeal airway. J Trauma 2000;49:967—8.

115. Muzzi DA, Losasso TJ, Cucchiara RF. Complication from a nasopharyngeal airway in a patient with a basilar skull fracture. Anesthesiology 1991;74:366—8.

116. Roberts K, Porter K. How do you size a nasopharyngeal airway. Resuscitation 2003;56:19—23.

117. Stoneham MD. The nasopharyngeal airway. Assessment of position by fibreoptic laryngoscopy. Anaesthesia 1993;48:575—80.

118. Moser DK, Dracup K, Doering LV. Effect of cardiopulmonary resuscitation training for parents of high-risk neonates on perceived anxiety, control, and burden. Heart Lung 1999;28:326—33.

119. Kandakai T, King K. Perceived self-efficacy in performing lifesaving skills: an assessment of the American Red Cross's Responding to Emergencies course. J Health Educ 1999;30:235—41.

120. Lester CA, Donnelly PD, Assar D. Lay CPR trainees: retraining, confidence and willingness to attempt resuscitation 4 years after training. Resuscitation 2000;45:77—82.

121. Pane GA, Salness KA. A survey of participants in a mass CPR training course. Ann Emerg Med 1987;16:1112—6.

122. Heilman KM, Muschenheim C. Primary cutaneous tuberculosis resulting from mouth-to-mouth respiration. N Engl J Med 1965;273:1035—6.

123. Christian MD, Loutfy M, McDonald LC, et al. Possible SARS coronavirus transmission during cardiopulmonary resuscitation. Emerg Infect Dis 2004;10:287—93.

124. Alexander R, Hodgson P, Lomax D, Bullen C. A comparison of the laryngeal mask airway and Guedel airway, bag and face mask for manual ventilation following formal training. Anaesthesia 1993;48:231—4.

125. Dorges V, Sauer C, Ocker H, Wenzel V, Schmucker P. Smaller tidal volumes during cardiopulmonary resuscitation: comparison of adult and paediatric self-inflatable bags with three different ventilatory devices. Resuscitation 1999;43:31—7.

126. Ocker H, Wenzel V, Schmucker P, Dorges V. Effectiveness of various airway management techniques in a bench model simulating a cardiac arrest patient. J Emerg Med 2001;20:7—12.

127. Stone BJ, Chantler PJ, Baskett PJ. The incidence of regurgitation during cardiopulmonary resuscitation: a comparison between the bag valve mask and laryngeal mask airway. Resuscitation 1998;38:3—6.

128. Hartsilver EL, Vanner RG. Airway obstruction with cricoid pressure. Anaesthesia 2000;55:208—11.

129. Aufderheide TP, Sigurdsson G, Pirrallo RG, et al. Hyperventilation-induced hypotension during cardiopulmonary resuscitation. Circulation 2004;109:1960—5.

130. Stallinger A, Wenzel V, Wagner-Berger H, et al. Effects of decreasing inspiratory flow rate during simulated basic life support ventilation of a cardiac arrest patient on lung and stomach tidal volumes. Resuscitation 2002;54:167—73.

131. Noordergraaf GJ, van Dun PJ, Kramer BP, et al. Can first responders achieve and maintain normocapnia when sequentially ventilating with a bag-valve device and two oxygen-driven resuscitators? A controlled clinical trial in 104 patients. Eur J Anaesthesiol 2004;21:367—72.

132. Jones JH, Murphy MP, Dickson RL, Somerville GG, Brizendine EJ. Emergency physician-verified out-of-hospital intubation: miss rates by paramedics. Acad Emerg Med 2004;11:707–9.

133. Pelucio M, Halligan L, Dhindsa H. Out-of-hospital experience with the syringe esophageal detector device. Acad Emerg Med 1997;4:563–8.

134. Sayre MR, Sakles JC, Mistler AF, Evans JL, Kramer AT, Pancioli AM. Field trial of endotracheal intubation by basic EMTs. Ann Emerg Med 1998;31:228–33.

135. Katz SH, Falk JL. Misplaced endotracheal tubes by paramedics in an urban emergency medical services system. Ann Emerg Med 2001;37:32–7.

136. Nolan JP, Prehospital. resuscitative airway care: should the gold standard be reassessed? Curr Opin Crit Care 2001;7:413–21.

137. Davies PR, Tighe SQ, Greenslade GL, Evans GH. Laryngeal mask airway and tracheal tube insertion by unskilled personnel. Lancet 1990;336:977–9.

138. Flaishon R, Sotman A, Ben-Abraham R, Rudick V, Varssano D, Weinbroum AA. Antichemical protective gear prolongs time to successful airway management: a randomized, crossover study in humans. Anesthesiology 2004;100:260–6.

139. Ho BY, Skinner HJ, Mahajan RP. Gastro-oesophageal reflux during day case gynaecological laparoscopy under positive pressure ventilation: laryngeal mask vs. tracheal intubation. Anaesthesia 1998;53:921–4.

140. Reinhart DJ, Simmons G. Comparison of placement of the laryngeal mask airway with endotracheal tube by paramedics and respiratory therapists. Ann Emerg Med 1994;24:260–3.

141. Rewari W, Kaul HL. Regurgitation and aspiration during gynaecological laparoscopy: comparison between laryngeal mask airway and tracheal intubation. J Anaesth Clin Pharmacol 1999;15:67–70.

142. Pennant JH, Walker MB. Comparison of the endotracheal tube and laryngeal mask in airway management by paramedical personnel. Anesth Analg 1992;74:531–4.

143. Maltby JR, Beriault MT, Watson NC, Liepert DJ, Fick GH. LMA-Classic and LMA-ProSeal are effective alternatives to endotracheal intubation for gynecologic laparoscopy. Can J Anaesth 2003;50:71–7.

144. Rumball CJ, MacDonald D, The PTL. Combitube, laryngeal mask, and oral airway: a randomized prehospital comparative study of ventilatory device effectiveness and cost-effectiveness in 470 cases of cardiorespiratory arrest. Prehosp Emerg Care 1997;1:1–10.

145. Verghese C, Prior-Willeard PF, Baskett PJ. Immediate management of the airway during cardiopulmonary resuscitation in a hospital without a resident anaesthesiologist. Eur J Emerg Med 1994;1:123–5.

146. Tanigawa K, Shigematsu A. Choice of airway devices for 12,020 cases of nontraumatic cardiac arrest in Japan. Prehosp Emerg Care 1998;2:96–100.

147. The use of the laryngeal mask airway by nurses during cardiopulmonary resuscitation: results of a multicentre trial. Anaesthesia 1994;49:3–7.

148. Grantham H, Phillips G, Gilligan JE. The laryngeal mask in prehospital emergency care. Emerg Med 1994;6:193–7.

149. Kokkinis K. The use of the laryngeal mask airway in CPR. Resuscitation 1994;27:9–12.

150. Leach A, Alexander CA, Stone B. The laryngeal mask in cardiopulmonary resuscitation in a district general hospital: a preliminary communication. Resuscitation 1993;25:245–8.

151. Staudinger T, Brugger S, Watschinger B, et al. Emergency intubation with the Combitube: comparison with the endotracheal airway. Ann Emerg Med 1993;22:1573–5.

152. Lefrancois DP, Dufour DG. Use of the esophageal tracheal combitube by basic emergency medical technicians. Resuscitation 2002;52:77–83.

153. Ochs M, Vilke GM, Chan TC, Moats T, Buchanan J. Successful prehospital airway management by EMT-Ds using the combitube. Prehosp Emerg Care 2000;4:333–7.

154. Vezina D, Lessard MR, Bussieres J, Topping C, Trepanier CA. Complications associated with the use of the esophageal–tracheal Combitube. Can J Anaesth 1998;45:76–80.

155. Richards CF. Piriform sinus perforation during esophageal–tracheal Combitube placement. J Emerg Med 1998;16:37–9.

156. Rumball C, Macdonald D, Barber P, Wong H, Smecher C. Endotracheal intubation and esophageal tracheal Combitube insertion by regular ambulance attendants: a comparative trial. Prehosp Emerg Care 2004;8:15–22.

157. Rabitsch W, Schellongowski P, Staudinger T, et al. Comparison of a conventional tracheal airway with the Combitube in an urban emergency medical services system run by physicians. Resuscitation 2003;57:27–32.

158. Cook TM, McCormick B, Asai T. Randomized comparison of laryngeal tube with classic laryngeal mask airway for anaesthesia with controlled ventilation. Br J Anaesth 2003;91:373–8.

159. Cook TM, McKinstry C, Hardy R, Twigg S. Randomized crossover comparison of the ProSeal laryngeal mask airway with the laryngeal tube during anaesthesia with controlled ventilation. Br J Anaesth 2003;91:678–83.

160. Asai T, Kawachi S. Use of the laryngeal tube by paramedic staff. Anaesthesia 2004;59:408–9.

161. Asai T, Moriyama S, Nishita Y, Kawachi S. Use of the laryngeal tube during cardiopulmonary resuscitation by paramedical staff. Anaesthesia 2003;58:393–4.

162. Genzwuerker HV, Dhonau S, Ellinger K. Use of the laryngeal tube for out-of-hospital resuscitation. Resuscitation 2002;52:221–4.

163. Kette F, Reffo I, Giordani G, et al. The use of laryngeal tube by nurses in out-of-hospital emergencies: preliminary experience. Resuscitation 2005;66:21–5.

164. Cook TM, Nolan JP, Verghese C, et al. Randomized crossover comparison of the proseal with the classic laryngeal mask airway in unparalysed anaesthetized patients. Br J Anaesth 2002;88:527–33.

165. Cook TM, Lee G, Nolan JP. The ProSealTM laryngeal mask airway: a review of the literature [Le masque larynge ProSealTM: un examen des publications]. Can J Anaesth 2005;52:739–60.

166. Cook TM, Gupta K, Gabbott DA, Nolan JP. An evaluation of the airway management device. Anaesthesia 2001;56:660–4.

167. Chiu CL, Wang CY. An evaluation of the modified airway management device. Anaesth Intensive Care 2004;32:77–80.

168. Cook TM, McCormick B, Gupta K, Hersch P, Simpson T. An evaluation of the PA(Xpress) pharyngeal airway—a new single use airway device. Resuscitation 2003;58:139–43.

169. Burgoyne L, Cyna A. Laryngeal mask vs intubating laryngeal mask: insertion and ventilation by inexperienced resuscitators. Anaesth Intensive Care 2001;29:604–8.

170. Choyce A, Avidan MS, Shariff A, Del Aguila M, Radcliffe JJ, Chan T. A comparison of the intubating and standard laryngeal mask airways for airway management by inexperienced personnel. Anaesthesia 2001;56:357–60.

171. Baskett PJ, Parr MJ, Nolan JP. The intubating laryngeal mask. Results of a multicentre trial with experience of 500 cases. Anaesthesia 1998;53:1174–9.

172. Gausche M, Lewis RJ, Stratton SJ, et al. Effect of out-of-hospital pediatric endotracheal intubation on survival and neurological outcome: a controlled clinical trial. JAMA 2000;283:783—970.

173. Guly UM, Mitchell RG, Cook R, Steedman DJ, Robertson CE. Paramedics and technicians are equally successful at managing cardiac arrest outside hospital. BMJ 1995;310:1091—4.

174. Stiell IG, Wells GA, Field B, et al. Advanced cardiac life support in out-of-hospital cardiac arrest. N Engl J Med 2004;351:647—56.

175. Garza AG, Gratton MC, Coontz D, Noble E, Ma OJ. Effect of paramedic experience on orotracheal intubation success rates. J Emerg Med 2003;25:251—6.

176. Li J. Capnography alone is imperfect for endotracheal tube placement confirmation during emergency intubation. J Emerg Med 2001;20:223—9.

177. Tanigawa K, Takeda T, Goto E, Tanaka K. Accuracy and reliability of the self-inflating bulb to verify tracheal intubation in out-of-hospital cardiac arrest patients. Anesthesiology 2000;93:1432—6.

178. Takeda T, Tanigawa K, Tanaka H, Hayashi Y, Goto E, Tanaka K. The assessment of three methods to verify tracheal tube placement in the emergency setting. Resuscitation 2003;56:153—7.

179. Baraka A, Khoury PJ, Siddik SS, Salem MR, Joseph NJ. Efficacy of the self-inflating bulb in differentiating esophageal from tracheal intubation in the parturient undergoing cesarean section. Anesth Analg 1997;84:533—7.

180. Davis DP, Stephen KA, Vilke GM. Inaccuracy in endotracheal tube verification using a Toomey syringe. J Emerg Med 1999;17:35—8.

181. Grmec S. Comparison of three different methods to confirm tracheal tube placement in emergency intubation. Intensive Care Med 2002;28:701—4.

182. American Heart Association in collaboration with International Liaison Committee on Resuscitation. Guidelines 2000 for Cardiopulmonary Resuscitation and Emergency Cardiovascular Care: International Consensus on Science. Part 6. Advanced Cardiovascular Life Support: Section 6. Pharmacology II: Agents to Optimize Cardiac Output and Blood Pressure. Circulation 2000;102(Suppl. I):I129—35.

183. Lindner KH, Strohmenger HU, Ensinger H, Hetzel WD, Ahnefeld FW, Georgieff M. Stress hormone response during and after cardiopulmonary resuscitation. Anesthesiology 1992;77:662—8.

184. Lindner KH, Haak T, Keller A, Bothner U, Lurie KG. Release of endogenous vasopressors during and after cardiopulmonary resuscitation. Heart 1996;75:145—50.

185. Morris DC, Dereczyk BE, Grzybowski M, et al. Vasopressin can increase coronary perfusion pressure during human cardiopulmonary resuscitation. Acad Emerg Med 1997;4:878—83.

186. Lindner KH, Prengel AW, Brinkmann A, Strohmenger HU, Lindner IM, Lurie KG. Vasopressin administration in refractory cardiac arrest. Ann Intern Med 1996;124:1061—4.

187. Lindner KH, Brinkmann A, Pfenninger EG, Lurie KG, Goertz A, Lindner IM. Effect of vasopressin on hemodynamic variables, organ blood flow, and acid—base status in a pig model of cardiopulmonary resuscitation. Anesth Analg 1993;77:427—35.

188. Lindner KH, Prengel AW, Pfenninger EG, et al. Vasopressin improves vital organ blood flow during closed-chest cardiopulmonary resuscitation in pigs. Circulation 1995;91:215—21.

189. Wenzel V, Lindner KH, Prengel AW, et al. Vasopressin improves vital organ blood flow after prolonged cardiac arrest with postcountershock pulseless electrical activity in pigs. Crit Care Med 1999;27:486—92.

190. Voelckel WG, Lurie KG, McKnite S, et al. Comparison of epinephrine and vasopressin in a pediatric porcine model of asphyxial cardiac arrest. Crit Care Med 2000;28:3777—83.

191. Babar SI, Berg RA, Hilwig RW, Kern KB, Ewy GA. Vasopressin versus epinephrine during cardiopulmonary resuscitation: a randomized swine outcome study. Resuscitation 1999;41:185—92.

192. Lindner KH, Dirks B, Strohmenger HU, Prengel AW, Lindner IM, Lurie KG. Randomised comparison of epinephrine and vasopressin in patients with out-of-hospital ventricular fibrillation. Lancet 1997;349:535—7.

193. Stiell IG, Hebert PC, Wells GA, et al. Vasopressin versus epinephrine for inhospital cardiac arrest: a randomised controlled trial. Lancet 2001;358:105—9.

194. Wenzel V, Krismer AC, Arntz HR, Sitter H, Stadlbauer KH, Lindner KH. A comparison of vasopressin and epinephrine for out-of-hospital cardiopulmonary resuscitation. N Engl J Med 2004;350:105—13.

195. Aung K, Htay T. Vasopressin for cardiac arrest: a systematic review and meta-analysis. Arch Intern Med 2005;165:17—24.

196. Callaham M, Madsen C, Barton C, Saunders C, Daley M, Pointer J. A randomized clinical trial of high-dose epinephrine and norepinephrine versus standard-dose epinephrine in prehospital cardiac arrest. JAMA 1992;268:2667—72.

197. Masini E, Planchenault J, Pezziardi F, Gautier P, Gagnol JP. Histamine-releasing properties of Polysorbate 80 in vitro and in vivo: correlation with its hypotensive action in the dog. Agents Actions 1985;16:470—7.

198. Somberg JC, Bailin SJ, Haffajee CI, et al. Intravenous lidocaine versus intravenous amiodarone (in a new aqueous formulation) for incessant ventricular tachycardia. Am J Cardiol 2002;90:853—9.

199. Somberg JC, Timar S, Bailin SJ, et al. Lack of a hypotensive effect with rapid administration of a new aqueous formulation of intravenous amiodarone. Am J Cardiol 2004;93:576—81.

200. Skrifvars MB, Kuisma M, Boyd J, et al. The use of undiluted amiodarone in the management of out-of-hospital cardiac arrest. Acta Anaesthesiol Scand 2004;48:582—7.

201. Petrovic T, Adnet F, Lapandry C. Successful resuscitation of ventricular fibrillation after low-dose amiodarone. Ann Emerg Med 1998;32:518—9.

202. Levine JH, Massumi A, Scheinman MM, et al. Intravenous amiodarone for recurrent sustained hypotensive ventricular tachyarrhythmias. Intravenous Amiodarone Multicenter Trial Group. J Am Coll Cardiol 1996;27:67—75.

203. Matsusaka T, Hasebe N, Jin YT, Kawabe J, Kikuchi K. Magnesium reduces myocardial infarct size via enhancement of adenosine mechanism in rabbits. Cardiovasc Res 2002;54:568—75.

204. Longstreth Jr WT, Fahrenbruch CE, Olsufka M, Walsh TR, Copass MK, Cobb LA. Randomized clinical trial of magnesium, diazepam, or both after out-of-hospital cardiac arrest. Neurology 2002;59:506—14.

205. Baraka A, Ayoub C, Kawkabani N. Magnesium therapy for refractory ventricular fibrillation. J Cardiothorac Vasc Anesth 2000;14:196—9.

206. Stiell IG, Wells GA, Hebert PC, Laupacis A, Weitzman BN. Association of drug therapy with survival in cardiac arrest: limited role of advanced cardiac life support drugs. Acad Emerg Med 1995;2:264—73.

207. Engdahl J, Bang A, Lindqvist J, Herlitz J. Can we define patients with no and those with some chance of sur-

vival when found in asystole out of hospital? Am J Cardiol 2000;86:610—4.

208. Engdahl J, Bang A, Lindqvist J, Herlitz J. Factors affecting short- and long-term prognosis among 1069 patients with out-of-hospital cardiac arrest and pulseless electrical activity. Resuscitation 2001;51:17—25.

209. Dumot JA, Burval DJ, Sprung J, et al. Outcome of adult cardiopulmonary resuscitations at a tertiary referral center including results of ''limited'' resuscitations. Arch Intern Med 2001;161:1751—8.

210. Tortolani AJ, Risucci DA, Powell SR, Dixon R. In-hospital cardiopulmonary resuscitation during asystole. Therapeutic factors associated with 24-hour survival. Chest 1989;96:622—6.

211. Viskin S, Belhassen B, Roth A, et al. Aminophylline for bradyasystolic cardiac arrest refractory to atropine and epinephrine. Ann Intern Med 1993;118:279—81.

212. Mader TJ, Gibson P. Adenosine receptor antagonism in refractory asystolic cardiac arrest: results of a human pilot study. Resuscitation 1997;35:3—7.

213. Mader TJ, Smithline HA, Gibson P. Aminophylline in undifferentiated out-of-hospital asystolic cardiac arrest. Resuscitation 1999;41:39—45.

214. Mader TJ, Smithline HA, Durkin L, Scriver G. A randomized controlled trial of intravenous aminophylline for atropine-resistant out-of-hospital asystolic cardiac arrest. Acad Emerg Med 2003;10:192—7.

215. Dybvik T, Strand T, Steen PA. Buffer therapy during out-of-hospital cardiopulmonary resuscitation. Resuscitation 1995;29:89—95.

216. Aufderheide TP, Martin DR, Olson DW, et al. Prehospital bicarbonate use in cardiac arrest: a 3-year experience. Am J Emerg Med 1992;10:4—7.

217. Delooz H, Lewi PJ. Are inter-center differences in EMS-management and sodium-bicarbonate administration important for the outcome of CPR? The Cerebral Resuscitation Study Group. Resuscitation 1989;17(Suppl.):S199—206.

218. Roberts D, Landolfo K, Light R, Dobson K. Early predictors of mortality for hospitalized patients suffering cardiopulmonary arrest. Chest 1990;97:413—9.

219. Suljaga-Pechtel K, Goldberg E, Strickon P, Berger M, Skovron ML. Cardiopulmonary resuscitation in a hospitalized population: prospective study of factors associated with outcome. Resuscitation 1984;12:77—95.

220. Weil MH, Trevino RP, Rackow EC. Sodium bicarbonate during CPR. Does it help or hinder? Chest 1985;88:487.

221. Bar-Joseph G, Abramson NS, Kelsey SF, Mashiach T, Craig MT, Safar P. Improved resuscitation outcome in emergency medical systems with increased usage of sodium bicarbonate during cardiopulmonary resuscitation. Acta Anaesthesiol Scand 2005;49:6—15.

222. Sandeman DJ, Alahakoon TI, Bentley SC. Tricyclic poisoning—successful management of ventricular fibrillation following massive overdose of imipramine. Anaesth Intensive Care 1997;25:542—5.

223. Lin SR. The effect of dextran and streptokinase on cerebral function and blood flow after cardiac arrest. An experimental study on the dog. Neuroradiology 1978;16:340—2.

224. Fischer M, Bottiger BW, Popov-Cenic S, Hossmann KA. Thrombolysis using plasminogen activator and heparin reduces cerebral no-reflow after resuscitation from cardiac arrest: an experimental study in the cat. Intensive Care Med 1996;22:1214—23.

225. Ruiz-Bailen M, Aguayo de Hoyos E, Serrano-Corcoles MC, Diaz-Castellanos MA, Ramos-Cuadra JA, Reina-Toral A. Efficacy of thrombolysis in patients with acute myocardial infarction requiring cardiopulmonary resuscitation. Intensive Care Med 2001;27:1050—7.

226. Lederer W, Lichtenberger C, Pechlaner C, Kroesen G, Baubin M. Recombinant tissue plasminogen activator during cardiopulmonary resuscitation in 108 patients with out-of-hospital cardiac arrest. Resuscitation 2001;50:71—6.

227. Tiffany PA, Schultz M, Stueven H. Bolus thrombolytic infusions during CPR for patients with refractory arrest rhythms: outcome of a case series. Ann Emerg Med 1998;31:124—6.

228. Abu-Laban RB, Christenson JM, Innes GD, et al. Tissue plasminogen activator in cardiac arrest with pulseless electrical activity. N Engl J Med 2002;346:1522—8.

229. Janata K, Holzer M, Kurkciyan I, et al. Major bleeding complications in cardiopulmonary resuscitation: the place of thrombolytic therapy in cardiac arrest due to massive pulmonary embolism. Resuscitation 2003;57:49—55.

230. Scholz KH, Hilmer T, Schuster S, Wojcik J, Kreuzer H, Tebbe U. Thrombolysis in resuscitated patients with pulmonary embolism. Dtsch Med Wochenschr 1990;115:930—5.

231. Lederer W, Lichtenberger C, Pechlaner C, Kinzl J, Kroesen G, Baubin M. Long-term survival and neurological outcome of patients who received recombinant tissue plasminogen activator during out-of-hospital cardiac arrest. Resuscitation 2004;61:123—9.

232. Gramann J, Lange-Braun P, Bodemann T, Hochrein H. Der Einsatz von Thrombolytika in der Reanimation als Ultima ratio zur Überwindung des Herztodes. Intensiv- und Notfallbehandlung 1991;16:134—7.

233. Klefisch F, et al. Praklinische ultima-ratio thrombolyse bei therapierefraktarer kardiopulmonaler reanimation. Intensivmedizin 1995;32:155—62.

234. Ruiz-Bailen M, Aguayo-de-Hoyos E, Serrano-Corcoles MC, et al. Thrombolysis with recombinant tissue plasminogen activator during cardiopulmonary resuscitation in fulminant pulmonary embolism. A case series. Resuscitation 2001;51:97—101.

235. Böttiger BW, Martin E. Thrombolytic therapy during cardiopulmonary resuscitation and the role of coagulation activation after cardiac arrest. Curr Opin Crit Care 2001;7:176—83.

236. Spöhr F, Böttiger BW. Safety of thrombolysis during cardiopulmonary resuscitation. Drug Saf 2003;26:367—79.

237. Langhelle A, Tyvold SS, Lexow K, Hapnes SA, Sunde K, Steen PA. In-hospital factors associated with improved outcome after out-of-hospital cardiac arrest. A comparison between four regions in Norway. Resuscitation 2003;56:247—63.

238. Calle PA, Buylaert WA, Vanhaute OA. Glycemia in the post-resuscitation period. The Cerebral Resuscitation Study Group. Resuscitation 1989;17(Suppl.):S181—8.

239. Longstreth Jr WT, Diehr P, Inui TS. Prediction of awakening after out-of-hospital cardiac arrest. N Engl J Med 1983;308:1378—82.

240. Longstreth Jr WT, Inui TS. High blood glucose level on hospital admission and poor neurological recovery after cardiac arrest. Ann Neurol 1984;15:59—63.

241. Longstreth Jr WT, Copass MK, Dennis LK, Rauch-Matthews ME, Stark MS, Cobb LA. Intravenous glucose after out-of-hospital cardiopulmonary arrest: a community-based randomized trial. Neurology 1993;43:2534—41.

242. Mackenzie CF. A review of 100 cases of cardiac arrest and the relation of potassium, glucose, and haemoglobin levels to survival. West Indian Med J 1975;24:39—45.

243. Mullner M, Sterz F, Binder M, Schreiber W, Deimel A, Laggner AN. Blood glucose concentration after cardiopulmonary resuscitation influences functional neurological

recovery in human cardiac arrest survivors. J Cereb Blood Flow Metab 1997;17:430—6.

244. Skrifvars MB, Pettila V, Rosenberg PH, Castren M. A multiple logistic regression analysis of in-hospital factors related to survival at six months in patients resuscitated from out-of-hospital ventricular fibrillation. Resuscitation 2003;59:319—28.

245. Ditchey RV, Lindenfeld J. Potential adverse effects of volume loading on perfusion of vital organs during closed-chest resuscitation. Circulation 1984;69:181—9.

246. Gentile NT, Martin GB, Appleton TJ, Moeggenberg J, Paradis NA, Nowak RM. Effects of arterial and venous volume infusion on coronary perfusion pressures during canine CPR. Resuscitation 1991;22:55—63.

247. Jameson SJ, Mateer JR, DeBehnke DJ. Early volume expansion during cardiopulmonary resuscitation. Resuscitation 1993;26:243—50.

248. Voorhees WD, Ralston SH, Kougias C, Schmitz PM. Fluid loading with whole blood or Ringer's lactate solution during CPR in dogs. Resuscitation 1987;15:113—23.

249. Banerjee S, Singhi SC, Singh S, Singh M. The intraosseous route is a suitable alternative to intravenous route for fluid resuscitation in severely dehydrated children. Indian Pediatr 1994;31:1511—20.

250. Brickman KR, Krupp K, Rega P, Alexander J, Guinness M. Typing and screening of blood from intraosseous access. Ann Emerg Med 1992;21:414—7.

251. Fiser RT, Walker WM, Seibert JJ, McCarthy R, Fiser DH. Tibial length following intraosseous infusion: a prospective, radiographic analysis. Pediatr Emerg Care 1997;13:186—8.

252. Ummenhofer W, Frei FJ, Urwyler A, Drewe J. Are laboratory values in bone marrow aspirate predictable for venous blood in paediatric patients? Resuscitation 1994;27:123—8.

253. Guy J, Haley K, Zuspan SJ. Use of intraosseous infusion in the pediatric trauma patient. J Pediatr Surg 1993;28:158—61.

254. Macnab A, Christenson J, Findlay J, et al. A new system for sternal intraosseous infusion in adults. Prehosp Emerg Care 2000;4:173—7.

255. Ellemunter H, Simma B, Trawoger R, Maurer H. Intraosseous lines in preterm and full term neonates. Arch Dis Child Fetal Neonatal Ed 1999;80:F74—5.

256. Prengel AW, Lindner KH, Hahnel JH, Georgieff M. Pharmacokinetics and technique of endotracheal and deep endobronchial lidocaine administration. Anesth Analg 1993;77:985—9.

257. Prengel AW, Rembecki M, Wenzel V, Steinbach G. A comparison of the endotracheal tube and the laryngeal mask airway as a route for endobronchial lidocaine administration. Anesth Analg 2001;92:1505—9.

258. Steinfath M, Scholz I, Schulte am Esch J, Laer S, Reymann A, Scholz H. The technique of endobronchial lidocaine administration does not influence plasma concentration profiles and pharmacokinetic parameters in humans. Resuscitation 1995;29:55—62.

259. Hahnel JH, Lindner KH, Schurmann C, Prengel A, Ahnefeld FW. Plasma lidocaine levels and PaO2 with endobronchial administration: dilution with normal saline or distilled water? Ann Emerg Med 1990;19:1314—7.

260. Del Guercio LRM, Feins NR, Cohn JD, Coumaraswamy RP, Wollmann SB, State D. Comparison of blood flow during external and internal cardiac massage in man. Circulation 1965;31(Suppl. 1):I171—80.

261. Feneley MP, Maier GW, Kern KB, et al. Influence of compression rate on initial success of resuscitation and 24 hour survival after prolonged manual cardiopulmonary resuscitation in dogs. Circulation 1988;77:240—50.

262. Halperin HR, Tsitlik JE, Guerci AD, et al. Determinants of blood flow to vital organs during cardiopulmonary resuscitation in dogs. Circulation 1986;73:539—50.

263. Kern KB, Sanders AB, Raife J, Milander MM, Otto CW, Ewy GA. A study of chest compression rates during cardiopulmonary resuscitation in humans: the importance of rate-directed chest compressions. Arch Intern Med 1992;152:145—9.

264. Ornato JP, Gonzalez ER, Garnett AR, Levine RL, McClung BK. Effect of cardiopulmonary resuscitation compression rate on end-tidal carbon dioxide concentration and arterial pressure in man. Crit Care Med 1988;16:241—5.

265. Swenson RD, Weaver WD, Niskanen RA, Martin J, Dahlberg S. Hemodynamics in humans during conventional and experimental methods of cardiopulmonary resuscitation. Circulation 1988;78:630—9.

266. Boczar ME, Howard MA, Rivers EP, et al. A technique revisited: hemodynamic comparison of closed- and open-chest cardiac massage during human cardiopulmonary resuscitation. Crit Care Med 1995;23:498—503.

267. Anthi A, Tzelepis GE, Alivizatos P, Michalis A, Palatianos GM, Geroulanos S. Unexpected cardiac arrest after cardiac surgery: incidence, predisposing causes, and outcome of open chest cardiopulmonary resuscitation. Chest 1998;113:15—9.

268. Pottle A, Bullock I, Thomas J, Scott L. Survival to discharge following Open Chest Cardiac Compression (OCCC). A 4-year retrospective audit in a cardiothoracic specialist centre—Royal Brompton and Harefield NHS Trust, United Kingdom. Resuscitation 2002;52:269—72.

269. Babbs CF. Interposed abdominal compression CPR: a comprehensive evidence based review. Resuscitation 2003;59:71—82.

270. Babbs CF, Nadkarni V. Optimizing chest compression to rescue ventilation ratios during one-rescuer CPR by professionals and lay persons: children are not just little adults. Resuscitation 2004;61:173—81.

271. Beyar R, Kishon Y, Kimmel E, Neufeld H, Dinnar U. Intrathoracic and abdominal pressure variations as an efficient method for cardiopulmonary resuscitation: studies in dogs compared with computer model results. Cardiovasc Res 1985;19:335—42.

272. Voorhees WD, Niebauer MJ, Babbs CF. Improved oxygen delivery during cardiopulmonary resuscitation with interposed abdominal compressions. Ann Emerg Med 1983;12:128—35.

273. Sack JB, Kesselbrenner MB, Jarrad A. Interposed abdominal compression-cardiopulmonary resuscitation and resuscitation outcome during asystole and electromechanical dissociation. Circulation 1992;86:1692—700.

274. Sack JB, Kesselbrenner MB, Bregman D. Survival from in-hospital cardiac arrest with interposed abdominal counterpulsation during cardiopulmonary resuscitation. JAMA 1992;267:379—85.

275. Mateer JR, Stueven HA, Thompson BM, Aprahamian C, Darin JC. Pre-hospital IAC-CPR versus standard CPR: paramedic resuscitation of cardiac arrests. Am J Emerg Med 1985;3:143—6.

276. Lindner KH, Pfenninger EG, Lurie KG, Schurmann W, Lindner IM, Ahnefeld FW. Effects of active compression—decompression resuscitation on myocardial and cerebral blood flow in pigs. Circulation 1993;88:1254—63.

277. Shultz JJ, Coffeen P, Sweeney M, et al. Evaluation of standard and active compression—decompression CPR in an acute human model of ventricular fibrillation. Circulation 1994;89:684—93.

278. Chang MW, Coffeen P, Lurie KG, Shultz J, Bache RJ, White CW. Active compression—decompression CPR improves vital organ perfusion in a dog model of ventricular fibrillation. Chest 1994;106:1250—9.

279. Orliaguet GA, Carli PA, Rozenberg A, Janniere D, Sauval P, Delpech P. End-tidal carbon dioxide during out-of-hospital cardiac arrest resuscitation: comparison of active compression—decompression and standard CPR. Ann Emerg Med 1995;25:48—51.

280. Tucker KJ, Galli F, Savitt MA, Kahsai D, Bresnahan L, Redberg RF. Active compression—decompression resuscitation: effect on resuscitation success after in-hospital cardiac arrest. J Am Coll Cardiol 1994;24:201—9.

281. Malzer R, Zeiner A, Binder M, et al. Hemodynamic effects of active compression—decompression after prolonged CPR. Resuscitation 1996;31:243—53.

282. Lurie KG, Shultz JJ, Callaham ML, et al. Evaluation of active compression—decompression CPR in victims of out-of-hospital cardiac arrest. JAMA 1994;271:1405—11.

283. Cohen TJ, Goldner BG, Maccaro PC, et al. A comparison of active compression—decompression cardiopulmonary resuscitation with standard cardiopulmonary resuscitation for cardiac arrests occurring in the hospital. N Engl J Med 1993;329:1918—21.

284. Schwab TM, Callaham ML, Madsen CD, Utecht TA. A randomized clinical trial of active compression—decompression CPR vs standard CPR in out-of-hospital cardiac arrest in two cities. JAMA 1995;273:1261—8.

285. Stiell I, H'ebert P, Well G, et al. Tne Ontario trial of active compression—decompression cardiopulmonary resuscitation for in-hospital and prehospital cardiac arrest. JAMA 1996;275:1417—23.

286. Mauer D, Schneider T, Dick W, Withelm A, Elich D, Mauer M. Active compression—decompression resuscitation: a prospective, randomized study in a two-tiered EMS system with physicians in the field. Resuscitation 1996;33:125—34.

287. Nolan J, Smith G, Evans R, et al. The United Kingdom pre-hospital study of active compression—decompression resuscitation. Resuscitation 1998;37:119—25.

288. Luiz T, Ellinger K, Denz C. Active compression—decompression cardiopulmonary resuscitation does not improve survival in patients with prehospital cardiac arrest in a physician-manned emergency medical system. J Cardiothorac Vasc Anesth 1996;10:178—86.

289. Plaisance P, Lurie KG, Vicaut E, et al. A comparison of standard cardiopulmonary resuscitation and active compression—decompression resuscitation for out-of-hospital cardiac arrest. French Active Compression—Decompression Cardiopulmonary Resuscitation Study Group. N Engl J Med 1999;341:569—75.

290. Lafuente-Lafuente C, Melero-Bascones M. Active chest compression—decompression for cardiopulmonary resuscitation. Cochrane Database Syst Rev 2004:CD002751.

291. Baubin M, Rabl W, Pfeiffer KP, Benzer A, Gilly H. Chest injuries after active compression—decompression cardiopulmonary resuscitation (ACD-CPR) in cadavers. Resuscitation 1999;43:9—15.

292. Rabl W, Baubin M, Broinger G, Scheithauer R. Serious complications from active compression—decompression cardiopulmonary resuscitation. Int J Legal Med 1996;109:84—9.

293. Hoke RS, Chamberlain D. Skeletal chest injuries secondary to cardiopulmonary resuscitation. Resuscitation 2004;63:327—38.

294. Plaisance P, Lurie KG, Payen D. Inspiratory impedance during active compression—decompression cardiopulmonary resuscitation: a randomized evaluation in patients in cardiac arrest. Circulation 2000;101:989—94.

295. Plaisance P, Soleil C, Lurie KG, Vicaut E, Ducros L, Payen D. Use of an inspiratory impedance threshold device on a facemask and endotracheal tube to reduce intrathoracic pressures during the decompression phase of active compression—decompression cardiopulmonary resuscitation. Crit Care Med 2005;33:990—4.

296. Wolcke BB, Mauer DK, Schoefmann MF, et al. Comparison of standard cardiopulmonary resuscitation versus the combination of active compression—decompression cardiopulmonary resuscitation and an inspiratory impedance threshold device for out-of-hospital cardiac arrest. Circulation 2003;108:2201—5.

297. Aufderheide T, Pirrallo R, Provo T, Lurie K. Clinical evaluation of an inspiratory impedance threshold device during standard cardiopulmonary resuscitation in patients with out-of-hospital cardiac arrest. Crit Care Med 2005;33:734—40.

298. Plaisance P, Lurie KG, Vicaut E, et al. Evaluation of an impedance threshold device in patients receiving active compression—decompression cardiopulmonary resuscitation for out of hospital cardiac arrest. Resuscitation 2004;61:265—71.

299. Sunde K, Wik L, Steen PA. Quality of mechanical, manual standard and active compression—decompression CPR on the arrest site and during transport in a manikin model. Resuscitation 1997;34:235—42.

300. Wik L, Bircher NG, Safar P. A comparison of prolonged manual and mechanical external chest compression after cardiac arrest in dogs. Resuscitation 1996;32:241—50.

301. Dickinson ET, Verdile VP, Schneider RM, Salluzzo RF. Effectiveness of mechanical versus manual chest compressions in out-of-hospital cardiac arrest resuscitation: a pilot study. Am J Emerg Med 1998;16:289—92.

302. McDonald JL. Systolic and mean arterial pressures during manual and mechanical CPR in humans. Ann Emerg Med 1982;11:292—5.

303. Ward KR, Menegazzi JJ, Zelenak RR, Sullivan RJ, McSwain Jr N. A comparison of chest compressions between mechanical and manual CPR by monitoring end-tidal PCO_2 during human cardiac arrest. Ann Emerg Med 1993;22:669—74.

304. Steen S, Liao Q, Pierre L, Paskevicius A, Sjoberg T. Evaluation of LUCAS, a new device for automatic mechanical compression and active decompression resuscitation. Resuscitation 2002;55:285—99.

305. Rubertsson S, Karlsten R. Increased cortical cerebral blood flow with LUCAS; a new device for mechanical chest compressions compared to standard external compressions during experimental cardiopulmonary resuscitation. Resuscitation 2005;65:357—63.

306. Nielsen N, Sandhall L, Schersten F, Friberg H, Olsson SE. Successful resuscitation with mechanical CPR, therapeutic hypothermia and coronary intervention during manual CPR after out-of-hospital cardiac arrest. Resuscitation 2005;65:111—3.

307. Timerman S, Cardoso LF, Ramires JA, Halperin H. Improved hemodynamic performance with a novel chest compression device during treatment of in-hospital cardiac arrest. Resuscitation 2004;61:273—80.

308. Halperin H, Berger R, Chandra N, et al. Cardiopulmonary resuscitation with a hydraulic-pneumatic band. Crit Care Med 2000;28:N203—6.

309. Halperin HR, Paradis N, Ornato JP, et al. Cardiopulmonary resuscitation with a novel chest compression device in a porcine model of cardiac arrest: improved hemodynamics and mechanisms. J Am Coll Cardiol 2004;44:2214—20.

310. Casner M, Anderson D, et al. Preliminary report of the impact of a new CPR assist device on the rate of return of spontaneous circulation in out of hospital cardiac arrest. Prehosp Emerg Med 2005;9:61—7.

311. Arntz HR, Agrawal R, Richter H, et al. Phased chest and abdominal compression—decompression versus conventional cardiopulmonary resuscitation in out-of-hospital cardiac arrest. Circulation 2001;104:768—72.

312. Rozenberg A, Incagnoli P, Delpech P, et al. Prehospital use of minimally invasive direct cardiac massage (MID-CM): a pilot study. Resuscitation 2001;50:257—62.

313. Dauchot P, Gravenstein JS. Effects of atropine on the electrocardiogram in different age groups. Clin Pharmacol Ther 1971;12:274—80.

314. Chamberlain DA, Turner P, Sneddon JM. Effects of atropine on heart-rate in healthy man. Lancet 1967;2:12—5.

315. Bernheim A, Fatio R, Kiowski W, Weilenmann D, Rickli H, Rocca HP. Atropine often results in complete atrioventricular block or sinus arrest after cardiac transplantation: an unpredictable and dose-independent phenomenon. Transplantation 2004;77:1181—5.

316. Klumbies A, Paliege R, Volkmann H. Mechanical emergency stimulation in asystole and extreme bradycardia. Z Gesamte Inn Med 1988;43:348—52.

317. Zeh E, Rahner E. The manual extrathoracal stimulation of the heart. Technique and effect of the precordial thump (author's transl). Z Kardiol 1978;67:299—304.

318. Chan L, Reid C, Taylor B. Effect of three emergency pacing modalities on cardiac output in cardiac arrest due to ventricular asystole. Resuscitation 2002;52:117—9.

319. Manz M, Pfeiffer D, Jung W, Lueritz B. Intravenous treatment with magnesium in recurrent persistent ventricular tachycardia. New Trends Arrhythmias 1991;7:437—42.

320. Tzivoni D, Banai S, Schuger C, et al. Treatment of torsade de pointes with magnesium sulfate. Circulation 1988;77:392—7.

321. Sticherling C, Tada H, Hsu W, et al. Effects of diltiazem and esmolol on cycle length and spontaneous conversion of atrial fibrillation. J Cardiovasc Pharmacol Ther 2002;7:81—8.

322. Shettigar UR, Toole JG, Appunn DO. Combined use of esmolol and digoxin in the acute treatment of atrial fibrillation or flutter. Am Heart J 1993;126:368—74.

323. Demircan C, Cikriklar HI, Engindeniz Z, et al. Comparison of the effectiveness of intravenous diltiazem and metoprolol in the management of rapid ventricular rate in atrial fibrillation. Emerg Med J 2005;22:411—4.

324. Wattanasuwan N, Khan IA, Mehta NJ, et al. Acute ventricular rate control in atrial fibrillation: IV combination of diltiazem and digoxin vs. IV diltiazem alone. Chest 2001;119:502—6.

325. Davey MJ, Teubner D. A randomized controlled trial of magnesium sulfate, in addition to usual care, for rate control in atrial fibrillation. Ann Emerg Med 2005;45:347—53.

326. Chiladakis JA, Stathopoulos C, Davlouros P, Manolis AS. Intravenous magnesium sulfate versus diltiazem in paroxysmal atrial fibrillation. Int J Cardiol 2001;79:287—91.

327. Camm AJ, Garratt CJ. Adenosine and supraventricular tachycardia. N Engl J Med 1991;325:1621—9.

328. Wang HE, O'Connor RE, Megargel RE, et al. The use of diltiazem for treating rapid atrial fibrillation in the out-of-hospital setting. Ann Emerg Med 2001;37:38—45.

329. Martinez-Marcos FJ, Garcia-Garmendia JL, Ortega-Carpio A, Fernandez-Gomez JM, Santos JM, Camacho C. Comparison of intravenous flecainide, propafenone, and amiodarone for conversion of acute atrial fibrillation to sinus rhythm. Am J Cardiol 2000;86:950—3.

330. Kalus JS, Spencer AP, Tsikouris JP, et al. Impact of prophylactic i.v. magnesium on the efficacy of ibutilide for conversion of atrial fibrillation or flutter. Am J Health Syst Pharm 2003;60:2308—12.

331. Langhelle A, Nolan J, Herlitz J, et al. Recommended guidelines for reviewing, reporting, and conducting research on post-resuscitation care: the Utstein style. Resuscitation 2005;66:271—83.

332. Menon DK, Coles JP, Gupta AK, et al. Diffusion limited oxygen delivery following head injury. Crit Care Med 2004;32:1384—90.

333. Buunk G, van der Hoeven JG, Meinders AE. Cerebrovascular reactivity in comatose patients resuscitated from a cardiac arrest. Stroke 1997;28:1569—73.

334. Buunk G, van der Hoeven JG, Meinders AE. A comparison of near-infrared spectroscopy and jugular bulb oximetry in comatose patients resuscitated from a cardiac arrest. Anaesthesia 1998;53:13—9.

335. Roine RO, Launes J, Nikkinen P, Lindroth L, Kaste M. Regional cerebral blood flow after human cardiac arrest. A hexamethylpropyleneamine oxime single photon emission computed tomographic study. Arch Neurol 1991;48:625—9.

336. Beckstead JE, Tweed WA, Lee J, MacKeen WL. Cerebral blood flow and metabolism in man following cardiac arrest. Stroke 1978;9:569—73.

337. Laurent I, Monchi M, Chiche JD, et al. Reversible myocardial dysfunction in survivors of out-of-hospital cardiac arrest. J Am Coll Cardiol 2002;40:2110—6.

338. Kern KB, Hilwig RW, Rhee KH, Berg RA. Myocardial dysfunction after resuscitation from cardiac arrest: an example of global myocardial stunning. J Am Coll Cardiol 1996;28:232—40.

339. Adrie C, Adib-Conquy M, Laurent I, et al. Successful cardiopulmonary resuscitation after cardiac arrest as a ''sepsis-like'' syndrome. Circulation 2002;106:562—8.

340. Mullner M, Sterz F, Binder M, et al. Arterial blood pressure after human cardiac arrest and neurological recovery. Stroke 1996;27:59—62.

341. Angelos MG, Ward KR, Hobson J, Beckley PD. Organ blood flow following cardiac arrest in a swine low-flow cardiopulmonary bypass model. Resuscitation 1994;27:245—54.

342. Rello J, Diaz E, Roque M, Valles J. Risk factors for developing pneumonia within 48 hours of intubation. Am J Respir Crit Care Med 1999;159:1742—6.

343. Krumholz A, Stern BJ, Weiss HD. Outcome from coma after cardiopulmonary resuscitation: relation to seizures and myoclonus. Neurology 1988;38:401—5.

344. Wijdicks EF, Parisi JE, Sharbrough FW. Prognostic value of myoclonus status in comatose survivors of cardiac arrest. Ann Neurol 1994;35:239—43.

345. Takino M, Okada Y. Hyperthermia following cardiopulmonary resuscitation. Intensive Care Med 1991;17:419—20.

346. Hickey RW, Kochanek PM, Ferimer H, Alexander HL, Garman RH, Graham SH. Induced hyperthermia exacerbates neurologic neuronal histologic damage after asphyxial cardiac arrest in rats. Crit Care Med 2003;31:531—5.

347. Takasu A, Saitoh D, Kaneko N, Sakamoto T, Okada Y. Hyperthermia: is it an ominous sign after cardiac arrest? Resuscitation 2001;49:273—7.

348. Zeiner A, Holzer M, Sterz F, et al. Hyperthermia after cardiac arrest is associated with an unfavorable neurologic outcome. Arch Intern Med 2001;161:2007—12.

349. Coimbra C, Boris-Moller F, Drake M, Wieloch T. Diminished neuronal damage in the rat brain by late treatment with the antipyretic drug dipyrone or cooling following cerebral ischemia. Acta Neuropathol (Berl) 1996;92: 447—53.

350. Coimbra C, Drake M, Boris-Moller F, Wieloch T. Long-lasting neuroprotective effect of postischemic hypothermia and treatment with an anti-inflammatory/antipyretic drug: evidence for chronic encephalopathic processes following ischemia. Stroke 1996;27:1578—85.

351. Colbourne F, Sutherland G, Corbett D. Postischemic hypothermia. A critical appraisal with implications for clinical treatment. Mol Neurobiol 1997;14:171—201.

352. Ginsberg MD, Sternau LL, Globus MY, Dietrich WD, Busto R. Therapeutic modulation of brain temperature: relevance to ischemic brain injury. Cerebrovasc Brain Metab Rev 1992;4:189—225.

353. Safar PJ, Kochanek PM. Therapeutic hypothermia after cardiac arrest. N Engl J Med 2002;346:612—3.

354. Hypothermia After Cardiac Arrest Study Group. Mild therapeutic hypothermia to improve the neurologic outcome after cardiac arrest. N Engl J Med 2002;346:549—56.

355. Bernard SA, Gray TW, Buist MD, et al. Treatment of comatose survivors of out-of-hospital cardiac arrest with induced hypothermia. N Engl J Med 2002;346:557—63.

356. Hachimi-Idrissi S, Corne L, Ebinger G, Michotte Y, Huyghens L. Mild hypothermia induced by a helmet device: a clinical feasibility study. Resuscitation 2001;51:275—81.

357. Bernard SA, Jones BM, Horne MK. Clinical trial of induced hypothermia in comatose survivors of out-of-hospital cardiac arrest. Ann Emerg Med 1997;30:146—53.

358. Bernard S, Buist M, Monteiro O, Smith K. Induced hypothermia using large volume, ice-cold intravenous fluid in comatose survivors of out-of-hospital cardiac arrest: a preliminary report. Resuscitation 2003;56:9—13.

359. Virkkunen I, Yli-Hankala A, Silfvast T. Induction of therapeutic hypothermia after cardiac arrest in prehospital patients using ice-cold Ringer's solution: a pilot study. Resuscitation 2004;62:299—302.

360. Al-Senani FM, Graffagnino C, Grotta JC, et al. A prospective, multicenter pilot study to evaluate the feasibility and safety of using the CoolGard System and Icy catheter following cardiac arrest. Resuscitation 2004;62:143—50.

361. Kliegel A, Losert H, Sterz F, et al. Cold simple intravenous infusions preceding special endovascular cooling for faster induction of mild hypothermia after cardiac arrest—a feasibility study. Resuscitation 2005;64:347—51.

362. Kim F, Olsufka M, Carlbom D, et al. Pilot study of rapid infusion of 2 L of 4 degrees C normal saline for induction of mild hypothermia in hospitalized, comatose survivors of out-of-hospital cardiac arrest. Circulation 2005;112:715—9.

363. Schmutzhard E, Engelhardt K, Beer R, et al. Safety and efficacy of a novel intravascular cooling device to control body temperature in neurologic intensive care patients: a prospective pilot study. Crit Care Med 2002;30:2481—8.

364. Diringer MN, Reaven NL, Funk SE, Uman GC. Elevated body temperature independently contributes to increased length of stay in neurologic intensive care unit patients. Crit Care Med 2004;32:1489—95.

365. Keller E, Imhof HG, Gasser S, Terzic A, Yonekawa Y. Endovascular cooling with heat exchange catheters: a new method to induce and maintain hypothermia. Intensive Care Med 2003;29:939—43.

366. Polderman KH, Peerdeman SM, Girbes AR. Hypophosphatemia and hypomagnesemia induced by cooling in patients with severe head injury. J Neurosurg 2001;94:697—705.

367. Polderman KH. Application of therapeutic hypothermia in the intensive care unit. Opportunities and pitfalls of a promising treatment modality—Part 2. Practical aspects and side effects. Intensive Care Med 2004;30: 757—69.

368. Agnew DM, Koehler RC, Guerguerian AM, et al. Hypothermia for 24 hours after asphyxic cardiac arrest in piglets provides striatal neuroprotection that is sustained 10 days after rewarming. Pediatr Res 2003;54: 253—62.

369. Hicks SD, DeFranco DB, Callaway CW. Hypothermia during reperfusion after asphyxial cardiac arrest improves functional recovery and selectively alters stress-induced protein expression. J Cereb Blood Flow Metab 2000;20:520—30.

370. Sterz F, Safar P, Tisherman S, Radovsky A, Kuboyama K, Oku K. Mild hypothermic cardiopulmonary resuscitation improves outcome after prolonged cardiac arrest in dogs. Crit Care Med 1991;19:379—89.

371. Xiao F, Safar P, Radovsky A. Mild protective and resuscitative hypothermia for asphyxial cardiac arrest in rats. Am J Emerg Med 1998;16:17—25.

372. Katz LM, Young A, Frank JE, Wang Y, Park K. Neurotensin-induced hypothermia improves neurologic outcome after hypoxic-ischemia. Crit Care Med 2004;32:806—10.

373. Abella BS, Zhao D, Alvarado J, Hamann K, Vanden Hoek TL, Becker LB. Intra-arrest cooling improves outcomes in a murine cardiac arrest model. Circulation 2004;109:2786—91.

374. Nolan JP, Morley PT, Vanden Hoek TL, Hickey RW. Therapeutic hypothermia after cardiac arrest. An advisory statement by the Advancement Life support Task Force of the International Liaison committee on Resuscitation. Resuscitation 2003;57:231—5.

375. Baird TA, Parsons MW, Phanh T, et al. Persistent post-stroke hyperglycemia is independently associated with infarct expansion and worse clinical outcome. Stroke 2003;34:2208—14.

376. Capes SE, Hunt D, Malmberg K, Pathak P, Gerstein HC. Stress hyperglycemia and prognosis of stroke in nondiabetic and diabetic patients: a systematic overview. Stroke 2001;32:2426—32.

377. Scott JF, Robinson GM, French JM, O'Connell JE, Alberti KG, Gray CS. Glucose potassium insulin infusions in the treatment of acute stroke patients with mild to moderate hyperglycemia: the Glucose Insulin in Stroke Trial (GIST). Stroke 1999;30:793—9.

378. Yip PK, He YY, Hsu CY, Garg N, Marangos P, Hogan EL. Effect of plasma glucose on infarct size in focal cerebral ischemia-reperfusion. Neurology 1991;41:899—905.

379. van den Berghe G, Wouters P, Weekers F, et al. Intensive insulin therapy in the critically ill patients. N Engl J Med 2001;345:1359—67.

380. Krinsley JS. Effect of an intensive glucose management protocol on the mortality of critically ill adult patients. Mayo Clin Proc 2004;79:992—1000.

381. Van den Berghe G, Wouters PJ, Bouillon R, et al. Outcome benefit of intensive insulin therapy in the critically ill: insulin dose versus glycemic control. Crit Care Med 2003;31:359—66.

382. Katz LM, Wang Y, Ebmeyer U, Radovsky A, Safar P. Glucose plus insulin infusion improves cerebral outcome after asphyxial cardiac arrest. Neuroreport 1998;9:3363—7.

383. Laver S, Farrow C, Turner D, Nolan J. Mode of death after admission to an intensive care unit following cardiac arrest. Intensive Care Med 2004;30:2126—8.

384. Zandbergen EG, de Haan RJ, Stoutenbeek CP, Koelman JH, Hijdra A. Systematic review of early prediction of poor outcome in anoxic-ischaemic coma. Lancet 1998;352:1808—12.

385. Booth CM, Boone RH, Tomlinson G, Detsky AS. Is this patient dead, vegetative, or severely neurologically impaired?

Assessing outcome for comatose survivors of cardiac arrest. Jama 2004;291:870—9.

386. Edgren E, Hedstrand U, Kelsey S, Sutton-Tyrrell K, Safar P. Assessment of neurological prognosis in comatose survivors of cardiac arrest. BRCT I Study Group. Lancet 1994;343:1055—9.

387. Tiainen M, Roine RO, Pettila V, Takkunen O. Serum neuron-specific enolase and S-100B protein in cardiac arrest patients treated with hypothermia. Stroke 2003;34:2881—6.

388. Fogel W, Krieger D, Veith M, et al. Serum neuron-specific enolase as early predictor of outcome after cardiac arrest. Crit Care Med 1997;25:1133—8.

389. Mussack T, Biberthaler P, Kanz KG, et al. Serum S-100B and interleukin-8 as predictive markers for comparative neurologic outcome analysis of patients after cardiac arrest and severe traumatic brain injury. Crit Care Med 2002;30:2669—74.

390. Mussack T, Biberthaler P, Kanz KG, Wiedemann E, Gippner-Steppert C, Jochum M. S-100b, sE-selectin, and sP-selectin for evaluation of hypoxic brain damage in patients after cardiopulmonary resuscitation: pilot study. World J Surg 2001;25:539—43 [discussion 44].

391. Rosen H, Karlsson JE, Rosengren L. CSF levels of neurofilament is a valuable predictor of long-term outcome after cardiac arrest. J Neurol Sci 2004;221:19—24.

392. Rosen H, Rosengren L, Herlitz J, Blomstrand C. Increased serum levels of the S-100 protein are associated with hypoxic brain damage after cardiac arrest. Stroke 1998;29:473—7.

393. Meynaar IA, Straaten HM, van der Wetering J, et al. Serum neuron-specific enolase predicts outcome in post-anoxic coma: a prospective cohort study. Intensive Care Med 2003;29:189—95.

394. Rosen H, Sunnerhagen KS, Herlitz J, Blomstrand C, Rosengren L. Serum levels of the brain-derived proteins S-100 and NSE predict long-term outcome after cardiac arrest. Resuscitation 2001;49:183—91.

395. Schreiber W, Herkner H, Koreny M, et al. Predictors of survival in unselected patients with acute myocardial infarction requiring continuous catecholamine support. Resuscitation 2002;55:269—76.

396. Schoerkhuber W, Kittler H, Sterz F, et al. Time course of serum neuron-specific enolase. A predictor of neurological outcome in patients resuscitated from cardiac arrest. Stroke 1999;30:1598—603.

397. Bottiger BW, Mobes S, Glatzer R, et al. Astroglial protein S-100 is an early and sensitive marker of hypoxic brain damage and outcome after cardiac arrest in humans. Circulation 2001;103:2694—8.

398. Martens P, Raabe A, Johnsson P, Serum. S-100 and neuron-specific enolase for prediction of regaining consciousness after global cerebral ischemia. Stroke 1998;29:2363—6.

399. Zingler VC, Krumm B, Bertsch T, Fassbender K, Pohlmann-Eden B. Early prediction of neurological outcome after car-

diopulmonary resuscitation: a multimodal approach combining neurobiochemical and electrophysiological investigations may provide high prognostic certainty in patients after cardiac arrest. Eur Neurol 2003;49:79—84.

400. Zandbergen EG, de Haan RJ, Hijdra A. Systematic review of prediction of poor outcome in anoxic-ischaemic coma with biochemical markers of brain damage. Intensive Care Med 2001;27:1661—7.

401. Synek VM. Validity of a revised EEG coma scale for predicting survival in anoxic encephalopathy. Clin Exp Neurol 1989;26:119—27.

402. Moller M, Holm B, Sindrup E, Nielsen BL. Electroencephalographic prediction of anoxic brain damage after resuscitation from cardiac arrest in patients with acute myocardial infarction. Acta Med Scand 1978;203:31—7.

403. Scollo-Lavizzari G, Bassetti C. Prognostic value of EEG in post-anoxic coma after cardiac arrest. Eur Neurol 1987;26:161—70.

404. Bassetti C, Karbowski K. Prognostic value of electroencephalography in non-traumatic comas. Schweiz Med Wochenschr 1990;120:1425—34.

405. Bassetti C, Bomio F, Mathis J, Hess CW. Early prognosis in coma after cardiac arrest: a prospective clinical, electrophysiological, and biochemical study of 60 patients. J Neurol Neurosurg Psychiatry 1996;61:610—5.

406. Rothstein TL. Recovery from near death following cerebral anoxia: a case report demonstrating superiority of median somatosensory evoked potentials over EEG in predicting a favorable outcome after cardiopulmonary resuscitation. Resuscitation 2004;60:335—41.

407. Berkhoff M, Donati F, Bassetti C. Postanoxic alpha (theta) coma: a reappraisal of its prognostic significance. Clin Neurophysiol 2000;111:297—304.

408. Kaplan PW, Genoud D, Ho TW, Jallon P. Etiology, neurologic correlations, and prognosis in alpha coma. Clin Neurophysiol 1999;110:205—13.

409. Yamashita S, Morinaga T, Ohgo S, et al. Prognostic value of electroencephalogram (EEG) in anoxic encephalopathy after cardiopulmonary resuscitation: relationship among anoxic period, EEG grading and outcome. Intern Med 1995;34:71—6.

410. Ajisaka H. Early electroencephalographic findings in patients with anoxic encephalopathy after cardiopulmonary arrest and successful resusitation. J Clin Neurosci 2004;11:616—8.

411. Rothstein TL, Thomas EM, Sumi SM. Predicting outcome in hypoxic-ischemic coma. A prospective clinical and electrophysiologic study. Electroencephalogr Clin Neurophysiol 1991;79:101—7.

412. Edgren E, Hedstrand U, Nordin M, Rydin E, Ronquist G. Prediction of outcome after cardiac arrest. Crit Care Med 1987;15:820—5.

413. Sorensen K, Thomassen A, Wernberg M. Prognostic significance of alpha frequency EEG rhythm in coma after cardiac arrest. J Neurol Neurosurg Psychiatry 1978;41:840—2.

Resuscitation (2005) **67S1**, S87—S96

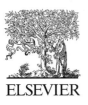

ELSEVIER

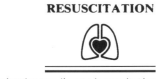

RESUSCITATION

www.elsevier.com/locate/resuscitation

European Resuscitation Council Guidelines for Resuscitation 2005
Section 5. Initial management of acute coronary syndromes

Hans-Richard Arntz, Leo Bossaert, Gerasimos S. Filippatos

Introduction

The incidence of acute myocardial infarction (AMI) is decreasing in many European countries.[1] Although in-hospital mortality from AMI has been reduced significantly by modern reperfusion therapy and improved secondary prophylaxis,[1] the overall 28-day mortality is virtually unchanged because about two thirds of those that die do so before arrival at hospital.[2] Thus, the best chance of improving survival after AMI is by improving treatment in the early, and particularly the out-of hospital, phase of the disease.

The term acute coronary syndrome (ACS) encompasses three different entities within the acute manifestation of coronary heart disease: ST elevation myocardial infarction (STEMI), non-ST elevation myocardial infarction (NSTEMI) and unstable angina pectoris (UAP) (Figure 5.1). The common pathophysiology of ACS is a ruptured or eroded atherosclerotic plaque.[3] Electrocardiographic characteristics (absence or presence of ST elevation) differentiate STEMI from the other forms of ACS. A NSTEMI or UAP may present with ST segment depression or non-specific ST segment wave abnormalities, or even a normal ECG. In the absence of ST elevation, an increase in the plasma concentration of cardiac markers, particularly troponin T or I as the most specific markers of myocardial cell necrosis, indicates NSTEMI.

Acute coronary syndromes are the commonest cause of malignant arrhythmias leading to sudden cardiac death. The therapeutic goals are to treat acute life-threatening conditions, such as ventricular fibrillation (VF) or extreme bradycardias, and to preserve left ventricular function and prevent heart failure by minimising the extent of any myocardial infarction. These guidelines address the first hours after onset of symptoms. Out-of-hospital treatment and initial therapy in the emergency department may vary according to local capabilities, resources and regulations. The data supporting out-of-hospital treatment are usually extrapolated from studies of initial treatment early after hospital admission; there are only few high-quality out-of-hospital studies. Comprehensive guidelines for the diagnosis and treatment of ACS with and without ST elevation have been published by the European Society of Cardiology and the American College of Cardiology/American Heart Association.[4,5] The current recommendations are in line with these guidelines.

Diagnostic tests in acute coronary syndromes

Since early treatment offers the greatest benefits, and myocardial ischaemia is the leading precipitant of sudden cardiac death, it is essential that the

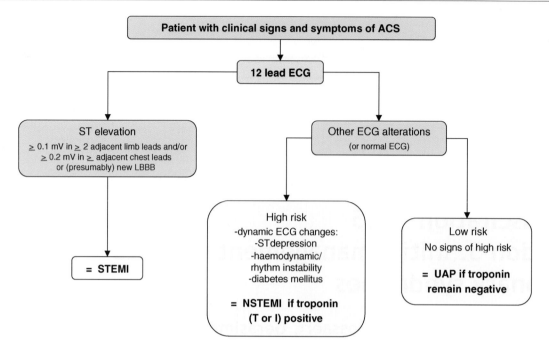

Figure 5.1 Classification of acute coronary syndromes.

public are aware of the typical symptoms associated with ACS. Patients at risk, and their families, should be able to recognise characteristic symptoms such as chest pain, which may radiate into other areas of the upper body, often accompanied by other symptoms including dyspnoea, sweating, nausea or vomiting and syncope. They should understand the importance of early activation of the emergency medical service (EMS) system and, ideally, should be trained in basic life support (BLS).

EMS dispatchers must be trained to recognize ACS symptoms and to ask targeted questions. When an ACS is suspected, an EMS crew trained in advanced life support (ALS) and capable of making the diagnosis and starting treatment should be alerted. The sensitivity, specificity and clinical impact of various diagnostic strategies have been evaluated for ACS/AMI. These include signs and symptoms, the 12-lead electrocardiogram (ECG) and biochemical markers of cardiac risk.

Signs and symptoms of ACS/AMI

Even though typical symptoms such as radiating chest pain, shortness of breath or sweating may be more intense and generally last longer in patients with AMI, they are not adequately specific for a reliable diagnosis of AMI. A 12-lead ECG, cardiac biomarkers and other diagnostic tests are required before ACS or AMI can be ruled out in the presence of a typical history. Atypical symptoms or unusual

presentations may occur in the elderly, in females, and in people with diabetes.[6,7]

12-lead ECG

A 12-lead ECG is the key investigation for assessment of an ACS. In case of STEMI, a 12-lead ECG can indicate the need for immediate reperfusion therapy (e.g., primary percutaneous coronary intervention (PCI) or prehospital thrombolysis). Recording of a 12-lead ECG out-of-hospital enables advanced notification to the receiving facility and expedites treatment decisions after hospital arrival; in many studies, the time from hospital admission to initiating reperfusion therapy is reduced by 10—60 min.[8—10] Recording and transmission of diagnostic quality ECGs to the hospital takes usually less than 5 min. Trained EMS personnel (emergency physicians, paramedics and nurses) can identify STEMI, defined by ST elevation of ≥0.1 mV elevation in at least two adjacent limb leads or >0.2 mV in two adjacent precordial leads, with high specificity and sensitivity comparable to diagnostic accuracy in the hospital.[11—13]

Biomarkers

In the presence of a suggestive history, the absence of ST elevation on the ECG, and elevated concentrations of biomarkers (troponin T and troponin I, CK, CK-MB, myoglobin) characterise non-STEMI and distinguish it from STEMI and unstable angina, respectively.[3] Elevated concentrations of troponin are particularly helpful in identifying patients at increased risk of adverse outcome.[14] However, the delay in release of biomarkers from damaged myocardium prevents their use in diagnosing myocardial infarction in the first 4—6 h after the onset of symptoms.[15]

Principles of acute treatment for ACS

Nitrates

Glyceryl trinitrate is an effective treatment for ischaemic chest pain (Figure 5.2) and has some beneficial haemodynamic effects, e.g., dilation of the venous capacitance vessels, coronary arteries and, to a minor degree, peripheral arteries. Glyceryl trinitrate may be considered if the systolic blood pressure is higher than 90 mmHg and the patient has ongoing ischaemic chest pain. Glyceryl trinitrate can be useful in the treatment of acute pulmonary congestion. Do not use nitrates in patients with hypotension (systolic blood pressure ≤90 mmHg), particularly if combined with bradycardia, nor in patients with inferior infarction and suspected right ventricular involvement. Use of nitrates under these circumstances may cause a precipitous decrease in blood pressure and cardiac output.

Morphine

Morphine is the analgesic of choice for nitrate-refractory pain. Being a dilator of venous capacitance vessels, it may have additional benefit in patients with pulmonary congestion. Give morphine in initial doses of 3—5 mg intravenously and repeat every few minutes until the patient is pain free.

Oxygen

Give supplementary oxygen ($4-8\,l\,min^{-1}$) to all patients with arterial oxygen saturation <90% and/or pulmonary congestion. Despite lack of proof for long-term benefit of supplementary oxygen,[16] give it to all patients with uncomplicated STEMI; it will benefit patients with unrecognised hypoxia.

Acetylsalicylic acid

Several large randomised controlled trials indicate decreased mortality when acetylsalicylic acid (ASA), 75—325 mg, is given to patients in hospital with ACS.[17,18] A few studies have suggested reduced mortality if ASA is given earlier.[19] Therefore, give ASA as soon as possible to all patients with suspected ACS unless the patient has a known true allergy to ASA. The initial dose of ASA to be chewed is 160—325 mg. Other forms of ASA (soluble, IV) may be as effective as chewed tablets.[20]

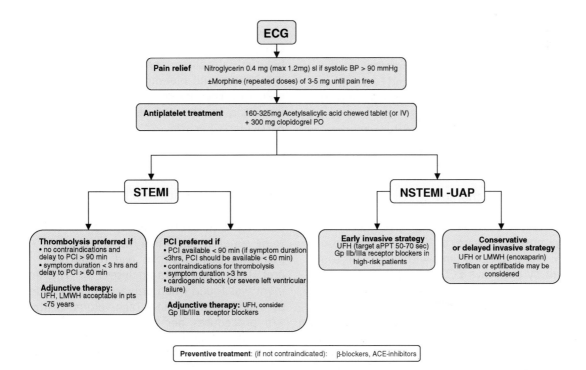

Figure 5.2 Early treatment of patients with signs/symptoms of ACS.

Reperfusion therapy

Reperfusion therapy is the most important advance in the treatment of AMI in the last 20 years. Large clinical trials have proven that fibrinolytic therapy in ACS patients with STEMI or new or presumed new LBBB, who present within 12 h of onset of symptoms, reduces short- and long-term mortality.[17,21–23] The benefit achieved with fibrinolytic therapy is profoundly time dependent; it is particularly effective if given within the first 3 h of the onset of symptoms.[17,21,22,24] The efficacy of primary PCI is also time-sensitive but less so than fibrinolysis.[25]

Out-of-hospital fibrinolysis

A meta-analysis of six trials involving 6434 patients documented a 17% decrease in the mortality among patients treated with out-of-hospital fibrinolysis compared with in-hospital fibrinolysis.[26] The average time gained by out-of-hospital fibrinolysis was 60 min, and the results were independent of the experience of the provider. Thus, giving fibrinolytics out-of-hospital to patients with STEMI or signs and symptoms of an ACS with presumed new LBBB is beneficial. Fibrinolytic therapy can be given safely by trained paramedics, nurses or physicians using an established protocol.[27–29] The efficacy is greatest within the first 3 h of the onset of symptoms. An effective and safe system for out-of-hospital thrombolytic therapy requires adequate facilities for the diagnosis and treatment of STEMI and its complications. Ideally, there should be a capability to communicate with experienced hospital doctors (e.g., emergency physicians or cardiologists).

Patients with symptoms of ACS and ECG evidence of STEMI (or presumably new LBBB or true posterior infarction) presenting directly to the emergency department should be given fibrinolytic therapy as soon as possible unless there is immediate access to primary PCI within 90 min.

Risks of fibrinolytic therapy

Healthcare professionals who give fibrinolytic therapy must be aware of its contraindications (Table 5.1) and risks. Patients with large AMIs (e.g., indicated by extensive ECG changes) are likely to derive the greatest benefit from fibrinolytic therapy. Benefits of fibrinolytic therapy are less impressive in inferior wall infarctions than in anterior infarctions. Older patients have an absolute higher risk of death, but the absolute benefit of fibrinolytic therapy is similar to that of younger patients. Patients over 75 years of age have an increased

Table 5.1 Contraindications for thrombolysis[a].

Absolute contraindications
Haemorrhagic stroke or stroke of unknown origin at any time
Ischaemic stroke in the preceding 6 months
Central nervous system damage or neoplasms
Recent major trauma/surgery/head injury (within the preceding 3 weeks)
Gastro-intestinal bleeding within the last month
Known bleeding disorder
Aortic dissection

Relative contraindications
Transient ischaemic attack in preceding 6 months
Oral anticoagulant therapy
Pregnancy within 1 week post partum
Non-compressible punctures
Traumatic resuscitation
Refractory hypertension (systolic blood pressure >180 mmHg
Advanced liver disease
Infective endocarditis
Active peptic ulcer

[a] According to the guidelines of the European Society of Cardiology.

risk of intracranial bleeding from fibrinolysis; thus, the absolute benefit of thrombolysis is reduced by this complication.[30] The risk of intracranial bleeding in patients with a systolic blood pressure of over 180 mmHg is increased; this degree of hypertension is a relative contraindication to fibrinolytic therapy. The intracranial bleeding risk also depends in part on which fibrinolytic drug is used; the total mortality is lower with the more fibrin-specific thrombolytics (alteplase, tenecteplase, reteplase), but the intracranial bleeding risk is lower with streptokinase. The risk of intracranial bleeding is also increased by the use of antithrombotic therapy, particularly heparin.

Primary percutaneous intervention

Coronary angioplasty with or without stent placement has become the first-line treatment for patients with STEMI, because it has been shown to be superior to fibrinolysis in the combined endpoints of death, stroke and reinfarction in several studies and meta-analyses.[31,32] This improvement was found when primary PCI was undertaken by a skilled person in a high-volume centre (i.e., >75 procedures per operator per year), with a delay of balloon inflation of not more than 90 min after first contact. In the randomised studies comparing primary PCI and fibrinolytic therapy, the typical delay from decision to the beginning of treatment with either primary PCI or fibrinolytic therapy was less than 60 min; however, in registries that reflect standard practice more realistically, the delay was often longer. One study[33] and one post hoc analysis[34] comparing fibrinolytic therapy with primary PCI showed no difference in survival if fibrinolytic therapy was initiated within 2 or 3 h of onset of symptoms.

All patients presenting with STEMI and symptoms of ACS and presumably new LBBB presenting within 12 h after onset of symptoms should be evaluated for reperfusion therapy (fibrinolytic therapy or PCI). Primary PCI is preferred in patients with symptom duration of over 3 h, if a skilled team can undertake it within 90 min after first patient contact, and in all patients who have contraindications to fibrinolytic therapy. If the duration of symptoms is less than 3 h, treatment is more time-sensitive and the superiority of out-of-hospital fibrinolytic therapy, immediate in-hospital fibrinolytic therapy or transfer for primary PCI is not yet established clearly.

Triage and interfacility transfer for primary PCI. The risk of death, reinfarction or stroke is reduced if patients with STEMI are transferred promptly from community hospitals to tertiary care facilities for primary PCI.[35] It is unclear whether immediate fibrinolytic therapy (in- or out-of-hospital) or transfer for primary PCI is superior for patients presenting with STEMI with a symptom duration of <2–3 h.[33,34] Transfer of STEMI patients for primary PCI is reasonable for those presenting later than 3 h but less than 12 h after onset of symptoms, provided that the transfer can be achieved rapidly. Optimally, primary PCI should occur within 90 min from the first contact with the healthcare provider deciding to treat or transfer.

Interfacility transfer for early PCI after fibrinolytic therapy. Older studies, that did not include modern adjunctive drugs and PCI techniques with stenting, do not support a strategy of fibrinolytic therapy combined with early PCI. In contrast, several recent smaller studies support a strategy of in-hospital fibrinolytic therapy in a peripheral hospital followed by transfer for PCI within 24 h of fibrinolytic therapy.[36,37] The timing of PCI after fibrinolytic therapy, the use of coronary stents and control-group interventions differ widely among these trials.

There is insufficient evidence to recommend routine transfer of patients for early PCI after successful fibrinolytic therapy. Transfer for early PCI after is recommended for patients in cardiogenic shock, particularly for those younger than 75 years and for those who are haemodynamically unstable or have persistent ischaemic symptoms after fibrinolytic therapy.

Cardiogenic shock

Cardiogenic shock (and to some extent, severe left ventricular failure) is one of the complications of ACS and has a mortality rate of more than 50%. Cardiogenic shock in STEMI is not a contraindication to fibrinolytic therapy, but PCI is preferable. Early revascularisation (i.e., primary or facilitated PCI or surgery) is indicated for those patients who develop shock within 36 h after symptom onset of AMI and are suitable for revascularisation.[38,39]

Suspect right ventricular infarction in patients with inferior infarction, clinical shock and clear lung fields. ST segment elevation ≥ 1 mm in lead V4R is a useful indicator of right ventricular infarction. These patients have an in-hospital mortality of up to 30%, and many benefit greatly from reperfusion therapy (fibrinolytic therapy and/or PCI). Avoid nitrates and other vasodilators, and treat hypotension with intravenous fluid.

Adjunctive treatment in reperfusion therapy in ACS

Heparin

Heparin is an indirect inhibitor of thrombin, which in combination with ASA is used as an adjunct with fibrinolytic therapy or primary PCI and as an important part of treatment of unstable angina and STEMI. Limitations of unfractionated heparin include its unpredictable anticoagulant effect in individual patients, the need for it to be given intravenously and the need to monitor aPTT. Moreover, heparin can induce thrombocytopenia. Low-molecular-weight heparin has a more predictable anticoagulant effect with lower rates of thrombocytopenia. It can be given subcutaneously in a weight-adjusted dose and does not require laboratory monitoring. Low-molecular-weight heparins may accumulate in patients with impaired renal function.

Unfractionated heparin versus low-molecular-weight heparin in NSTEMI

In comparison with unfractionated heparin (UFH), low-molecular-weight heparin (LMWH) (enoxaparin) reduces the combined endpoint of mortality, myocardial infarction and the need for urgent revascularisation, if given within the first 24–36 h of onset of symptoms of NSTEMI/UAP.[40–42] Although LMWH increases the incidence of minor bleeding, in comparison with UFH, the incidence of serious bleeding is not increased. Early treatment with LMWH (enoxaparin) is the preferred therapy for patients with NSTEMI/UAP in addition to ASA, whenever a non-interventional strategy is planned. Consider UFH if reperfusion is planned in the first 24—36 h after symptom onset. Optimal target value of aPPT is 50—70 s. Avoid switching between UFH and LMWH, because it may increase bleeding complications.[43]

Unfractionated heparin versus low-molecular-weight heparin in STEMI

Two large randomised controlled thrombolysis studies comparing LMWH with UFH demonstrated a reduced frequency of ischaemic complications when given to patients with STEMI within 6 h of the onset of symptoms.[44,45] This must be balanced against the increase in intracranial haemorrhage in patients over 75 years of age who receive LMWH.[45] There is no evidence to support giving LMWH to patients with STEMI proceeding to an invasive strategy. Thus, LMWH is an acceptable alternative to UFH as an ancillary therapy for patients younger than 75 years without significant renal dysfunction who are treated with fibrinolytic therapy. UFH is recommended as an ancillary therapy to fibrinolytic therapy in elderly patients and any STEMI patient for whom revascularisation is planned. The optimal target value of aPPT is 50—70 s. The use of heparin (preferably LMWH) depends partly on which fibrinolytic drug is used. Heparin is needed after shorter-acting drugs because of the rebound hypercoagulable state that occurs after a few hours, but not after streptokinase because the fibrinolytic effect of streptokinase lasts for about 48 h.

Glycoprotein IIb/IIIa inhibitors

The platelet glycoprotein (Gp) IIb/IIIa receptor is the final common pathway to platelet aggregation. The synthetic substances eptifibatide and tirofiban modulate this receptor activity reversibly, whereas the receptor antibody abciximab blocks it irreversibly.

Gp IIb/IIIa inhibitors in NSTEMI/unstable angina. The incidences of death and recurrent ischaemia are reduced when Gp IIb/IIIa inhibitors are added to standard therapy including ASA and heparin in high-risk patients with UAP/NSTEMI treated with mechanical reperfusion.[46] High-risk features include persistent pain, haemodynamic or rhythm instability, diabetes, acute or dynamic ECG changes and any elevation in cardiac troponins. Tirofiban or eptifibatide failed to reduce death or recur-

rent ischaemia in patients with UA/NSTEMI without mechanical perfusion, but showed a reduction in 30-day mortality in a later meta-analysis.[46] In patients with UA/NSTEMI, abciximab, given in addition to standard therapy without mechanical intervention, resulted in a trend towards a worse outcome.[47] Therefore, in high-risk patients, give Gp IIb/IIIa inhibitors in addition to standard therapy in patients for whom revascularisation therapy is planned. If revascularisation therapy is not planned, tirofiban and eptifibatide can be given to high-risk NSTEMI/UAP patients in conjunction with ASA and LMWH. Do not give abciximab if PCI is not planned.

Gp IIb/IIIa inhibitors in STEMI. Gp IIb/IIIa receptor blockers in combination with a reduced dose of fibrinolytics do not reduce mortality in patients with STEMI, but increase bleeding risk in patients over 75 years of age.[44,48] Abciximab reduces mortality when given to patients with STEMI and planned primary PCI, but is not beneficial in patients not proceeding to primary PCI.[46] Prehospital use of abciximab may improve the patency of the infarct-related artery with regard to PCI.[49] There is no benefit in giving tirofiban in addition to standard therapy out of hospital or in the emergency department.[50] Abciximab may be helpful in reducing short-term mortality and short-term reinfarction in patients treated with PCI without fibrinolytic therapy. Abciximab is not recommended in combination with fibrinolytics in patients with STEMI.

Clopidogrel

Clopidogrel inhibits the platelet ADP receptor irreversibly, which further reduces platelet aggregation in addition to that produced by ASA. Compared with ASA, there is no increased risk of bleeding with clopidogrel.[51] If given in addition to heparin and ASA within 4 h of presentation, clopidogrel improves outcome in patients with high-risk ACS.[52,53] There is a significant reduction in adverse ischaemic events at 28 days after elective PCI when clopidogrel is given at least 6 h before intervention.[54] A recent trial documented a significant reduction in the composite endpoint of an occluded infarct-related artery (TIMI flow grade 0 or 1) on angiography or death or recurrent myocardial infarction before angiography, when clopidogrel (300 mg loading dose, followed by 75 mg daily dose up to 8 days in hospital) is given to patients up to 75 years of age with STEMI who are treated with fibrinolytic therapy, ASA and heparin.[55]

Give a 300-mg oral loading dose of clopidogrel early, as well as standard care, to patients with ACS if they have an increase in serum cardiac biomarkers and/or new ECG changes consistent with ischaemia when a medical approach or PCI is planned. Give clopidogrel to patients with STEMI up to 75 years of age receiving fibrinolytic therapy, ASA and heparin. Clopidogrel, 300 mg, can be given instead of ASA to patients with a suspected ACS who have a true allergy to or gastrointestinal intolerance of ASA.

Primary and secondary prevention interventions

Start preventive interventions, at the latest, at the initial admission with a confirmed diagnosis of ACS. Give a beta-blocker as soon as possible unless contraindicated or poorly tolerated. Treat all patients with a statin (HRG co-enzyme A reductase inhibitor) unless contraindicated or poorly tolerated. Start an ACE inhibitor in all patients with STEMI, all patients with STEMI and left ventricular systolic impairment, and consider it in all other patients with STEMI unless contraindicated or poorly tolerated. In patients unable to tolerate an ACE inhibitor, an angiotensin receptor blocker may be used as a substitute in those patients with left ventricular systolic impairment.

Beta-blockers

Several studies, undertaken mainly in the pre-reperfusion era, indicate decreased mortality and incidence of reinfarction and cardiac rupture as well as a lower incidence of VF and supraventricular arrhythmia in patients treated early with a beta-blocker.[56,57] Intravenous beta-blockade may also reduce mortality in patients undergoing primary PCI who are not on oral beta-blockers.[58]

Haemodynamically stable patients presenting with an ACS should be given intravenous beta-blockers promptly, followed by regular oral therapy unless contraindicated or poorly tolerated. Contraindications to beta-blockers include hypotension, bradycardia, second- or third-degree AV block, moderate to severe congestive heart failure and severe reactive airway disease. Give a beta-blocker irrespective of the need for early revascularisation therapy.

Anti-arrhythmics

Apart from the use of a beta-blocker as recommended above, there is no evidence to support the use of anti-arrhythmic prophylaxis after ACS. VF accounts for most of the early deaths from ACS; the incidence of VF is highest in the first

hours after onset of symptoms.[59,60] This explains why numerous studies have been performed with the aim of demonstrating the prophylactic effect of anti-arrhythmic therapy. The effects of anti-arrhythmic drugs (lidocaine, magnesium, disopyramide, mexiletine, verapamil) given prophylactically to patients with ACS have been studied.[61–63] Prophylaxis with lidocaine reduces the incidence of VF but may increase mortality.[58] Routine treatment with magnesium in patients with AMI does not improve mortality.[64] Arrhythmia prophylaxis using disopyramide, mexiletine or verapamil, given within the first hours of an ACS, does not improve mortality.[63] In contrast, intravenous beta-blockers reduced the incidence of VF when given to patients with ACS.[56,57]

Angiotensin-converting enzyme inhibitors and angiotensin-II receptor blockers

Oral angiotensin-converting inhibitors (ACE) inhibitors reduce mortality when given to patients with acute myocardial infarction with or without early reperfusion therapy.[65,66] The beneficial effects are most pronounced in patients presenting with anterior infarction, pulmonary congestion or left ventricular ejection fraction <40%.[66] Do not give ACE inhibitors if the systolic blood pressure is less than 100 mmHg at admission or if there is a known contraindication to these drugs.[66] A trend towards higher mortality has been documented if an intravenous ACE inhibitor is started within the first 24 h after onset of symptoms.[67] Therefore, give an oral ACE inhibitor within 24 h after symptom onset in patients with AMI regardless of whether early reperfusion therapy is planned, particularly in those patients with anterior infarction, pulmonary congestion or left ventricular ejection fraction below 40%. Do not give intravenous ACE inhibitors within 24 h of onset of symptoms. Give an angiotensin receptor blocker (ARB) to patients intolerant of ACE inhibitors.

Statins

Statins reduce the incidence of major adverse cardiovascular events when given within a few days after onset of ACS. Start statin therapy within 24 h of onset of symptoms of ACS. If patients are already receiving statin therapy, do not stop it.[68]

References

1. Tunstall-Pedoe H, Vanuzzo D, Hobbs M, et al. Estimation of contribution of changes in coronary care to improving

survival, event rates, and coronary heart disease mortality across the WHO MONICA Project populations. Lancet 2000;355:688—700.

2. Lowel H, Meisinger C, Heier M, et al. Sex specific trends of sudden cardiac death and acute myocardial infarction: results of the population-based KORA/MONICA-Augsburg register 1985 to 1998. Dtsch Med Wochenschr 2002;127:2311—6.

3. European Society Cardiology. Myocardial infarction redefined—a consensus document of The Joint European Society of Cardiology/American College of Cardiology Committee for the redefinition of myocardial infarction. J Am Coll Cardiol 2000;36:959—69.

4. Van de Werf F, Ardissino D, Betriu A, et al. Management of acute myocardial infarction in patients presenting with ST-segment elevation. The Task Force on the Management of Acute Myocardial Infarction of the European Society of Cardiology. Eur Heart J 2003;24:28—66.

5. Antman EM, Anbe DT, Armstrong PW, et al. ACC/AHA guidelines for the management of patients with ST-elevation myocardial infarction—executive summary: a report of the American College of Cardiology/American Heart Association Task Force on Practice Guidelines (Writing Committee to Revise the 1999 Guidelines for the Management of Patients With Acute Myocardial Infarction). Circulation 2004;110:588—636.

6. Douglas PS, Ginsburg GS. The evaluation of chest pain in women. N Engl J Med 1996;334:1311—5.

7. Solomon CG, Lee TH, Cook EF, et al. Comparison of clinical presentation of acute myocardial infarction in patients older than 65 years of age to younger patients: the Multicenter Chest Pain Study experience. Am J Cardiol 1989;63:772—6.

8. Kereiakes DJ, Gibler WB, Martin LH, Pieper KS, Anderson LC. Relative importance of emergency medical system transport and the prehospital electrocardiogram on reducing hospital time delay to therapy for acute myocardial infarction: a preliminary report from the Cincinnati Heart Project. Am Heart J 1992;123(Pt 1):835—40.

9. Canto JG, Rogers WJ, Bowlby LJ, French WJ, Pearce DJ, Weaver WD. The prehospital electrocardiogram in acute myocardial infarction: is its full potential being realized? National Registry of Myocardial Infarction 2 Investigators. J Am Coll Cardiol 1997;29:498—505.

10. Aufderheide TP, Hendley GE, Thakur RK, et al. The diagnostic impact of prehospital 12-lead electrocardiography. Ann Emerg Med 1990;19:1280—7.

11. Foster DB, Dufendach JH, Barkdoll CM, Mitchell BK. Prehospital recognition of AMI using independent nurse/paramedic 12-lead ECG evaluation: impact on in-hospital times to thrombolysis in a rural community hospital. Am J Emerg Med 1994;12:25—31.

12. Millar-Craig MW, Joy AV, Adamowicz M, Furber R, Thomas B. Reduction in treatment delay by paramedic ECG diagnosis of myocardial infarction with direct CCU admission. Heart 1997;78:456—61.

13. Brinfield K. Identification of ST elevation AMI on prehospital 12 lead ECG; accuracy of unaided paramedic interpretation. J Emerg Med 1998;16:22S.

14. Antman EM, Tanasijevic MJ, Thompson B, et al. Cardiac-specific troponin I levels to predict the risk of mortality in patients with acute coronary syndromes. N Engl J Med 1996;335:1342—9.

15. Schuchert A, Hamm C, Scholz J, Klimmeck S, Goldmann B, Meinertz T. Prehospital testing for troponin T in patients with suspected acute myocardial infarction. Am Heart J 1999;138:45—8.

16. Rawles JM, Kenmure AC. Controlled trial of oxygen in uncomplicated myocardial infarction. BMJ 1976;1:1121—3.

17. Randomised trial of intravenous streptokinase, oral aspirin, both, or neither among 17,187 cases of suspected acute myocardial infarction: ISIS-2. ISIS-2 (Second International Study of Infarct Survival) Collaborative Group. Lancet 1988;2:349—60.

18. Gurfinkel EP, Manos EJ, Mejail RI, et al. Low molecular weight heparin versus regular heparin or aspirin in the treatment of unstable angina and silent ischemia. J Am Coll Cardiol 1995;26:313—8.

19. Freimark D, Matetzky S, Leor J, et al. Timing of aspirin administration as a determinant of survival of patients with acute myocardial infarction treated with thrombolysis. Am J Cardiol 2002;89:381—5.

20. Husted SE, Kristensen SD, Vissinger H, Morn B, Schmidt EB, Nielsen HK. Intravenous acetylsalicylic acid—dose-related effects on platelet function and fibrinolysis in healthy males. Thromb Haemost 1992;68:226—9.

21. Indications for fibrinolytic therapy in suspected acute myocardial infarction: collaborative overview of early mortality and major morbidity results from all randomised trials of more than 1000 patients. Fibrinolytic Therapy Trialists' (FTT) Collaborative Group. Lancet 1994;343:311—22.

22. Effectiveness of intravenous thrombolytic treatment in acute myocardial infarction. Gruppo Italiano per lo Studio della Streptochinasi nell'Infarto Miocardico (GISSI). Lancet 1986;1:397—402.

23. The GUSTO investigators. An international randomized trial comparing four thrombolytic strategies for acute myocardial infarction. N Engl J Med 1993;329:673—82.

24. Boersma E, Maas AC, Deckers JW, Simoons ML. Early thrombolytic treatment in acute myocardial infarction: reappraisal of the golden hour. Lancet 1996;348:771—5.

25. De Luca G, van't Hof AW, de Boer MJ, et al. Time-to-treatment significantly affects the extent of ST-segment resolution and myocardial blush in patients with acute myocardial infarction treated by primary angioplasty. Eur Heart J 2004;25:1009—13.

26. Morrison LJ, Verbeek PR, McDonald AC, Sawadsky BV, Cook DJ. Mortality and prehospital thrombolysis for acute myocardial infarction: a meta-analysis. JAMA 2000;283:2686—92.

27. Welsh RC, Goldstein P, Adgey J, et al. Variations in prehospital fibrinolysis process of care: insights from the Assessment of the Safety and Efficacy of a New Thrombolytic 3 Plus international acute myocardial infarction pre-hospital care survey. Eur J Emerg Med 2004;11:134—40.

28. Weaver W, Cerqueira M, Hallstrom A, et al. Prehospital-initiated vs hospital-initiated thrombolytic therapy: the Myocardial Infacrtion Triage and Intervention Trial (MITI). JAMA 1993;270:1203—10.

29. European Myocardial Infarction Project Group (EMIP). Prehospital thrombolytic therapy in patients with suspected acute myocardial infarction. The European Myocardial Infarction Project Group. N Engl J Med 1993;329:383—9.

30. White HD. Debate: should the elderly receive thrombolytic therapy, or primary angioplasty? Current Control Trials Cardiovasc Med 2000;1:150—4.

31. Weaver WD, Simes RJ, Betriu A, et al. Comparison of primary coronary angioplasty and intravenous thrombolytic therapy for acute myocardial infarction: a quantitative review. JAMA 1997;278:2093—8.

32. Keeley EC, Boura JA, Grines CL. Primary angioplasty versus intravenous thrombolytic therapy for acute myocardial infarction: a quantitative review of 23 randomised trials. Lancet 2003;361:13—20.

33. Widimsky P, Budesinsky T, Vorac D, et al. Long distance transport for primary angioplasty vs immediate thrombolysis in acute myocardial infarction. Final results of the ran-

domized national multicentre trial—PRAGUE-2. Eur Heart J 2003;24:94—104.

34. Steg PG, Bonnefoy E, Chabaud S, et al. Impact of time to treatment on mortality after prehospital fibrinolysis or primary angioplasty: data from the CAPTIM randomized clinical trial. Circulation 2003;108:2851—6.

35. Dalby M, Bouzamondo A, Lechat P, Montalescot G. Transfer for primary angioplasty versus immediate thrombolysis in acute myocardial infarction: a meta-analysis. Circulation 2003;108:1809—14.

36. Scheller B, Hennen B, Hammer B, et al. Beneficial effects of immediate stenting after thrombolysis in acute myocardial infarction. J Am Coll Cardiol 2003,42.634—41.

37. Fernandez-Aviles F, Alonso JJ, Castro-Beiras A, et al. Routine invasive strategy within 24 h of thrombolysis versus ischaemia-guided conservative approach for acute myocardial infarction with ST-segment elevation (GRACIA-1): a randomised controlled trial. Lancet 2004;364:1045—53.

38. Hochman JS, Sleeper LA, Webb JG, et al. Early revascularization in acute myocardial infarction complicated by cardiogenic shock. SHOCK Investigators. Should we emergently revascularize occluded coronaries for cardiogenic shock. N Engl J Med 1999;341:625—34.

39. Hochman JS, Sleeper LA, White HD, et al. One-year survival following early revascularization for cardiogenic shock. JAMA 2001;285:190—2.

40. Antman EM, McCabe CH, Gurfinkel EP, et al. Enoxaparin prevents death and cardiac ischemic events in unstable angina/non-Q-wave myocardial infarction. Results of the thrombolysis in myocardial infarction (TIMI) 11B trial. Circulation 1999;100:1593—601.

41. Cohen M, Demers C, Gurfinkel EP, et al. A comparison of low-molecular-weight heparin with unfractionated heparin for unstable coronary artery disease. Efficacy and Safety of Subcutaneous Enoxaparin in Non-Q-Wave Coronary Events Study Group. N Engl J Med 1997;337:447—52.

42. Petersen JL, Mahaffey KW, Hasselblad V, et al. Efficacy and bleeding complications among patients randomized to enoxaparin or unfractionated heparin for antithrombin therapy in non-ST-Segment elevation acute coronary syndromes: a systematic overview. JAMA 2004;292:89—96.

43. Ferguson JJ, Califf RM, Antman EM, et al. Enoxaparin vs unfractionated heparin in high-risk patients with non-ST-segment elevation acute coronary syndromes managed with an intended early invasive strategy: primary results of the SYNERGY randomized trial. JAMA 2004;292:45—54.

44. Van de Werf FJ, Armstrong PW, Granger C, Wallentin L. Efficacy and safety of tenecteplase in combination with enoxaparin, abciximab, or unfractionated heparin: the ASSENT-3 randomised trial in acute myocardial infarction. Lancet 2001;358:605—13.

45. Wallentin L, Goldstein P, Armstrong PW, et al. Efficacy and safety of tenecteplase in combination with the low-molecular-weight heparin enoxaparin or unfractionated heparin in the prehospital setting: the Assessment of the Safety and Efficacy of a New Thrombolytic Regimen (ASSENT)-3 PLUS randomized trial in acute myocardial infarction. Circulation 2003;108:135—42.

46. Boersma E, Harrington RA, Moliterno DJ, et al. Platelet glycoprotein IIb/IIIa inhibitors in acute coronary syndromes: a meta-analysis of all major randomised clinical trials. Lancet 2002;359:189—98 [erratum appears in Lancet 2002 Jun 15;359(9323):2120].

47. Simoons ML. Effect of glycoprotein IIb/IIIa receptor blocker abciximab on outcome in patients with acute coronary syndromes without early coronary revascularisation: the GUSTO IV-ACS randomised trial. Lancet 2001;357:1915—24.

48. Topol EJ. Reperfusion therapy for acute myocardial infarction with fibrinolytic therapy or combination reduced fibrinolytic therapy and platelet glycoprotein IIb/IIIa inhibition: the GUSTO V randomised trial. Lancet 2001;357:1905—14.

49. Montalescot G, Borentain M, Payot L, Collet JP, Thomas D. Early vs late administration of glycoprotein IIb/IIIa inhibitors in primary percutaneous coronary intervention of acute ST-segment elevation myocardial infarction: a meta-analysis. JAMA 2004;292:362—6.

50. van't Hof AW, Ernst N, de Boer MJ, et al. Facilitation of primary coronary angioplasty by early start of a glycoprotein 2b/3a inhibitor: results of the ongoing tirofiban in myocardial infarction evaluation (On-TIME) trial. Eur Heart J 2004;25:837—46.

51. A randomised, blinded, trial of clopidogrel versus aspirin in patients at risk of ischaemic events (CAPRIE). CAPRIE Steering Committee. Lancet 1996;348:1329—39.

52. Yusuf S, Zhao F, Mehta SR, Chrolavicius S, Tognoni G, Fox KK. Effects of clopidogrel in addition to aspirin in patients with acute coronary syndromes without ST-segment elevation. N Engl J Med 2001;345:494—502.

53. Mehta SR, Yusuf S, Peters RJ, et al. Effects of pretreatment with clopidogrel and aspirin followed by long-term therapy in patients undergoing percutaneous coronary intervention: the PCI-CURE study. Lancet 2001;358:527—33.

54. Steinhubl SR, Berger PB, Mann IIIrd JT, et al. Early and sustained dual oral antiplatelet therapy following percutaneous coronary intervention: a randomized controlled trial. JAMA 2002;288:2411—20.

55. Sabatine MS, Cannon CP, Gibson CM, et al. Addition of clopidogrel to aspirin and fibrinolytic therapy for myocardial infarction with ST-segment elevation. N Engl J Med 2005;352:1179—89.

56. The MIAMI Trial Research Group. Metoprolol in acute myocardial infarction (MIAMI): a randomised placebo-controlled international trial. Eur Heart J 1985;6:199—226.

57. Randomised trial of intravenous atenolol among 16 027 cases of suspected acute myocardial infarction: ISIS-1. First International Study of Infarct Survival Collaborative Group. Lancet 1986;2:57—66.

58. Halkin A, Grines CL, Cox DA, et al. Impact of intravenous beta-blockade before primary angioplasty on survival in patients undergoing mechanical reperfusion therapy for acute myocardial infarction. J Am Coll Cardiol 2004;43:1780—7.

59. Campbell RW, Murray A, Julian DG. Ventricular arrhythmias in first 12 h of acute myocardial infarction: natural history study. Br Heart J 1981;46:351—7.

60. O'Doherty M, Tayler DI, Quinn E, Vincent R, Chamberlain DA. Five hundred patients with myocardial infarction monitored within one hour of symptoms. BMJ 1983;286:1405—8.

61. Teo KK, Yusuf S, Furberg CD. Effects of prophylactic antiarrhythmic drug therapy in acute myocardial infarction. An overview of results from randomized controlled trials. JAMA 1993;270:1589—95.

62. Sadowski ZP, Alexander JH, Skrabucha B, et al. Multicenter randomized trial and a systematic overview of lidocaine in acute myocardial infarction. Am Heart J 1999;137:792—8.

63. McAlister FA, Teo KK. Antiarrhythmic therapies for the prevention of sudden cardiac death. Drugs 1997;54:235—52.

64. ISIS-4: a randomised factorial trial assessing early oral captopril, oral mononitrate, and intravenous magnesium sulphate in 58,050 patients with suspected acute myocardial infarction. ISIS-4 (Fourth International Study of Infarct Survival) Collaborative Group. Lancet 1995;345:669—85.

65. Teo KK, Yusuf S, Pfeffer M, et al. Effects of long-term treatment with angiotensin-converting-enzyme inhibitors in the presence or absence of aspirin: a systematic review. Lancet 2002;360:1037—43.

66. ACE Inhibitor MI Collaborative Group. Indications for ACE inhibitors in the early treatment of acute myocardial infarction: systematic overview of individual data from 100,000 patients in randomized trials. ACE Inhibitor Myocardial Infarction Collaborative Group. Circulation 1998;97:2202—12.

67. Swedberg K, Held P, Kjekshus J, Rasmussen K, Ryden L, Wedel H. Effects of the early administration of enalapril on mortality in patients with acute myocardial infarction. Results of the Cooperative New Scandinavian Enalapril Survival Study II (CONSENSUS II). N Engl J Med 1992;327:678—84.

68. Heeschen C, Hamm CW, Laufs U, Snapinn S, Bohm M, White HD. Withdrawal of statins increases event rates in patients with acute coronary syndromes. Circulation 2002;105:1446—52.

Resuscitation (2005) **67S1**, S97—S133

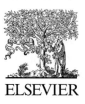

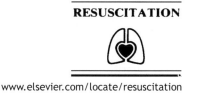

RESUSCITATION

www.elsevier.com/locate/resuscitation

European Resuscitation Council Guidelines for Resuscitation 2005
Section 6. Paediatric life support

Dominique Biarent, Robert Bingham, Sam Richmond, Ian Maconochie, Jonathan Wyllie, Sheila Simpson, Antonio Rodriguez Nunez, David Zideman

Introduction

The process

The European Resuscitation Council (ERC) issued guidelines for paediatric life support (PLS) in 1994, 1998 and 2000.[1–4] The last edition was based on the International Consensus on Science published by the American Heart Association in collaboration with the International Liaison Committee on Resuscitation (ILCOR), undertaking a series of evidence-based evaluations of the science of resuscitation which culminated in the publication of the Guidelines 2000 for Cardiopulmonary Resuscitation and Emergency Cardiovascular Care in August 2000.[5,6] This process was repeated in 2004/2005, and the resulting Consensus on Science and Treatment Recommendations were published simultaneously in *Resuscitation, Circulation* and *Pediatrics* in November 2005.[7,8] The PLS Working Party of the ERC has considered this document and the supporting scientific literature, and has recommended changes to the ERC PLS Guidelines. These are presented in this paper.

Guidelines changes

The approach to changes has been to alter the guidelines in response to convincing new scientific evidence and, where possible, to simplify them in order to assist teaching and retention. As before, there remains a paucity of good-quality evidence on paediatric resuscitation specifically and some conclusions have had to be drawn from animal work and extrapolated adult data.

The current guidelines have a strong focus on simplification based on the knowledge that many children receive no resuscitation at all because rescuers fear doing harm. This fear is fuelled by the knowledge that resuscitation guidelines for children are different. Consequently, a major area of study was the feasibility of applying the same guidance for all adults and children. Bystander resuscitation improves outcome significantly,[9,10] and there is good evidence from paediatric animal models that even doing chest compressions or expired air ventilation alone may be better than doing nothing at all.[11] It follows that outcomes could be improved if bystanders, who would otherwise do nothing, were encouraged to begin resuscitation, even if they do not follow an algorithm targeted specifically at children. There are, however, distinct differences between the predominantly adult arrest of cardiac origin and asphyxial arrest, which is most common in children,[12] so a separate paediatric algorithm is justified for those with a duty to respond to paediatric emergencies (usually healthcare professionals), who are also in a position to receive enhanced training.

Compression:ventilation ratios

The ILCOR treatment recommendation was that the compression:ventilation ratio should be based on whether one or more than one rescuers were present. ILCOR recommends that lay rescuers, who usually learn only single rescuer techniques, should be taught to use a ratio of 30 compressions to 2 ventilations, which is the same as the adult guidelines and enables anyone trained in BLS techniques to resuscitate children with minimal additional information. Two or more rescuers with a duty to respond should learn a different ratio (15:2), as this has been validated by animal and manikin studies.[13–17] This latter group, who would normally be healthcare professionals, should receive enhanced training targeted specifically at the resuscitation of children. Although there are no data to support the superiority of any particular ratio in children, ratios of between 5:1 and 15:2 have been studied in manikins, and animal and mathematical models, and there is increasing evidence that the 5:1 ratio delivers an inadequate number of compressions.[14,18] There is certainly no justification for having two separate ratios for children aged greater or less than 8 years, so a single ratio of 15:2 for multiple rescuers with a duty to respond is a logical simplification.

It would certainly negate any benefit of simplicity if lay rescuers were taught a different ratio for use if there were two of them, but those with a duty to respond can use the 30:2 ratio if they are alone, particularly if they are not achieving an adequate number of compressions because of difficulty in the transition between ventilation and compression.

Age definitions

The adoption of single compression:ventilation ratios for children of all ages, together with the change in advice on the lower age limit for the use of automated external defibrillators (AEDs), renders the previous guideline division between children above and below 8 years of age unnecessary. The differences between adult and paediatric resuscitation are based largely on differing aetiology, as primary cardiac arrest is more common in adults whereas children usually suffer from sec-

ondary cardiac arrest. The onset of puberty, which is the physiological end of childhood, is the most logical landmark for the upper age limit for use of paediatric guidance. This has the advantage of being simple to determine, in contrast to an age limit in years, as age may be unknown at the start of resuscitation. Clearly, it is inappropriate and unnecessary to establish the onset of puberty formally; if rescuers believe the victim to be a child they should use the paediatric guidelines. If a misjudgement is made and the victim turns out to be a young adult, little harm will accrue, as studies of aetiology have shown that the paediatric pattern of arrest continues into early adulthood.[19] An infant is a child under 1 year of age; a child is between 1 year and puberty. It is necessary to differentiate between infants and older children, as there are some important differences between these two groups.

Chest compression technique

The modification to age definitions enables a simplification of the advice on chest compression. Advice for determining the landmarks for infant compression is now the same as for older children, as there is evidence that the previous recommendation could result in compression over the upper abdomen.[20] Infant compression technique remains the same: two-finger compression for single rescuers and two-thumb, encircling technique for two or more rescuers,[21–25] but for older children there is no division between the one- or two-hand technique.[26] The emphasis is on achieving an adequate depth of compression with minimal interruptions, using one or two hands according to rescuer preference.

Automated external defibrillators

Case reports published since International Guidelines 2000 have reported safe and successful use of AEDs in children less than 8 years of age.[27,28] Furthermore, recent studies have shown that AEDs are capable of identifying arrhythmias in children accurately and that, in particular, they are extremely unlikely to advise a shock inappropriately.[29,30] Consequently, advice on the use of AEDs has been revised to include all children aged greater than 1 year.[31] Nevertheless, if there is any possibility that an AED may need to be used in children, the purchaser should check that the performance of the particular model has been tested against paediatric arrhythmias.

Many manufacturers now supply purpose-made paediatric pads or programmes, which typically attenuate the output of the machine to 50–75 J.[32]

These devices are recommended for children aged 1—8 years.[33,34] If no such system or manually adjustable machine is available, an unmodified adult AED may be used in children older than 1 year.[35] There is currently insufficient evidence to support a recommendation for or against the use of AEDs in children aged less than 1 year.

Manual defibrillators

The 2005 Consensus Conference treatment recommendation for paediatric ventricular fibrillation (VF) or paediatric pulseless ventricular tachycardia (VT) is to defibrillate promptly. In adult ALS, the recommendation is to give a single shock and then resume CPR immediately without checking for a pulse or reassessing the rhythm (see Section 3). As a consequence of this single-shock strategy, when using a monophasic defibrillator in adults a higher initial energy dose than used previously is recommended (360 J versus 200 J) (see Section 3). The ideal energy dose for safe and effective defibrillation in children is unknown, but animal models and small paediatric series show that doses larger than 4 J kg^{-1} defibrillate effectively with negligible side effects.[27,34,36,37] Biphasic shocks are at least as effective and produce less post-shock myocardial dysfunction than monophasic shocks.[33,34,37—40] For simplicity of sequence and consistency with adult BLS and ALS, we recommend a single-shock strategy using a non-escalating dose of 4 J kg^{-1} (monophasic or biphasic) for defibrillation in children.

Foreign-body airway obstruction sequence

The guidance for managing foreign-body airway obstruction (FBAO) in children has been simplified and brought into closer alignment to the adult sequence. These changes are discussed in detail at the end of this section.

In the following text the masculine includes the feminine and 'child' refers to both infants and children unless noted otherwise.

6a Paediatric basic life support

Sequence of action

Rescuers who have been taught adult BLS and have no specific knowledge of paediatric resuscitation may use the adult sequence, with the exception that they should perform 5 initial breaths followed by approximately 1 min of CPR before they go for help (Figure 6.1; also see adult BLS guideline).

Paediatric Basic Life Support (Healthcare professionals with a duty to respond)

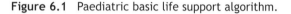

UNRESPONSIVE?

↓

Shout for help

↓

Open airway

↓

NOT BREATHING NORMALLY?

↓

5 rescue breaths

↓

STILL UNRESPONSIVE?
(no signs of a circulation)

↓

15 chest compressions
2 rescue breaths

After 1 minute call resuscitation team then continue CPR

Figure 6.1 Paediatric basic life support algorithm.

The following sequence is to be observed by those with a duty to respond to paediatric emergencies (usually health professionals).

1. Ensure the safety of rescuer and child.
2. Check the child's responsiveness.
   - Gently stimulate the child and ask loudly: ''Are you all right?''
   - Do not shake infants or children with suspected cervical spinal injuries.

3a If the child responds by answering or moving
   - leave the child in the position in which you find him (provided he is not in further danger)
   - check his condition and get help if needed
   - reassess him regularly

3b If the child does not respond
   - shout for help;
   - open the child's airway by tilting the head and lifting the chin, as follows:
     o initially with the child in the position in which you find him, place your hand on his forehead and gently tilt his head back;
     o at the same time, with your fingertip(s) under the point of the child's chin, lift the chin. Do not push on the soft tissues under the chin as this may block the airway;
     o if you still have difficulty in opening the airway, try the jaw thrust method. Place the first two fingers of each hand behind each side of the child's mandible and push the jaw forward;
     o both methods may be easier if the child is turned carefully onto his back.

If you suspect that there may have been an injury to the neck, try to open the airway using chin lift or jaw thrust alone. If this is unsuccessful, add head tilt a small amount at a time until the airway is open.

4. Keeping the airway open, look, listen and feel for normal breathing by putting your face close to the child's face and looking along the chest.

- Look for chest movements.
- Listen at the child's nose and mouth for breath sounds.
- Feel for air movement on your cheek.

Look, listen and feel for no more than 10 s before deciding.

5a If the child is breathing normally
- turn the child on his side into the recovery position (see below)
- check for continued breathing

5b If the child is *not* breathing or is making agonal gasps (infrequent, irregular breaths)
- carefully remove any obvious airway obstruction;
- give five initial rescue breaths;
- while performing the rescue breaths, note any gag or cough response to your action. These responses or their absence will form part of your assessment of signs of a circulation, which will be described later.

Rescue breaths for a child over 1 year are performed as follows (Figure 6.2).

- Ensure head tilt and chin lift.

- Pinch the soft part of the nose closed with the index finger and thumb of your hand on his forehead.
- Open his mouth a little, but maintain the chin upwards.
- Take a breath and place your lips around the mouth, making sure that you have a good seal.
- Blow steadily into the mouth over about 1—1.5 s, watching for chest rise.
- Maintain head tilt and chin lift, take your mouth away from the victim and watch for his chest to fall as air is expelled.
- Take another breath and repeat this sequence five times. Identify effectiveness by seeing that the child's chest has risen and fallen in a similar fashion to the movement produced by a normal breath.

Rescue breaths for an infant are performed as follows (Figure 6.3).

- Ensure a neutral position of the head and a chin lift.
- Take a breath and cover the mouth and nasal apertures of the infant with your mouth, making sure you have a good seal. If the nose and mouth cannot be covered in the older infant, the rescuer may attempt to seal only the infant's nose or mouth with his mouth (if the nose is used, close the lips to prevent air escape).
- Blow steadily into the infant's mouth and nose over 1—1.5 s, sufficient to make the chest visibly rise.
- Maintain head tilt and chin lift, take your mouth away from the victim and watch for his chest to fall as air is expelled.
- Take another breath and repeat this sequence five times.

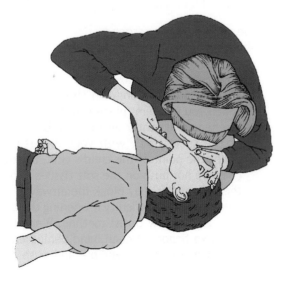

Figure 6.2 Mouth-to-mouth ventilation— child. © 2005 ERC.

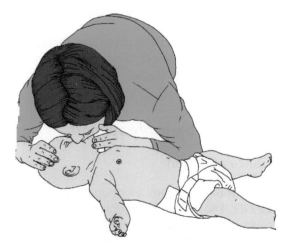

Figure 6.3 Mouth-to-mouth and nose ventilation— infant. © 2005 ERC.

If you have difficulty achieving an effective breath, the airway may be obstructed.

- Open the child's mouth and remove any visible obstruction. Do not perform a blind finger sweep.
- Ensure that there is adequate head tilt and chin lift but also that the neck is not over-extended.
- If head tilt and chin lift have not opened the airway, try the jaw thrust method.
- Make up to five attempts to achieve effective breaths; if still unsuccessful, move on to chest compressions.

6. Assess the child's circulation. Take no more than 10 s to
   - look for signs of a circulation. This includes any movement, coughing or normal breathing (not agonal gasps, which are infrequent, irregular breaths);
   - check the pulse (if you are a health care provider) but ensure you take no more than 10 s.

If the child is aged over 1 year, feel for the carotid pulse in the neck.

In an infant, feel for the brachial pulse on the inner aspect of the upper arm.

7a If you are confident that you can detect signs of a circulation within 10 s
   - continue rescue breathing, if necessary, until the child starts breathing effectively on his own
   - turn the child onto his side (into the recovery position) if he remains unconscious
   - re-assess the child frequently
7b If there are no signs of a circulation, or no pulse or a slow pulse (less than $60 \, \text{min}^{-1}$ with poor perfusion), or you are not sure
   - start chest compressions
   - combine rescue breathing and chest compressions

Chest compressions are performed as follows. For all children, compress the lower third of the sternum. To avoid compressing the upper abdomen, locate the xiphisternum by finding the angle where the lowest ribs join in the middle. Compress the sternum one finger's breadth above this; the compression should be sufficient to depress the sternum by approximately one third of the depth of the chest. Release the pressure and repeat at a rate of about $100 \, \text{min}^{-1}$. After 15 compressions, tilt the head, lift the chin, and give two effective breaths. Continue compressions and breaths in a ratio of 15:2. Lone rescuers may use a ratio of 30:2, particularly if having difficulty with the transition between compression and ventilation. Although the

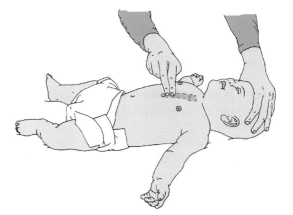

Figure 6.4 Chest compression — infant. © 2005 ERC.

rate of compressions will be $100 \, \text{min}^{-1}$, the actual number delivered per minute will be less than 100 because of pauses to give breaths. The best method for compression varies slightly between infants and children.

To perform chest compression in infants, the lone rescuer compresses the sternum with the tips of two fingers (Figure 6.4). If there are two or more rescuers, use the encircling technique. Place both thumbs flat side by side on the lower third of the sternum (as above) with the tips pointing towards the infant's head. Spread the rest of both hands with the fingers together to encircle the lower part of the infant's rib cage with the tips of the fingers supporting the infant's back. Press down on the lower sternum with the two thumbs to depress it approximately one third of the depth of the infant's chest.

To perform chest compression in children over 1 year of age, place the heel of one hand over the lower third of the sternum (as above) (Figures 6.5 and 6.6). Lift the fingers to ensure that pressure is not applied over the child's ribs. Position yourself vertically above the victim's chest and, with your arm straight, compress the sternum to depress it by approximately one third of the depth of the chest. In larger children or for small rescuers, this is achieved most easily by using both hands with the fingers interlocked.

8. Continue resuscitation until
   - the child shows signs of life (spontaneous respiration, pulse, movement)
   - qualified help arrives
   - you become exhausted

When to call for assistance

It is vital for rescuers to get help as quickly as possible when a child collapses.

- When more than one rescuer is available, one starts resuscitation while another rescuer goes for assistance.
- If only one rescuer is present, undertake resuscitation for about 1 min before going for assistance. To minimise interruption in CPR, it may be possible to carry an infant or small child while summoning help.
- The only exception to performing 1 min of CPR before going for help is in the case of a child with a witnessed, sudden collapse when the rescuer is alone. In this case cardiac arrest is likely to be arrhythmogenic in origin and the child will need defibrillation. Seek help immediately if there is no one to go for you.

Recovery position

An unconscious child whose airway is clear, and who is breathing spontaneously, should be turned on his side into the recovery position. There are several

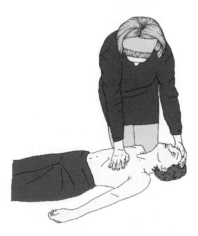

Figure 6.5 Chest compression with one hand — child. © 2005 ERC.

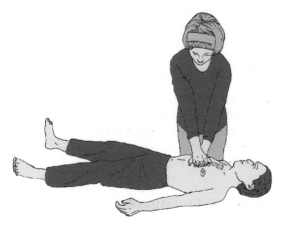

Figure 6.6 Chest compression with two hands — child. © 2005 ERC.

recovery positions; each has its advocates. There are important principles to be followed.

- Place the child in as near true lateral position as possible, with his mouth dependent to enable free drainage of fluid.
- The position should be stable. In an infant this may require the support of a small pillow or a rolled-up blanket placed behind the back to maintain the position.
- Avoid any pressure on the chest that impairs breathing.
- It should be possible to turn the child onto his side and to return him back easily and safely, taking into consideration the possibility of cervical spine injury.
- Ensure the airway can be observed and accessed easily.
- The adult recovery position is suitable for use in children.

Foreign-body airway obstruction (FBAO)

No new evidence on this subject was presented during the 2005 Consensus Conference. Back blows, chest thrusts and abdominal thrusts all increase intrathoracic pressure and can expel foreign bodies from the airway. In half of the episodes, more than one technique is needed to relieve the obstruction.[41] There are no data to indicate which measure should be used first or in which order they should be applied. If one is unsuccessful, try the others in rotation until the object is cleared.

The International Guidelines 2000 algorithm is difficult to teach and knowledge retention poor. The FBAO algorithm for children has been simplified and aligned with the adult version (Figure 6.7). This should improve skill retention and encourage people, who might otherwise have been reluctant, to perform FBAO manoeuvres on children.

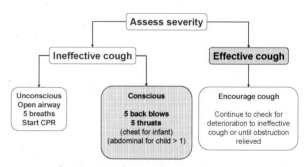

Figure 6.7 Paediatric foreign body airway obstruction algorithm.

The most significant difference from the adult algorithm is that abdominal thrusts should not be used to treat choking infants. Although abdominal thrusts have caused injuries in all age groups, the risk is particularly high in infants and very young children. This is because of the horizontal position of the ribs, which leaves the upper abdominal viscera much more exposed to trauma. For this reason, the guidelines for the treatment of FBAO are different between infants and children.

Recognition of FBAO

When a foreign body enters the airway, the child reacts immediately by coughing in an attempt to expel it. A spontaneous cough is likely to be more effective and safer than any manoeuvre a rescuer might perform. However, if coughing is absent or ineffective and the object completely obstructs the airway, the child will rapidly become asphyxiated. Active interventions to relieve FBAO are therefore required only when coughing becomes ineffective, but they then need to be commenced rapidly and confidently.

The majority of choking events in infants and children occur during play or eating episodes when a carer is usually present; thus, the events are frequently witnessed and interventions are usually initiated when the child is conscious.

Foreign-body airway obstruction is characterized by the sudden onset of respiratory distress associated with coughing, gagging or stridor. Similar signs and symptoms may be associated with other causes of airway obstruction, such as laryngitis or epiglottitis, which require different management. Suspect FBAO if the onset was very sudden and there are no other signs of illness and if there are clues to alert the rescuer, e.g. a history of eating or playing with small items immediately before the onset of symptoms.

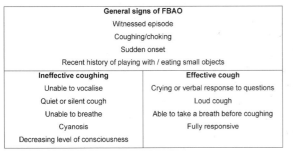

General signs of FBAO	
Witnessed episode	
Coughing/choking	
Sudden onset	
Recent history of playing with / eating small objects	
Ineffective coughing	**Effective cough**
Unable to vocalise	Crying or verbal response to questions
Quiet or silent cough	Loud cough
Unable to breathe	Able to take a breath before coughing
Cyanosis	Fully responsive
Decreasing level of consciousness	

Relief of FBAO

1. Safety and summoning assistance

Safety is paramount: rescuers must not place themselves in danger and should consider the safest

treatment of the choking child.

- If the child is coughing effectively, no external manoeuvre is necessary. Encourage the child to cough, and monitor continually.
- If the child's coughing is (or is becoming) ineffective, shout for help immediately and determine the child's conscious level.

2. Conscious child with FBAO

- If the child is still conscious but has absent or ineffective coughing, give back blows.
- If back blows do not relieve the FBAO, give chest thrusts to infants or abdominal thrusts to children. These manoeuvres create an 'artificial cough' to increase intrathoracic pressure and dislodge the foreign body.

Back blows. Back blows in the infant are performed as follows.

- Support the infant in a head downwards, prone position, to enable gravity to assist removal of the foreign body.
- A seated or kneeling rescuer should be able to support the infant safely across their lap.
- Support the infant's head by placing the thumb of one hand at the angle of the lower jaw, and one or two fingers from the same hand at the same point on the other side of the jaw.
- Do not compress the soft tissues under the infant's jaw, as this will exacerbate the airway obstruction.
- Deliver up to five sharp back blows with the heel of one hand in the middle of the back between the shoulder blades.
- The aim is to relieve the obstruction with each blow rather than to give all five blows.

Back blows in the child over 1 year of age are performed as follows.

- Back blows are more effective if the child is positioned head down.
- A small child may be placed across the rescuer's lap, as with the infant.
- If this is not possible, support the child in a forward-leaning position and deliver the back blows from behind.

If back blows fail to dislodge the object, and the child is still conscious, use chest thrusts for infants or abdominal thrusts for children. Do not use abdominal thrusts (Heimlich manoeuvre) in infants.

Chest thrusts for infants.

- Turn the infant into a head-downwards supine position. This is achieved safely by placing the free arm along the infant's back and encircling the occiput with the hand.
- Support the infant down your arm, which is placed down (or across) your thigh.
- Identify the landmark for chest compressions (lower sternum approximately a finger's breadth above the xiphisternum).
- Give five chest thrusts; these are similar to chest compressions but sharper and delivered at a slower rate.

Abdominal thrusts for children over 1 year.

- Stand or kneel behind the child; place your arms under the child's arms and encircle his torso.
- Clench your fist and place it between the umbilicus and xiphisternum.
- Grasp this hand with the other hand and pull sharply inwards and upwards.
- Repeat up to five times.
- Ensure that pressure is not applied to the xiphoid process or the lower rib cage; this might cause abdominal trauma.

Following the chest or abdominal thrusts, reassess the child. If the object has not been expelled and the victim is still conscious, continue the sequence of back blows and chest (for infant) or abdominal (for children) thrusts. Call out, or send, for help if it is still not available. Do not leave the child at this stage.

If the object is expelled successfully, assess the child's clinical condition. It is possible that part of the object may remain in the respiratory tract and cause complications. If there is any doubt, seek medical assistance. Abdominal thrusts may cause internal injuries, and all victims so treated should be examined by a medical practitioner.[42]

3. Unconscious child with FBAO

If the child with FBAO is, or becomes, unconscious, place him on a firm, flat surface. Call out, or send, for help if it is still not available. Do not leave the child at this stage; proceed as follows.

- Open the mouth and look for any obvious object. If an object is seen, make an attempt to remove it with a single finger sweep. Do not attempt blind or repeated finger sweeps; these can impact the object more deeply into the pharynx and cause injury.
- Open the airway using a head tilt and/or chin lift and attempt five rescue breaths. Assess the effectiveness of each breath; if a breath does not make the chest rise, reposition the head before making the next attempt.
- Attempt five rescue breaths and, if there is no response (moving, coughing, spontaneous breaths), proceed to chest compressions without further assessment of the circulation.
- Follow the sequence for single-rescuer CPR (step 7b above) for approximately 1 min before summoning the EMS (if this has not already been done by someone else).
- When the airway is opened for attempted delivery of rescue breaths, look to see if the foreign body can be seen in the mouth.
- If an object is seen, attempt to remove it with a single finger sweep.
- If it appears the obstruction has been relieved, open and check the airway as above; deliver rescue breaths if the child is not breathing.
- If the child regains consciousness and exhibits spontaneous effective breathing, place him in a safe position lying on his side and monitor breathing and conscious level while awaiting the arrival of the EMS.

6b Paediatric advanced life support

Prevention of cardiopulmonary arrest

In children, secondary cardiopulmonary arrests, caused by either circulatory or respiratory failure, are more frequent than primary arrests caused by arrhythmias.[9,12,43–46] So-called 'asphyxial arrests' or respiratory arrests are also more common in young adulthood (e.g., trauma, drowning, poisoning).[47,48] The outcome from cardiopulmonary arrests in children is poor; identification of the antecedent stages of cardiac or respiratory failure is a priority, as effective early intervention may be life saving.

The order of assessment and intervention for any seriously ill or injured child follows the ABC principles.

- A indicates airway (Ac for airway and cervical spine stabilisation for the injured child).
- B indicates breathing.
- C indicates circulation.

Interventions are made at each step of the assessment as abnormalities are identified; the next step of the assessment is not started until the preceding abnormality has been managed and corrected if possible.

Diagnosing respiratory failure: assessment of A and B

The first steps in the assessment of the seriously ill or injured child are the management of the airway and breathing. Abnormalities in airway patency and breathing lead to respiratory failure. Signs of respiratory failure are

- respiratory rate outside the normal range for the child's age—either too fast or too slow
- initially increasing work of breathing which may progress to inadequate/decreased work of breathing, additional noises such as stridor, wheeze or grunting, or the loss of breath sounds
- cyanosis (without/with supplemental oxygen)

There may be associated signs in other organ systems affected by inadequate ventilation and oxygenation; these are detectable in the C steps of assessment, such as

- increasing tachycardia progressing to bradycardia (this latter sign being an ominous indicator of the loss of compensatory mechanisms)
- alteration in the level of consciousness

Diagnosing circulatory failure: assessment of C

Shock is characterised by a mismatch between metabolic tissue demand and delivery of oxygen and nutrients by the circulation.[49] Physiological compensatory mechanisms lead to changes in the heart rate, in the systemic vascular resistance (which commonly increases as an adaptive response) and in tissue and organ perfusion. Signs of circulatory failure are

- increased heart rate (bradycardia is an ominous sign, heralding physiological decompensation)
- decreased systemic blood pressure
- decreased peripheral perfusion (prolonged capillary refill time, decreased skin temperature, pale or mottled skin)
- weak or absent peripheral pulses
- decreased or increased preload
- decreased urine output and metabolic acidosis

Other systems may be affected, for example

- respiratory rate may be increased initially, becoming bradypnoeic with decompensated shock

- level of consciousness may decrease because of poor cerebral perfusion

Diagnosing cardiopulmonary arrest

Signs of cardiopulmonary arrest include

- unresponsiveness
- apnoea or gasping respiratory pattern
- absent circulation
- pallor or deep cyanosis

In the absence of 'signs of life', search for a central pulse or cardiac sounds (by direct chest auscultation) for a maximum of 10 s, before starting CPR. If there is any doubt, start CPR.[50–53]

Management of respiratory and circulatory failure

A and B

Open the airway and ensure adequate ventilation and oxygenation.

- Deliver high-flow oxygen.
- Achieving adequate ventilation and oxygenation may include the use of airway adjuncts, bag-mask ventilation (BMV), use of a laryngeal mask airway (LMA), securing a definitive airway by tracheal intubation and positive pressure ventilation.
- In rare, extreme circumstances, a surgical airway may be required.

C

Establish cardiac monitoring.

- Secure vascular access to the circulation. This may be via peripheral or central intravenous (IV) or by intraosseous (IO) cannulation.
- Give a fluid bolus and/or inotropes as required.

Assess and re-assess the child continuously, each time commencing at Airway before Breathing, thereafter moving onto the Circulation

Airway

Open the airway using basic life support techniques. Oropharyngeal and nasopharyngeal airways adjuncts can help maintain the airway. Use the oropharyngeal airway only in the unconscious child, in whom there is no gag reflex. Use the appropriate size, to avoid pushing the tongue backward and obstructing the epiglottis, or directly compressing the glottic area. The soft palate in the child can be damaged by insertion of the oropharygneal airway; avoid this by inserting the oropharygneal airway under direct vision and passing it over a tongue depressor or laryngoscope. The nasopharyngeal airway is tolerated better in the conscious child (who has an effective gag reflex), but should not be used if there is a basal skull fracture or a coagulopathy. These simple airway adjuncts do not protect the airway from aspiration of secretions, blood or stomach contents.

Laryngeal mask airway

The LMA is an acceptable initial airway device for providers experienced in its use. It may be particularly helpful in airway obstruction caused by upper airway abnormalities. The LMA does not, however, protect the airway from aspiration of secretions, blood or stomach contents, and therefore close observation is required. LMA use is associated with a higher incidence of complications in small children compared with adults.[54]

Tracheal intubation

Tracheal intubation is the most secure and effective way to establish and maintain the airway, prevent gastric distension, protect the lungs against pulmonary aspiration, enable optimal control of the airway pressure and provide positive end expiratory pressure (PEEP). The oral route is preferable during resuscitation. Oral intubation is usually quicker and is associated with fewer complications than nasal placement. The judicious use of anaesthetics, sedatives and neuromuscular blocking drugs is indicated in the conscious child to avoid multiple intubation attempts or intubation failure.[55–65] The anatomy of a child's airway differs significantly from that of an adult; hence, intubation of a child requires special training and experience. Check that tracheal tube placement is correct by clinical examination and end tidal capnography. The tracheal tube must be secured, and monitoring of the vital signs is essential.[66]

It is also essential to plan an alternative airway management technique in case the trachea cannot be intubated.

Rapid sequence induction and intubation. The child who is in cardiopulmonary arrest and deep coma does not require sedation or analgesia to be intubated; otherwise, intubation must be preceded by oxygenation, rapid sedation, analgesia and the use of neuromuscular blocking drugs to minimise intubation complications and failure.[63] The intuba-

tor must be experienced and familiar with rapid-sequence induction drugs.

Tracheal tube sizes. The tracheal tube internal diameters (ID) for different ages are

- for neonates, 2.5–3.5 mm according to the formula (gestational age in weeks 10)
- for infants, 4 or 4.5 mm
- for children older than 1 year, according to the formula [(age in years/4) + 4]

Tracheal tube size estimation according the length of the child's body as measured by resuscitation tapes is more accurate than using the above formulae.[67]

Cuffed versus uncuffed tracheal tubes. In the prehospital setting, an uncuffed tracheal tube may be preferable when using sizes of up to 5.5 mm ID (i.e., for children up to 8 years). In hospital, a cuffed tracheal tube may be useful in certain circumstances, e.g. in cases of poor lung compliance, high airway resistance or large glottic air leak.[68–70] The correctly sized cuffed tracheal tube is as safe as an uncuffed tube for infants and children (not for neonates), provided attention is paid to its placement, size and cuff inflation pressure; excessive cuff pressure can lead to ischaemic necrosis of the surrounding laryngeal tissue and stenosis. Maintain the cuff inflation pressure below 20 cmH$_2$O and check it regularly.[71]

Confirmation of correct tracheal tube placement. Displaced, misplaced or obstructed tubes occur frequently in the intubated child and are associated with increased risk of death.[72,73] No single technique is 100% reliable for distinguishing oesophageal from tracheal intubation.[74–76] Assessment of the correct tracheal tube position is made by

- observation of the tube passing beyond the vocal cords
- observation of symmetrical chest wall movement during positive pressure ventilation
- observation of mist in the tube during the expiratory phase of ventilation
- absence of gastric distension
- equal air entry heard on bilateral auscultation of both axillae and apices of the chest
- absence of air entry into the stomach on auscultation
- detection of end-tidal CO$_2$ if the child has a perfusing rhythm (this may be seen with effective CPR)
- improvement or stabilisation of SpO$_2$ to the expected range

- improvement of heart rate towards the age-expected value (or remaining within the normal range)

If the child is in cardiopulmonary arrest and exhaled CO_2 is not detected, or if there is any doubt, confirm tracheal tube position by direct laryngoscopy. After correct placement and confirmation, secure the tracheal tube and reassess its position. Maintain the child's head in neutral position; flexion of the head drives the tube further into the trachea whereas extension may pull it out of the airway.[77] Confirm the position of the tracheal tube at mid trachea by plain chest radiograph; the tracheal tube tip should be at the level of the 2nd or 3rd thoracic vertebra.

DOPES is a useful acronym for the causes of sudden deterioration in an intubated child

- D: displacement of the tracheal tube
- O: obstruction of the tracheal tube
- P: pneumothorax
- E: equipment failure (source of gas, BMV, ventilator, etc.)
- S: stomach (gastric distension may alter diaphragm mechanics)

Breathing

Oxygenation

Use oxygen at the highest concentration (i.e., 100%) during resuscitation. Once circulation is restored, give sufficient oxygen to maintain peripheral oxygen saturation at or above 95%.[78,79]

Studies in neonates suggest some advantages to using room air during resuscitation, but the evidence as yet is inconclusive (see Section 6c).[80–83] In the older child, there is no evidence for any such advantages, so use 100% oxygen for resuscitation.

Ventilation

Healthcare providers commonly provide excessive ventilation to victims of cardiopulmonary or respiratory arrest, and this may be detrimental. Hyperventilation causes increased thoracic pressure, decreased cerebral and coronary perfusion, and poorer survival rates in animals and adults.[84–89] The ideal tidal volume should achieve modest chest wall rise. Use a ratio of 15 chest compressions to 2 ventilations (a lone rescuer may use 30:2); the correct compression rate is $100\,min^{-1}$.

Once the airway is protected by tracheal intubation, continue positive pressure ventilation at 12–20 breaths min^{-1} without interrupting chest compressions. Take care to ensure that lung infla-

tion is adequate during chest compressions. When circulation is restored, or if the child still has a perfusing rhythm, ventilate at 12–20 breaths min^{-1} to achieve a normal pCO_2. Hyperventilation is harmful.

Bag-mask ventilation. BMV is effective and safe for a child requiring assisted ventilation for a short period, i.e. in the prehospital setting or in an emergency department.[73,90–92] Assess the effectiveness of BMV by observing adequate chest rise, monitoring heart rate, auscultating for breath sounds and measuring peripheral oxygen saturation (SpO_2). Any healthcare provider dealing with children must be able to deliver BMV effectively.

Prolonged ventilation. If prolonged ventilation is required, the benefits of a secured airway probably outweigh the potential risks associated with tracheal intubation.

Monitoring of breathing and ventilation

End tidal CO_2. Monitoring end-tidal CO_2 with a colorimetric detector or capnometer confirms tracheal tube placement in the child weighing more than 2 kg, and may be used in pre- and in-hospital settings, as well as during any transportation of the child.[93–97] A colour change or the presence of a capnographic waveform indicates that the tube is in the tracheobronchial tree, both in the presence of a perfusing rhythm and during cardiopulmonary arrest. Capnography does not rule out intubation of the right mainstem bronchus. The absence of exhaled CO_2 during cardiopulmonary arrest may not be caused by tube misplacement, since a low or absent end-tidal CO_2 may reflect low or absent pulmonary blood flow.[98–101]

Oesophageal detector devices. The self-inflating bulb or aspirating syringe (oesophageal detector device, ODD) may be used for the secondary confirmation of tracheal tube placement in children with a perfusing rhythm.[102,103] There are no studies on the use of ODD in children who are in cardiopulmonary arrest.

Pulse oximetry. Clinical evaluation of the oxygen level is unreliable; therefore monitor the child's peripheral oxygen saturation continuously by pulse oximetry. Pulse oximetry can be unreliable under certain conditions, e.g. if the child is in shock, in cardiopulmonary arrest or has poor peripheral perfusion. Although pulse oximetry is relatively simple, it is a poor guide to tracheal tube displacement; capnography detects tracheal tube dislodgement more rapidly than pulse oximetry.[104]

Circulation

Vascular access

Vascular access is essential to give drugs and fluids and obtain blood samples. Venous access can be difficult to establish during resuscitation of an infant or child.[105] Limit the maximum number of attempts to obtain IV access to three; thereafter, insert an IO needle.[106]

Intraosseous access. IO access is a rapid, safe, and effective route to give drugs, fluids and blood products.[107–113] The onset of action and time to achieve adequate plasma drug concentrations are similar to those provided by central venous access.[114,115] Bone marrow samples can be used to cross-match for blood type or group,[116] for chemical analysis,[117,118] and for blood gas measurement (the values are comparable to central venous blood gases).[117,119,120] Flush each drug with a bolus of normal saline to ensure dispersal beyond the marrow cavity and to achieve faster distribution to the central circulation. Inject large boluses of fluid using manual pressure. Intraosseous access can be maintained until definitive IV access has been established.

Intravenous access. Peripheral IV access provides plasma concentrations of drugs and clinical responses equivalent to central or IO access.[121–125] Central lines provide more secure long-term access[121,122,124,125] but offer no advantages during resuscitation, compared with IO or peripheral IV access.

Tracheal tube access

IV and IO access are better than the tracheal route for giving drugs.[126] Lipid-soluble drugs, such as lidocaine, atropine, adrenaline and naloxone are absorbed via the lower airway.[127–131] Optimal tracheal tube drug doses are unknown because of the great variability of alveolar drug absorption, but the following dosages have been recommended as guidance

- adrenaline, $100\,mcg\,kg^{-1}$
- lidocaine, $2-3\,mg\,kg^{-1}$
- atropine, $30\,mcg\,kg^{-1}$

The optimal dose of naloxone is not known.

Dilute the drug in 5 ml of normal saline and follow administration with five ventilations.[132–134] Do not give non-lipid soluble medications (e.g., glucose, bicarbonate, calcium) via the tracheal tube because they will damage the airway mucosa.

Fluids and drugs

Volume expansion is indicated when a child shows signs of shock in the absence of volume overload.[135] If systemic perfusion is inadequate, give a bolus of $20\,ml\,kg^{-1}$ of an isotonic crystalloid, even if the systemic blood pressure is normal. Following every bolus, re-assess the child's clinical state using ABC, to decide whether a further bolus or other treatment is required.

There are insufficient data to make recommendations about the use of hypertonic saline for shock associated with head injuries or hypovolaemia.[136] There are also insufficient data to recommend delayed fluid resuscitation in the hypotensive child with blunt trauma.[137] Avoid dextrose-containing solutions unless there is hypoglycaemia.[138–141] However, hypoglycaemia must actively be sought and avoided, particularly in the small child or infant.

Adenosine

Adenosine is an endogenous nucleotide which causes a brief atrioventricular (AV) block and impairs accessory bundle re-entry at the level of the AV node. Adenosine is recommended for the treatment of supraventricular tachycardia (SVT).[142] It is safe to use, as it has a short half-life (10 s); give it intravenously via upper limb or central veins, to minimise the time taken to reach the heart. Give adenosine rapidly, followed by a flush of 3–5 ml of normal saline.[143]

Adrenaline (epinephrine)

Adrenaline is an endogenous catecholamine with potent alpha, beta-1 and beta-1 adrenergic actions. It is the essential medication in cardiopulmonary arrest, and is placed prominently in the treatment algorithms for non-shockable and shockable rhythms. Adrenaline induces vasoconstriction, increases diastolic pressure and thereby improves coronary artery perfusion pressure, enhances myocardial contractility, stimulates spontaneous contractions and increases the amplitude and frequency of VF, so increasing the likelihood of successful defibrillation. The recommended IV/IO dose of adrenaline in children is $10\,mcg\,kg^{-1}$. The dose of adrenaline given via the tracheal tube is ten times this ($100\,mcg\,kg^{-1}$).[127,144–146] If needed, give further doses of adrenaline every 3–5 min. The use of higher doses of adrenaline via the IV or IO route is not recommended routinely, as it does not improve survival or neurological outcome after cardiopulmonary arrest.[147–150]

Once spontaneous circulation is restored, a continuous infusion of adrenaline may be required. Its haemodynamic effects are dose related; there is also considerable variability between children in response, therefore, titrate the infusion dose to the desired effect. High infusion rates may cause excessive vasoconstriction, compromising extremity, mesenteric, and renal blood flow. High-dose adrenaline may cause severe hypertension and tachyarrhythmias.[151]

To avoid tissue damage it is essential to give adrenaline through a secure intravascular line (IV or IO). Adrenaline and other catecholamines are inactivated by alkaline solutions and should never be mixed with sodium bicarbonate.[152]

Amiodarone

Amiodarone is a non-competitive inhibitor of adrenergic receptors; it depresses conduction in myocardial tissue and therefore slows AV conduction and prolongs the QT interval and the refractory period. Except when given for the treatment of refractory VF/pulseless VT, amiodarone must be injected slowly (over 10–20 min) with systemic blood pressure and ECG monitoring to avoid fast-infusion-related hypotension. This side effect is less common with the aqueous solution.[153] Other rare but significant adverse effects are bradycardia and polymorphic VT.[154]

Atropine

Atropine accelerates sinus and atrial pacemakers by blocking the parasympathetic response. It may also increase AV conduction. Small doses (<100 mcg) may cause paradoxical bradycardia.[155]

Calcium

Calcium is essential for myocardial contraction[156,157] but routine use of calcium does not improve the outcome from cardiopulmonary arrest.[158–160]

Glucose

Neonatal, child and adult data show that both hyperglycaemia and hypoglycaemia are associated with poor outcome after cardiopulmonary arrest,[161–163] but it is uncertain if this is causative or merely an association.[164] Check blood or plasma glucose concentration and monitor closely in any ill or injured child, including after cardiac arrest. Do not give glucose-containing fluids during CPR unless hypoglycaemia is present. Avoid hyperglycaemia and hypoglycaemia following return of spontaneous circulation (ROSC).

Magnesium

There is no evidence for giving magnesium routinely during cardiopulmonary arrest.[165] Magnesium treatment is indicated in the child with documented hypomagnesaemia or with torsades de pointes VF, regardless of the cause.[166]

Sodium bicarbonate

Giving sodium bicarbonate routinely during cardiopulmonary arrest and CPR or after ROSC is not recommended.[167,168] After effective ventilation and chest compressions have been achieved and adrenaline given, sodium bicarbonate may be considered for the child who has had a prolonged cardiopulmonary arrest and severe metabolic acidosis. Sodium bicarbonate may also be considered in the case of haemodynamic instability and co-existing hyperkalaemia, or in the management of tricyclic overdose. Excessive quantities of sodium bicarbonate may impair tissue oxygen delivery, produce hypokalaemia, hypernatraemia and hyperosmolality and inactivate catecholamines.

Lidocaine

Lidocaine is less effective than amiodarone for defibrillation-resistant VF/VT in adults,[169] and therefore is not the first-line treatment in defibrillation-resistant VF/VT in children.

Procainamide

Procainamide slows intra-atrial conduction and prolongs the QRS and QT intervals; it can be used in SVT[170,171] or VT[172] resistant to other medications, in the haemodynamically stable child. However, paediatric data are sparse and procainamide should be used cautiously.[173,174] Procainamide is a potent vasodilator and can cause hypotension; infuse it slowly with careful monitoring.[170,175,176]

Vasopressin

Vasopressin is an endogenous hormone that acts at specific receptors, mediating systemic vasoconstriction (via V1 receptor) and the reabsorption of water in the renal tubule (by the V2 receptor).[177] The use of vasopressin for the treatment of cardiac arrest in adults is discussed in detail in Section 4e. There is currently insufficient evidence to support or refute the use of vasopressin as an alternative to, or in combination with, adrenaline in any cardiac arrest rhythm in adults. Thus, there is currently insufficient evidence to recommend the routine use of vasopressin in the child with cardiopulmonary arrest.[178–180]

Defibrillators

Defibrillators are either automatically (such as the AED) or manually operated, and may be capable of delivering either monophasic or biphasic shocks. Manual defibrillators capable of delivering the full energy requirements from neonates upwards must be available within hospitals and in other health-care facilities caring for children at risk of car-diopulmonary arrest. Automated external defibril-lators are preset for all variables, including the energy dose.

Pad/paddle size for defibrillation. The largest possible available paddles should be chosen to pro-vide good contact with the chest wall. The ideal size is unknown, but there should be good separa-tion between the pads.[181,182] Recommended sizes are

- 4.5 cm diameter for infants and children weighing <10 kg
- 8–12 cm diameter for children >10 kg (older than 1 year)

To decrease skin and thoracic impedance, an electrically conducting interface is required between the skin and the paddles. Preformed gel pads or self-adhesive defibrillation electrodes are effective. Do not use ultrasound gel, saline-soaked gauze, alcohol-soaked gauze/pads or ultrasound gel.

Position of the paddles. Apply the paddles firmly to the bare chest in the anterolateral position, one paddle placed below the right clavicle and the other in the left axilla (Figure 6.8). If the paddles are too large, and there is a danger of charge arcing across the paddles, one should be placed on the upper back, below the left scapula, and the other on the front, to the left of the sternum. This is known as the anteroposterior position.

Optimal paddle force. To decrease transthoracic impedance during defibrillation, apply a force of 3 kg for children weighing <10 kg, and 5 kg for larger children.[183,184]

Energy dose in children. The ideal energy dose for safe and effective defibrillation is unknown.

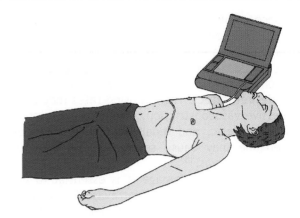

Figure 6.8 Paddle positions for defibrillation — child. © 2005 ERC.

Biphasic shocks are at least as effective and pro-duce less post-shock myocardial dysfunction than monophasic shocks.[33,34,37–40] Animal models show better results with paediatric doses of 3–4 J kg^{-1} than with lower doses,[34,37] or adult doses.[35] Doses larger than 4 J kg^{-1} (as much as 9 J kg^{-1}) have defib-rillated children effectively with negligible side effects.[27,36] When using a manual defibrillator, use 4 J kg^{-1} (biphasic or monophasic waveform) for the first and subsequent shocks.

If no manual defibrillator is available, use an AED that can recognise paediatric shockable rhythms.[29,30,185] This AED should be equipped with a dose attenuator which decreases the delivered energy to a lower dose more suitable for children aged 1–8 years (50–75 J).[31] If such an AED in not available, in an emergency use a standard AED and the preset adult energy levels. For children weigh-ing more than 25 kg (above 8 years), use a standard AED with standard paddles. There is currently insuf-ficient evidence to support a recommendation for or against the use of AEDs in children less than 1 year.

Management of cardiopulmonary arrest

A B C

Commence and continue with basic life support (Figure 6.9).

A and B

Oxygenate and ventilate with BMV.

- Provide positive pressure ventilation with a high inspired oxygen concentration.
- Give five rescue breaths followed by external chest compression and positive pressure ventila-

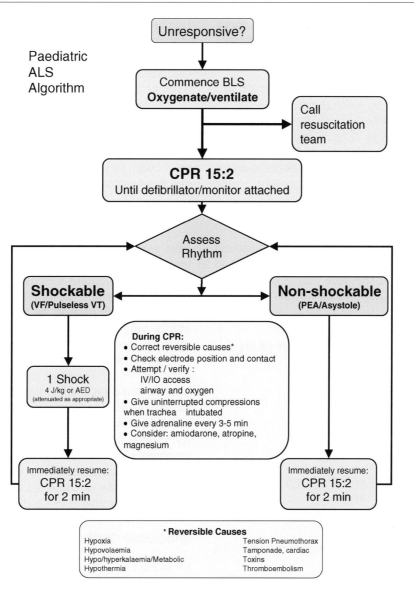

Figure 6.9 Paediatric advanced life support algorithm.

tion in the ratio of 15:2 (lone rescuer may use 30:2).

- Avoid rescuer fatigue by changing the rescuer performing chest compressions frequently.
- Establish cardiac monitoring.

C

Assess cardiac rhythm and signs of circulation (±check for a central pulse for no more than 10 s).

Asystole, pulseless electrical activity (PEA)—non-shockable

- Give adrenaline, 10 mcg kg^{-1} IV or IO, and repeat every 3—5 min.

- If no vascular access is available and a tracheal tube is in situ, give adrenaline, 100 mcg kg^{-1}, via this route until IV/IO access is obtained.
- Identify and treat any reversible causes (4Hs & 4Ts).

VF/pulseless VT—shockable

- Attempt defibrillation immediately (4 J kg^{-1} for all shocks).
- Resume CPR as soon as possible.
- After 2 min, check the cardiac rhythm on the monitor.
- Give second shock if still in VF/pulseless VT.

- Immediately resume CPR for 2 min and check monitor; if no change, give adrenaline followed immediately by a 3rd shock.
- CPR for 2 min.
- Give amiodarone if still in VF/pulseless VT followed immediately by a 4th shock.
- Give adrenaline every 3—5 min during CPR.
- If the child remains in VF/pulseless VT, continue to alternate shocks with 2 min of CPR.
- If signs of life become evident, check the monitor for an organised rhythm; if this is present, check for a central pulse.
- Identify and treat any reversible causes (4Hs & 4Ts).
- If defibrillation was successful but VF/pulseless VT recurs, resume CPR, give amiodarone and defibrillate again at the dose that was effective previously. Start a continuous infusion of amiodarone.

Reversible causes of cardiac arrest (4 Hs and 4 Ts)

- Hypoxia
- Hypovolaemia
- Hyper/hypokalaemia
- Hypothermia
- Tension pneumothorax
- Tamponade (coronary or pulmonary)
- Toxic/therapeutic disturbances
- Thrombosis (coronary or pulmonary)

Sequence of events in cardiopulmonary arrest

- When a child becomes unresponsive, without signs of life (no breathing, cough or any detectable movement), start CPR immediately.
- Provide BMV with 100% oxygen.
- Commence monitoring. Send for a manual or automatic external defibrillator (AED) to identify and treat shockable rhythms as quickly as possible.

In the less common circumstance of a witnessed sudden collapse, early activation of emergency services and getting an AED may be more appropriate; start CPR as soon as possible.

Rescuers must perform CPR with minimal interruption until attempted defibrillation.

Cardiac monitoring

Position the cardiac monitor leads or defibrillation paddles as soon as possible, to enable differentiation between a shockable and a non-shockable cardiac rhythm. Invasive monitoring of systemic blood pressure may help to improve effectiveness of chest compression,[186] but must not delay the provision of basic or advanced resuscitation.

Shockable rhythms comprise pulseless VT and VF. These rhythms are more likely in the child who presents with sudden collapse. Non-shockable rhythms comprise PEA, bradycardia (<60 beats min^{-1} with no signs of circulation) and asystole. PEA and bradycardia often have wide QRS complexes.

Non-shockable rhythms

Most cardiopulmonary arrests in children and adolescents are of respiratory origin.[19,44,187—189] A period of immediate CPR is therefore mandatory in this age group, before searching for an AED or manual defibrillator, as their immediate availability will not improve the outcome of a respiratory arrest.[11,13] Bystander CPR is associated with a better neurological outcome in adults and children.[9,10,190] The most common ECG patterns in infants, children and adolescents with cardiopulmonary arrest are asystole and PEA. PEA is characterised by organised, wide complex electrical activity, usually at a slow rate, and absent pulses. PEA commonly follows a period of hypoxia or myocardial ischaemia, but occasionally can have a reversible cause (i.e., one of the 4 H's and 4 T'S) that led to a sudden impairment of cardiac output.

Shockable rhythms

VF occurs in 3.8—19% of cardiopulmonary arrests in children[9,45,188,189]; the incidence of VF/pulseless VT increases with age.[185,191] The primary determinant of survival from VF/pulseless VT cardiopulmonary arrest is the time to defibrillation. Prehospital defibrillation within the first 3 min of witnessed adult VF arrest results in >50% survival. However, the success of defibrillation decreases dramatically as the time to defibrillation increases; for every minute delay in defibrillation (without any CPR), survival decreases by 7—10%. Survival after more than 12 min of VF in adult victims is <5%.[192] Cardiopulmonary resuscitation provided before defibrillation for response intervals longer than 5 min improved outcome in some studies,[193,194] but not in others.[195]

Drugs in shockable rhythms

Adrenaline is given every 3—5 min by the IV or IO route in preference to the tracheal tube route. Amiodarone is indicated in defibrillation-resistant

VF/pulseless VT. Experimental and clinical experience with amiodarone in children is scarce; evidence from adult studies[169,196,197] demonstrates increased survival to hospital admission, but not to hospital discharge. One paediatric case series demonstrates the effectiveness of amiodarone for life-threatening ventricular arrhythmias.[198] Therefore, IV amiodarone has a role in the treatment of defibrillation refractory or recurrent VF/pulseless VT in children.

Arrhythmias

Unstable arrhythmias

Check the central pulse of any child with an arrhythmia; if the pulse is absent, proceed to treating the child as being in cardiopulmonary arrest. If the child has a central pulse, evaluate his haemodynamic status. Whenever the haemodynamic status is compromised, the first steps are as follows.

- Open the airway.
- Assist ventilation and give oxygen.
- Attach ECG monitor or defibrillator and assess the cardiac rhythm.
- Evaluate if the rhythm is slow or fast for the child's age.
- Evaluate if the rhythm is regular or irregular.
- Measure QRS complex (narrow complexes, <0.08 s duration; large complexes, >0.08 s).
- The treatment options are dependent on the child's haemodynamic stability.

Bradycardia

Bradycardia is caused commonly by hypoxia, acidosis and severe hypotension; it may progress to cardiopulmonary arrest. Give 100% oxygen, and positive pressure ventilation if required, to any child presenting with bradyarrhythmia and circulatory failure.

If a poorly perfused child has a heart rate <60 beats min^{-1}, and does not respond rapidly to ventilation with oxygen, start chest compressions and give adrenaline. If the bradycardia is caused by vagal stimulation, provide ventilation with 100% oxygen and give atropine, before giving adrenaline.

A cardiac pacemaker is useful only in cases of AV block or sinus node dysfunction unresponsive to oxygenation, ventilation, chest compressions and other medications; the pacemaker is not effective in asystole or arrhythmias caused by hypoxia or ischaemia.[199]

Tachycardia

Narrow complex tachycardia. If supraventricular tachycardia (SVT) is the likely rhythm, vagal manoeuvres (Valsalva or diving reflex) may be used in haemodynamically stable children. The manoeuvres can be used in unstable children if they do not delay chemical or electrical cardioversion.[200] If the child is haemodynamically unstable, omit vagal manoeuvres and attempt electrical cardioversion immediately. Adenosine is usually effective in converting SVT into sinus rhythm. Adenosine is given by rapid IV injection as closely as practical to the heart (see above), followed immediately by a bolus of normal saline.

Electrical cardioversion (synchronised with R wave) is indicated in the haemodynamically compromised child, in whom vascular access is not available, or in whom adenosine has failed to convert the rhythm. The first energy dose for electrical cardioversion of SVT is 0.5—1 J kg^{-1} and the second dose is 2 J kg^{-1}. If unsuccessful, give amiodarone or procainamide under guidance from a paediatric cardiologist or intensivist before the third attempt.

Amiodarone has been shown to be effective in the treatment of SVT in several paediatric studies.[198,201—207] However, since most studies of the use of amiodarone in narrow-complex tachycardias have been for junctional ectopic tachycardia in postoperative children, the applicability of its use in all cases of SVT may be limited. If the child is haemodynamically stable, early consultation with an expert is recommended before giving amiodarone.

Wide complex tachycardia. In children, wide-QRS-complex tachycardia is more likely to be supraventricular than ventricular in origin.[208] However, wide-QRS-complex tachycardia, although uncommon, must be considered to be VT in haemodynamically unstable children until proven otherwise. VT occurs most often in the child with underlying heart disease (e.g., after cardiac surgery, cardiomyopathy, myocarditis, electrolyte disorders, prolonged QT interval, central intracardiac catheter). Synchronised cardioversion is the treatment of choice for unstable VT with a pulse. Consider antiarrhythmic therapy if a second cardioversion dose is unsuccessful or if VT recurs. Amiodarone has been shown to be safe and effective in treating paediatric arrhythmias.[198,202,203,209]

Stable arrhythmias

Contact an expert before initiating therapy, while maintaining the child's ABC. Depending on the child's clinical history, presentation and ECG diagnosis, a child with stable, wide-QRS-complex tachycardia may be treated for SVT and be given vagal manoeuvres or adenosine. Otherwise, consider amiodarone as a treatment option; similarly, consider amiodarone if the diagnosis of VT is confirmed by ECG. Procainamide may also be considered in stable SVT refractory to vagal manoeuvres and adenosine[210–212] as well as in stable VT.[172,213,214] Do not give procainamide with amiodarone.

Post-arrest management

Myocardial dysfunction is common after cardiopulmonary resuscitation.[215,216] Vasoactive drugs may improve the child's post-arrest haemodynamic values, but the drugs must be titrated according to the clinical condition. They must be given continuously through an IV line.

Temperature control and management

Hypothermia is common in the child following cardiopulmonary resuscitation.[217] Central hypothermia (32–34 °C) may be beneficial, whereas fever may be detrimental to the injured brain of survivors. Although there are no paediatric studies, mild hypothermia has an acceptable safety profile in adults[218,219] and neonates;[220–224] it could increase the number of neurologically intact survivors.

A child who regains a spontaneous circulation but remains comatose after cardiopulmonary arrest may benefit from being cooled to a core temperature of 32–34 °C for 12–24 h. The successfully resuscitated child with hypothermia and ROSC should not be actively rewarmed unless the core temperature is below 32 °C. Following a period of mild hypothermia, rewarm the child slowly at 0.25–0.5 °C h^{-1}.

There are several methods to induce, monitor and maintain body temperature in children. External and/or internal cooling techniques can be used to initiate cooling.[225–227] Shivering can be prevented by deep sedation and neuromuscular blockade. Complications can occur and include an increased risk of infection, cardiovascular instability, coagulopathy, hyperglycaemia and electrolyte abnormalities.[228,229]

The optimum target temperature, rate of cooling, duration of hypothermia and rate of rewarming after deliberate cooling have yet to be determined; currently, no specific protocol for children can be recommended.

Fever is common following cardiopulmonary resuscitation; it is associated with a poor neurological outcome,[230–232] the risk of which increases with each degree of body temperature greater than 37 °C.[230] There are limited experimental data suggesting that the treatment of fever with antipyretics and/or physical cooling reduces neuronal damage.[233,234] Antipyretics and accepted drugs to treat fever are safe; therefore, use them to treat fever aggressively.

Prognosis of cardiopulmonary arrest

There are no simple guidelines to determine when resuscitative efforts become futile. After 20 min of resuscitation, the team leader of the resuscitation team should consider whether or not to stop.[187,235–239] The relevant considerations in the decision to continue the resuscitation include the cause of arrest,[45,240] pre-existing conditions, whether the arrest was witnessed, the duration of untreated cardiopulmonary arrest (''no flow''), the effectiveness and duration of CPR (''low flow''), the promptness of extracorporeal life support for a reversible disease process[241–243] and associated special circumstances (e.g, icy water drowning,[9,244] exposure to toxic drugs).

Parental presence

The majority of parents would like to be present during resuscitation and when any procedure is carried out on their child.[245–255]. Parents witnessing their child's resuscitation can see that everything possible has been attempted.[256–260] Furthermore, they may have the opportunity to say goodbye to their child; allowing parents to be at the side of their child has been shown to help them gain a realistic view of the attempted resuscitation and the child's death.[261] Families who were present at their child's death showed less anxiety and depression, better adjustment and had an improved grieving process when assessed several months later.[260] Parental presence in the resuscitation room may help healthcare providers maintain their professional behaviour while also helping them to see the child as a human being and a family member.[261]

Family presence guidelines

A dedicated member of the resuscitation team should be present with the parents to explain the process in an empathetic manner, ensuring that the parents do not interfere with or distract the resuscitation. If the presence of the parents is impeding the progress of the resuscitation, they should be sensitively asked to leave. When appropriate, physical contact with the child should be allowed and, wherever possible, the parents should be allowed to be with their dying child at the final moment.[256,261-264]

The leader of the resuscitation team, not the parents, will decide when to stop the resuscitation; this should be expressed with sensitivity and understanding. After the event the team should be debriefed, to enable any concerns to be expressed and for the team to reflect on their clinical practice in a supportive environment.

6c Resuscitation of babies at birth

Introduction

The following guidelines for resuscitation at birth have been developed during the process that culminated in the 2005 International Consensus Conference on Emergency Cardiovascular Care (ECC) and Cardiopulmonary Resuscitation (CPR) Science with Treatment Recommendations.[265] They are an extension of the guidelines already published by the ERC,[2] and take into account recommendations made by other national[266] and international organisations.[267]

The guidelines that follow do not define the only way that resuscitation at birth should be achieved; they merely represent a widely accepted view of how resuscitation at birth can be carried out both safely and effectively.

Preparation

Relatively few babies need any resuscitation at birth. Of those that do need help, the overwhelming majority will require only assisted lung aeration. A small minority may need a brief period of chest compressions in addition to lung aeration. Of 100,000 babies born in Sweden in 1 year, only 10 per 1000 (1%) babies weighing 2.5 kg or more appeared to need resuscitation at delivery.[268] Of those babies receiving resuscitation, 8 per 1000 responded to mask inflation and only 2 per 1000 appeared to need intubation.[268] The same study tried to assess the unexpected need for resuscitation at birth, and found that for low-risk babies, i.e. those born after 32 weeks' gestation and following an apparently normal labour, about 2 per 1000

(0.2%) appeared to need resuscitation at delivery. Of these, 90% responded to mask inflation alone, whereas the remaining 10% appeared not to respond to mask inflation and therefore were intubated at birth.

Resuscitation or specialist help at birth is more likely to be needed by babies with intrapartum evidence of significant fetal compromise, babies delivering before 35 weeks' gestation, babies delivering vaginally by the breech and multiple pregnancies. Although it is often possible to predict the need for resuscitation before a baby is born, this is not always the case. Therefore, personnel trained in newborn life support should be easily available at every delivery and, should there be any need for resuscitation, the care of the baby should be their sole responsibility. One person experienced in tracheal intubation of the newborn should also be easily available for normal low-risk deliveries and, ideally, in attendance for deliveries associated with a high risk for neonatal resuscitation. Local guidelines indicating who should attend deliveries should be developed based on current practice and clinical audit.

An organised programme educating in the standards and skills required for resuscitation of the newborn is therefore essential for any institution in which deliveries occur.

Planned home deliveries

The recommendations for those who should attend a planned home delivery vary from country to country, but the decision to undergo a planned home delivery, once agreed by the medical and midwifery staff, should not compromise the standard of initial resuscitation at birth. There will inevitably be some limitations to resuscitation of a newborn baby in the home because of the distance from further assistance, and this must be made clear to the mother at the time plans for home delivery are made. Ideally, two trained professionals should be present at all home deliveries;[269] one of these must be fully trained and experienced in providing mask ventilation and chest compressions in the newborn.

Equipment and environment

Resuscitation at birth is often a predictable event. It is therefore simpler to prepare the environment and the equipment before delivery of the baby than is the case in adult resuscitation. Resuscitation should ideally take place in a warm, well-lit, draught-free area with a flat resuscitation surface placed below a radiant heater and other resuscitation equipment immediately available. All equipment must be checked daily.

When a birth takes place in a non-designated delivery area, the recommended minimum set of equipment includes a device for safe, assisted lung aeration of an appropriate size for the newborn, warm dry towels and blankets, a clean (sterile) instrument for cutting the umbilical cord and clean gloves for the attendant. It may also be helpful to have a suction device with a suitably sized suction catheter and a tongue depressor (or laryngoscope), to enable the oropharynx to be examined.

Temperature control

Naked, wet, newborn babies cannot maintain their body temperature in a room that feels comfortably warm for adults. Compromised babies are particularly vulnerable.[270] Exposure of the newborn to cold stress will lower arterial oxygen tension[271] and increase metabolic acidosis.[272] Prevent heat loss by

- protecting the baby from draughts
- keeping the delivery room warm
- drying the term baby immediately after delivery. Cover the head and body of the baby, apart from the face, with a warm towel to prevent further heat loss. Alternatively, place the baby skin to skin with the mother and cover both with a towel
- placing the baby on a warm surface under a pre-heated radiant warmer if resuscitation is needed

In very preterm babies (especially below 28 weeks' gestation), drying and wrapping may not be sufficiently effective. A more effective method of keeping these babies warm is to cover the head and body of the baby (apart from the face) with plastic wrapping, without drying the baby beforehand, and then to place the baby so covered under radiant heat.

Initial assessment

The Apgar scoring system was not designed to identify prospectively babies needing resuscitation.[273] Several studies have also suggested that it is highly subjective.[274] However, components of the score, namely respiratory rate, heart rate and colour, if assessed rapidly, can identify babies needing resuscitation.[275] Furthermore, repeated assessment of these components can indicate whether the baby is responding or whether further efforts are needed.

Respiratory activity

Check whether the baby is breathing. If so, evaluate the rate, depth and symmetry of respiration, together with any abnormal breathing pattern such as gasping or grunting.

Heart rate

This is best evaluated by listening to the apex beat with a stethoscope. Feeling the pulse in the base of the umbilical cord is often effective but can be misleading; cord pulsation is only reliable if found to be more than 100 beats min^{-1}.[276]

Colour

A healthy baby is born blue but becomes pink within 30 s of the onset of effective breathing. Observe whether the baby is centrally pink, cyanosed or pale. Peripheral cyanosis is common and does not, by itself, indicate hypoxaemia.

Tone

A very floppy baby is likely to be unconscious and is likely to need respiratory support.

Tactile stimulation

Drying the baby usually produces enough stimulation to induce effective respiration. Avoid more vigorous methods of stimulation. If the baby fails to establish spontaneous and effective respirations following a brief period of stimulation, further support will be required.

Classification according to initial assessment

On the basis of the initial assessment, the babies can usually be divided into four groups.

Group 1:　　　vigorous breathing or crying
　　　　　　　good tone
　　　　　　　rapidly becoming pink
　　　　　　　heart rate higher than 100 beats min^{-1}

This baby requires no intervention other than drying, wrapping in a warm towel and, where appropriate, handing to the mother. The baby will remain warm through skin-to-skin contact with mother under a cover, and may be put to the breast at this stage.

Group 2:   breathing inadequately or apnoeic
                    remaining centrally blue
                    normal or reduced tone
                    heart rate less than 100 beats min^{-1}

This baby may respond to tactile stimulation and/or facial oxygen, but may need mask inflation.

Group 3:   breathing inadequately or apnoeic
                    blue or pale
                    floppy
                    heart rate less than 100 beats min^{-1}

This baby may improve with mask inflation but may also require chest compressions.

Group 4:   breathing inadequately or apnoeic
                    pale
                    floppy
                    no detectable heart rate

This baby will require immediate airway control, lung inflation and ventilation. Once this has been successfully accomplished, the baby may also need chest compressions and perhaps drugs.

There remains a very rare group of babies who, though breathing adequately and with a good heart rate, remain blue. This group includes a range of possible diagnoses such as diaphragmatic hernia, surfactant deficiency, congenital pneumonia, pneumothorax or cyanotic congenital heart disease.

Newborn life support

Commence newborn life support (Figure 6.10) if assessment demonstrates that the baby has failed to establish adequate regular normal breathing, or has a heart rate of less than 100 beats min^{-1}. Opening the airway and aerating the lungs is usually all that is necessary. Furthermore, more complex interventions will be futile unless these two first steps have been successfully completed.

Airway

The baby should be on his or her back with the head in a neutral position (Figure 6.11). A 2-cm thickness of the blanket or towel placed under the baby's shoulder may be helpful in maintaining proper head position. In floppy babies, application of jaw thrust or the use of an appropriately sized oropharyngeal airway may be helpful in opening the airway.

Suction is needed only if there is particulate matter or blood obstructing the airway. Aggressive pharyngeal suction can delay the onset of spontaneous breathing and cause laryngeal spasm and vagal

bradycardia.[277] The presence of thick meconium in a non-vigorous baby is the only indication for considering immediate suction. If suction is required, it is best done under direct vision. Connect a 12—14 FG suction catheter, or a Yankauer sucker, to a suction source not exceeding −100 mmHg.

Breathing

There is currently insufficient evidence to specify the concentration of oxygen to be used when starting resuscitation. After initial steps at birth, if respiratory efforts are absent or inadequate, lung aeration is the priority (Figure 6.12). The primary measure of adequate initial lung inflation is a prompt improvement in heart rate; assess chest wall movement if the heart rate does not improve.

For the first few breaths maintain the initial inflation pressure for 2—3 s. This will help lung expansion. Most babies needing resuscitation at birth will respond with a rapid increase in heart rate within 30 s of lung inflation. If the heart rate increases but the baby is not breathing adequately, continue ventilation at a rate of about 30 breaths min^{-1}, allowing approximately 1 s for each inflation, until there is adequate spontaneous breathing.

Adequate passive ventilation is usually indicated by either a rapidly increasing heart rate or a heart rate that is maintained faster than 100 beats min^{-1}. If the baby does not respond in this way, the most likely reason is inadequate airway control or ventilation. Look for passive chest movement in time with inflation efforts; if these are present, then lung aeration has been achieved. If these are absent, then airway control and lung aeration have not been confirmed. Without adequate lung aeration chest compressions will be ineffective; therefore, confirm lung aeration before progressing to circulatory support. Some practitioners will ensure lung aeration by tracheal intubation, but this requires training and experience to be achieved effectively. If this skill is not available and the heart rate is decreasing, re-evaluate airway position and deliver aeration breaths while summoning a colleague with intubation skills.

Continue ventilatory support until the baby has established normal regular breathing.

Circulatory support

Circulatory support with chest compressions is effective only if the lungs have first been successfully inflated. Give chest compressions if the heart rate is less than 60 beats min^{-1} despite adequate ventilation. The optimal technique is to place the

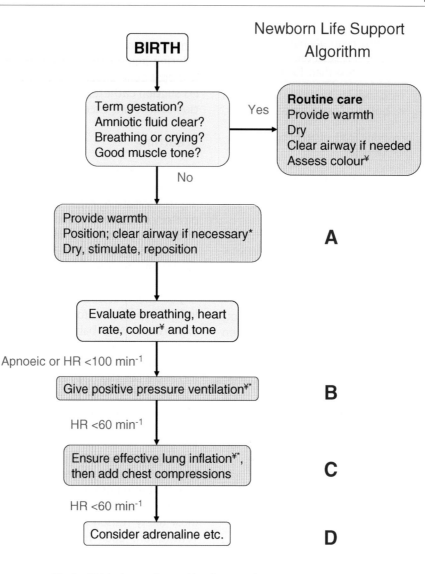

Newborn Life Support Algorithm

BIRTH

Term gestation?
Amniotic fluid clear?
Breathing or crying?
Good muscle tone?

Yes → **Routine care**
Provide warmth
Dry
Clear airway if needed
Assess colour¥

No

Provide warmth
Position; clear airway if necessary*
Dry, stimulate, reposition   **A**

Evaluate breathing, heart
rate, colour¥ and tone

Apnoeic or HR <100 min⁻¹

Give positive pressure ventilation¥*   **B**

HR <60 min⁻¹

Ensure effective lung inflation¥*,
then add chest compressions   **C**

HR <60 min⁻¹

Consider adrenaline etc.   **D**

*Tracheal intubation may be considered at several steps
¥Consider supplemental oxygen at any stage if cyanosis persists

Figure 6.10 Newborn life support algorithm.

two thumbs side by side over the lower third of the sternum, with the fingers encircling the torso and supporting the back (Figure 6.13).[21,22,25,278,279] The lower third of the sternum is compressed to a

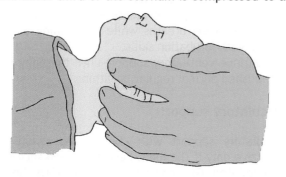

Figure 6.11 Newborn head in neutral position. © 2005 Resuscitation Council (UK).

depth of approximately one third of the anterior-posterior diameter of the chest. A compression to relaxation ratio with a slightly shorter compression than relaxation phase offers theoretical advantages for blood flow in the very young infant.[280] Do not lift the thumbs off the sternum during the relaxation phase, but allow the chest wall to return to its relaxed position between compressions. Use a 3:1 ratio of compressions to ventilations, aiming to achieve approximately 120 events min⁻¹, i.e. approximately 90 compressions and 30 breaths. However, the quality of the compressions and breaths are more important than the rate.[281]

Check the heart rate after about 30 s and periodically thereafter. Discontinue chest compressions when the spontaneous heart rate is faster then 60 beats min⁻¹.

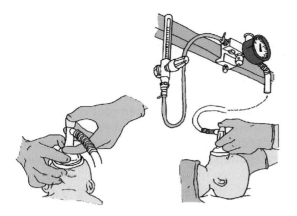

Figure 6.12　Airway and ventilation — newborn. © 2005 Resuscitation Council (UK).

Drugs

Drugs are rarely indicated in resuscitation of the newborn infant. Bradycardia in the newborn infant is usually caused by inadequate lung inflation or profound hypoxia, and establishing adequate ventilation is the most important step to correct it. However, if the heart rate remains less than 60 beats min^{-1} despite adequate ventilation and chest compressions, drugs may be needed. These drugs are presumed to exert their effect by their action on the heart and are being given because cardiac function is inadequate. It is therefore necessary to give them as close to the heart as possible, ideally via a rapidly inserted umbilical venous catheter (Figure 6.14).

Adrenaline

Despite the lack of human data, it is reasonable to continue to use adrenaline when adequate ventilation and chest compressions have failed to increase the heart rate above 60 beats min^{-1}. Use the IV route as soon as venous access is established. The recommended IV dose is 10–30 mcg kg^{-1}. The tracheal route is not recommended (see below) but, if

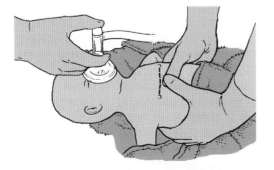

Figure 6.13　Ventilation and chest compression — newborn. © 2005 Resuscitation Council (UK).

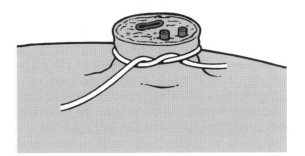

Figure 6.14　Newborn umbilical cord showing the arteries and veins. © 2005 Resuscitation Council (UK).

it is used, it is highly likely that doses of 30 mcg kg^{-1} or less are ineffective. Try a higher dose (up to 100 mcg kg^{-1}). The safety of these higher tracheal doses has not been studied. Do not give high IV doses.

Bicarbonate

If effective spontaneous cardiac output is not restored despite adequate ventilation and adequate chest compressions, reversing intracardiac acidosis may improve myocardial function and achieve a spontaneous circulation. Give 1–2 mmol kg^{-1} IV.

Fluids

Consider volume expansion when there has been suspected blood loss or the infant appears to be in shock (pale, poor perfusion, weak pulse) and has not responded adequately to other resuscitative measures. In the absence of suitable blood (i.e., irradiated and leucocyte-depleted group O Rh-negative blood) isotonic crystalloid rather than albumin is the solution of choice for restoring intravascular volume in the delivery room. Give a bolus of 10–20 ml kg^{-1}.

Stopping resuscitation

Local and national committees will determine the indications for stopping resuscitation. However, data from infants without signs of life from birth lasting at least 10 min or longer show either high mortality or severe neurodevelopmental disability. After 10 min of continuous and adequate resuscitation efforts, discontinuation of resuscitation may be justified if there are no signs of life.

Communication with the parents

It is vitally important that the team caring for the newborn baby informs the parents of the baby's progress. At delivery adhere to the routine local plan and, if possible, hand the baby to the mother at the earliest opportunity. If resuscitation is required, inform the parents of the procedures being undertaken and why they are required.

Decisions to discontinue resuscitation ideally should involve senior paediatric staff. Whenever possible, the decision to attempt resuscitation of an extremely preterm baby should be taken in close consultation with the parents and senior paediatric and obstetric staff. Where a difficulty has been foreseen, for example in the case of severe congenital malformation, the options and prognosis should be discussed with the parents, midwives, obstetricians and birth attendants before delivery.

All discussions and decisions should be carefully recorded in the mother's notes before delivery and also in the baby's records after birth.

Specific questions addressed at the 2005 Consensus Conference

Maintaining normal temperature in preterm infants

Significantly, preterm babies are likely to become hypothermic despite careful application of the traditional techniques for keeping them warm (drying, wrapping and placing under radiant heat).[282] Several randomised controlled trials and observational studies have shown that placing preterm babies under radiant heat and then covering the babies with food-grade plastic wrapping, without drying them, significantly improves temperature on admission to intensive care compared with traditional techniques.[283–285] The baby's temperature must be monitored closely because of the small but described risk of hyperthermia with this technique.[286] All resuscitation procedures, including intubation, chest compression and insertion of lines, can be achieved with the plastic cover in place.

Infants born to febrile mothers have been reported to have a higher incidence of perinatal respiratory depression, neonatal seizures, early mortality and cerebral palsy.[286–288] Animal studies indicate that hyperthermia during or following ischaemia is associated with a progression of cerebral injury.[233,289] Hyperthermia should be avoided.

Meconium

Five years ago, a large randomised controlled study showed that attempting to intubate and aspirate inhaled meconium from the tracheas of vigorous infants at birth was not beneficial.[290] A more recent large multicentre randomised controlled study has now shown that suctioning meconium from the baby's nose and mouth before delivery of the baby's chest (intrapartum suctioning) does not reduce the incidence or severity of meconium aspiration syndrome.[291] Intrapartum suctioning is therefore no longer recommended. Intubation and suction of meconium from the trachea of non-vigorous infants born through meconium-stained liquor is still recommended.

Air or 100% oxygen

Several studies in recent years have raised concerns about the potential adverse effects of 100% oxygen on respiratory physiology and cerebral circulation, and the potential tissue damage from oxygen free radicals. There are also concerns about tissue damage from oxygen deprivation during and following asphyxia. Studies examining blood pressure, cerebral perfusion, and various biochemical measures of cell damage in asphyxiated animals resuscitated with 100% versus 21% oxygen, have shown conflicting results.[292–296] One study of preterm infants (below 33 weeks' gestation) exposed to 80% oxygen found lower cerebral blood flow when compared with those stabilised with 21% oxygen.[297] Some animal data indicate the opposite effect, i.e. reduced blood pressure and cerebral perfusion with air versus 100% oxygen.[292] Meta-analysis of four human studies demonstrated a reduction in mortality and no evidence of harm in infants resuscitated with air versus those resuscitated with 100% oxygen. However, there are several significant concerns about the methodology of these studies, and these results should be interpreted with caution.[80,298]

At present, the standard approach to resuscitation is to use 100% oxygen. Some clinicians may elect to start resuscitation with an oxygen concentration less than 100%, including some who may start with air. Evidence suggests that this approach may be reasonable. However, where possible, ensure supplemental oxygen is available for use if there is no rapid improvement following successful lung aeration. If supplemental oxygen is not readily available, ventilate the lungs with air. Supplemental oxygen is recommended for babies who are breathing but have central cyanosis.

Monitoring the oxygen saturation of babies undergoing resuscitation may be useful, but studies have shown that term healthy newborns may take more than 10 min to achieve a preductal oxygen saturation above 95% and nearly an hour to achieve this post-ductally.[299–301] Giving a variable concentration of oxygen guided by pulse oximetry may improve the ability to achieve 'normal' oxygen saturation values while more quickly avoiding 'hyperoxia', but the definition of these two terms in the baby at birth are undetermined. Oxygen is a drug, and oxidant injury is theoretically more likely in preterm infants.

Initial breaths and assisted ventilation

In term infants, spontaneous or assisted initial inflations create a functional residual capacity (FRC).[302–309] The optimum pressure, inflation time and flow required to establish an effective FRC have not been determined. Average initial peak inflating pressures of 30–40 cmH$_2$O (inflation time undefined) usually ventilate unresponsive term infants successfully.[305–307,309] Assisted ventilation rates of 30–60 breaths min^{-1} are used commonly, but the relative efficacy of various rates has not been investigated.

The primary measure of adequate initial ventilation is prompt increase in heart rate; assess passive chest wall movement if the heart rate does not increase. The initial peak inflating pressures needed are variable and unpredictable, and should be individualised to achieve an increase in heart rate or movement of the chest with each breath. Where pressure is being monitored, an initial inflation pressure of 20 cmH$_2$O may be effective, but 30–40 cmH$_2$O or higher may be required in some term babies. If pressure is not being monitored but merely limited by a non-adjustable 'blow-off' valve, use the minimum inflation required to achieve an increase in heart rate. There is insufficient evidence to recommend an optimum inflation time. In summary, provide artificial ventilation at 30–60 breaths min^{-1} to achieve or maintain a heart rate higher than 100 beats min^{-1} promptly.

Assisted ventilation of preterm infants

Animal studies show that preterm lungs are easily damaged by large volume inflations immediately after birth,[310] and that maintaining a positive end-expiratory pressure (PEEP) immediately after birth protects against lung damage. PEEP also improves lung compliance and gas exchange.[311,312] Human case series show that most apnoeic preterm infants can be ventilated with an initial inflation pressure of 20–25 cmH$_2$O, though some infants appear to require a higher pressure.[313,314]

When ventilating preterm infants, very obvious passive chest wall movement may indicate excessive tidal volumes and should be avoided. Monitoring of pressure may help to provide consistent inflations and avoid high pressures. If positive-pressure ventilation is required, an initial inflation pressure of 20–25 cmH$_2$O is adequate for most preterm infants. If a prompt increase in heart rate or chest movement is not obtained, higher pressures may be needed. If continued positive-pressure ventilation is required, PEEP may be beneficial. Continuous positive airway pressure (CPAP) in spontaneously breathing preterm infants following resuscitation may also be beneficial.[314]

Devices

Effective ventilation can be achieved with either a flow-inflating or self-inflating bag or with a T-piece mechanical device designed to regulate pressure.[315–317] The blow-off valves of self-inflating bags are flow dependent, and pressures generated may exceed the value specified by the manufacturer.[318] Target inflation pressures and long inspiratory times are achieved more consistently in mechanical models when using T-piece devices than when using bags,[319] although the clinical implications are not clear. More training is required to provide an appropriate pressure using flow-inflating bags compared with self-inflating bags.[320] A self-inflating bag, a flow-inflating bag or a T-piece mechanical device, all designed to regulate pressure or limit pressure applied to the airway, can be used to ventilate a newborn.

Laryngeal mask airways (LMAs) are effective for ventilating newborn near-term and full-term infants.[321,322] There are few data on the use of these devices in small preterm infants.[323,324] Three case series show that the LMA can provide effective ventilation in a time frame consistent with current resuscitation guidelines, although the babies being studied were not being resuscitated.[322,325,326] A randomised controlled trial found no clinically significant difference between the LMA and tracheal intubation when bag-mask ventilation was unsuccessful.[321] It is unclear whether the conclusions of this study can be generalized, since the LMA was inserted by experienced providers. Case reports suggest that when bag-mask ventilation has been unsuccessful and tracheal intubation is unfeasible or unsuccessful, the LMA may provide effective ventilation.[327–329] There is insufficient evidence to support the routine use of the LMA as the primary airway device for resuscitation at birth.

Table 6.1 Calculation of tracheal tube size and depth of insertion[a]

Child's weight (kg)	Gestation (weeks)	Tube size (mm ID)	Depth of insertion (cm)[a]
<1	<28	2.5	6.5–7
1–2	28–34	3.0	7–8
2–3	34–38	3.0/3.5	8–9
>3	>38	3.5/4.0	>9

[a] Depth of insertion from the upper lip can be estimated as insertion depth at lip (cm) = weight in kg + 6 cm.

There are also reservations concerning its effectiveness in the following situations

- when chest compressions are required
- for very low birth weight (VLBW) babies
- when the amniotic fluid is meconium stained

Confirming tracheal tube placement

Tracheal intubation may be considered at several points during neonatal resuscitation

- when suctioning to remove meconium or other tracheal blockage is required
- if bag-mask ventilation is ineffective or prolonged
- when chest compressions are performed
- in special circumstances (e.g., congenital diaphragmatic hernia or birth weight below 1000 g)

The use and timing of tracheal intubation will depend on the skill and experience of the available resuscitators.

Following tracheal intubation and intermittent positive pressure, a prompt increase in heart rate is the best indicator that the tube is in the tracheobronchial tree.[330] Exhaled CO_2 detection is effective for confirmation of tracheal tube placement in infants, including VLBW infants.[331–334] Detection of exhaled CO_2 in patients with adequate cardiac output confirms placement of the tube within the trachea, whereas failure to detect exhaled CO_2 strongly suggests oesophageal intubation.[331,333] Poor or absent pulmonary blood flow or tracheal obstruction may prevent detection of exhaled CO_2 despite correct tracheal tube placement. Tracheal tube placement is identified correctly in nearly all patients who are not in cardiac arrest[99]; however, in critically ill infants with poor cardiac output, inability to detect exhaled CO_2 despite correct placement may lead to unnecessary extubation. Other clinical indicators of correct tracheal tube placement include evaluation of condensed humidified gas during exhalation and presence or absence of chest movement, but these have not been evaluated systematically in newborn babies.

Tracheal tube placement (Table 6.1) must be assessed visually during intubation and, in most cases, will be confirmed by a rapid increase in heart rate on ventilating via the tracheal tube. If the heart rate remains slow, incorrect tube placement is the most likely cause. Check tube placement either visually or by detection of exhaled CO_2.

Route and dose of adrenaline

There are no placebo-controlled studies that have evaluated the use of adrenaline at any stage in human neonatal resuscitation. A paediatric study[148] and newborn animal studies[335,336] showed no benefit and a trend toward reduced survival and worse neurological status after high-dose IV adrenaline (100 mcg kg^{-1}) during resuscitation. Animal and adult human studies demonstrate that, when given via the trachea, considerably higher doses of adrenaline than currently recommended are required to achieve adequate plasma concentrations.[337–339] One neonatal animal study using the currently recommended dose of tracheal adrenaline (10 mcg kg^{-1}) showed no benefit.[126] One neonatal cohort study of nine preterm babies requiring resuscitation showed that tracheal adrenaline was absorbed, but these workers used 7–25 times the dose recommended currently.[340]

Post-resuscitation care

Babies who have required resuscitation may deteriorate. Once adequate ventilation and circulation are established, the infant should be maintained in or transferred to an environment in which close monitoring and anticipatory care can be provided.

Glucose

Hypoglycaemia was associated with adverse neurological outcome in a neonatal animal model of asphyxia and resuscitation.[341] Newborn animals which were hypoglycaemic at the time of an anoxic or hypoxic-ischaemic insult had larger areas of cerebral infarction and/or decreased survival compared with controls.[342,343] One clinical study demonstrated an association between hypoglycaemia and poor neurological outcome following perinatal asphyxia.[344] No clinical neonatal studies have investigated the relationship between hyperglycaemia and neurological outcome, although in adults hyperglycaemia is associated with a worse outcome.[345] The range of blood glucose concentration that is associated with the least brain injury following asphyxia and resuscitation cannot be defined on available evidence. Infants who require significant resuscitation should be monitored and treated to maintain blood glucose within the normal range.

Induced hypothermia

In a multicentre trial involving newborns with suspected asphyxia (indicated by need for resuscitation at birth, metabolic acidosis and early encephalopathy), selective head cooling ($34.5\,^{\circ}$C) was associated with a non-significant reduction in the number of survivors with severe disability at 18 months, but a significant benefit in the subgroup with moderate encephalopathy as judged by amplitude-integrated electroencephalogram.[220] Infants with severe electroencephalographic suppression and seizures did not benefit from treatment.[346] A second, small, controlled pilot study in asphyxiated infants with early induced systemic hypothermia resulted in fewer deaths and disabilities at 12 months. Modest hypothermia is associated with bradycardia and elevated blood pressure that do not usually require treatment, but a rapid increase in body temperature may cause hypotension.[347] Profound hypothermia (core temperature below $33\,^{\circ}$C) may cause arrhythmia, bleeding, thrombosis and sepsis, but studies so far have not reported these complications in infants treated with modest hypothermia.[220,348]

There are insufficient data to recommend routine use of modest systemic or selective cerebral hypothermia following resuscitation of infants with suspected asphyxia. Further clinical trials are needed to determine which infants benefit most and which method of cooling is most effective.

Withholding or discontinuing resuscitation

Mortality and morbidity for newborns varies according to region and to availability of resources.[349] Social science studies indicate that parents desire a larger role in decisions to resuscitate and to continue life support in severely compromised babies.[350] There is considerable variability among providers about the benefits and disadvantages of aggressive therapies in such babies.[351,352]

Withholding resuscitation

It is possible to identify conditions associated with high mortality and poor outcome, where withholding resuscitation may be considered reasonable, particularly when there has been the opportunity for discussion with parents.[282,353] A consistent and coordinated approach to individual cases by the obstetric and neonatal teams and the parents is an important goal. Withholding resuscitation and discontinuation of life-sustaining treatment during or following resuscitation are considered by many to be ethically equivalent, and clinicians should not be hesitant to withdraw support when the possibility of functional survival is highly unlikely. The following guidelines must be interpreted according to current regional outcomes.

- Where gestation, birth weight and/or congenital anomalies are associated with almost certain early death, and unacceptably high morbidity is likely among the rare survivors, resuscitation is not indicated. Examples from the published literature include extreme prematurity (gestational age <23 weeks and/or birthweight <400 g), and anomalies such as anencephaly and confirmed trisomy 13 or 18.
- Resuscitation is nearly always indicated in conditions associated with a high survival rate and acceptable morbidity. This will generally include babies with gestational age of 25 weeks or above (unless there is evidence of fetal compromise such as intrauterine infection or hypoxia-ischaemia) and those with most congenital malformations.
- In conditions associated with uncertain prognosis, where there is borderline survival and a relatively high rate of morbidity, and where the anticipated burden to the child is high, parental desires regarding resuscitation should be supported.

Withdrawing resuscitation efforts

Data from infants without signs of life from birth, lasting at least 10 min or longer, show either high mortality or severe neurodevelopmental disability.[354,355] After 10 min of uninterrupted and adequate resuscitation efforts, discontinuation of resuscitation may be justified if there are no signs of life.

References

1. Zideman D, Bingham R, Beattie T, et al. Guidelines for paediatric life support: a Statement by the Paediatric Life Support Working Party of the European Resuscitation Council. Resuscitation 1994;27:91—105.

2. European Resuscitation Council. Paediatric life support: (including the recommendations for resuscitation of babies at birth). Resuscitation 1998;37:95—6.

3. Phillips B, Zideman D, Garcia-Castrillo L, Felix M, Shwarz-Schwierin U. European Resuscitation Council Guidelines 2000 for Basic Paediatric Life Support. A statement from the Paediatric Life Support Working Group and approved by the Executive Committee of the European Resuscitation Council. Resuscitation 2001;48:223—9.

4. Phillips B, Zideman D, Garcia-Castrillo L, Felix M, Shwarz-Schwierin V. European Resuscitation Council Guidelines 2000 for Advanced Paediatric Life Support. A statement from Paediatric Life Support Working Group and approved by the Executive Committee of the European Resuscitation Council. Resuscitation 2001;48:231—4.

5. American Heart Association in collaboration with International Liaison Committee on Resuscitation. Guidelines for Cardiopulmonary Resuscitation and Emergency Cardiovascular Care—an international consensus on science. Resuscitation 2000;46:3—430.

6. American Heart Association in collaboration with International Liaison Committee on Resuscitation. Guidelines 2000 for Cardiopulmonary Resuscitation and Emergency Cardiovascular Care: International Consensus on Science. Circulation 2000;102(Suppl. I):I-1—I-370.

7. International Liaison Committee on Resuscitation. 2005 International Consensus on Cardiopulmonary Resuscitation and Emergency Cardiovascular Care Science with Treatment Recommendations. Resuscitation 2005;67:157—341.

8. International Liaison Committee on Resuscitation. 2005 International Consensus on Cardiopulmonary Resuscitation and Emergency Cardiovascular Care Science with Treatment Recommendations. Circulation, in press.

9. Kuisma M, Suominen P, Korpela R. Paediatric out-of-hospital cardiac arrests: epidemiology and outcome. Resuscitation 1995;30:141—50.

10. Kyriacou DN, Arcinue EL, Peek C, Kraus JF. Effect of immediate resuscitation on children with submersion injury. Pediatrics 1994;94:137—42.

11. Berg RA, Hilwig RW, Kern KB, Ewy GA. Bystander'' chest compressions and assisted ventilation independently improve outcome from piglet asphyxial pulseless ''cardiac arrest''. Circulation 2000;101:1743—8.

12. Young KD, Seidel JS. Pediatric cardiopulmonary resuscitation: a collective review. Ann Emerg Med 1999;33:195—205.

13. Berg RA, Hilwig RW, Kern KB, Babar I, Ewy GA. Simulated mouth-to-mouth ventilation and chest compressions (bystander cardiopulmonary resuscitation) improves outcome in a swine model of prehospital pediatric asphyxial cardiac arrest. Crit Care Med 1999;27:1893—9.

14. Dorph E, Wik L, Steen PA. Effectiveness of ventilation-compression ratios 1:5 and 2:15 in simulated single rescuer paediatric resuscitation. Resuscitation 2002;54:259—64.

15. Turner I, Turner S, Armstrong V. Does the compression to ventilation ratio affect the quality of CPR: a simulation study. Resuscitation 2002;52:55—62.

16. Babbs CF, Kern KB. Optimum compression to ventilation ratios in CPR under realistic, practical conditions: a physiological and mathematical analysis. Resuscitation 2002;54:147—57.

17. Babbs CF, Nadkarni V. Optimizing chest compression to rescue ventilation ratios during one-rescuer CPR by professionals and lay persons: children are not just little adults. Resuscitation 2004;61:173—81.

18. Whyte SD, Wyllie JP. Paediatric basic life support: a practical assessment. Resuscitation 1999;41:153—217.

19. Safranek DJ, Eisenberg MS, Larsen MP. The epidemiology of cardiac arrest in young adults. Ann Emerg Med 1992;21:1102—6.

20. Clements F, McGowan J. Finger position for chest compressions in cardiac arrest in infants. Resuscitation 2000;44:43—6.

21. Houri PK, Frank LR, Menegazzi JJ, Taylor R. A randomized, controlled trial of two-thumb vs two-finger chest compression in a swine infant model of cardiac arrest. Prehosp Emerg Care 1997;1:65—7.

22. David R. Closed chest cardiac massage in the newborn infant. Pediatrics 1988;81:552—4.

23. Dorfsman ML, Menegazzi JJ, Wadas RJ, Auble TE. Two-thumb vs two-finger chest compression in an infant model of prolonged cardiopulmonary resuscitation. Acad Emerg Med 2000;7:1077—82.

24. Whitelaw CC, Slywka B, Goldsmith LJ. Comparison of a two-finger versus two-thumb method for chest compressions by healthcare providers in an infant mechanical model. Resuscitation 2000;43:213—6.

25. Menegazzi JJ, Auble TE, Nicklas KA, Hosack GM, Rack L, Goode JS. Two-thumb versus two-finger chest compression during CRP in a swine infant model of cardiac arrest. Ann Emerg Med 1993;22:240—3.

26. Stevenson AG, McGowan J, Evans AL, Graham CA. CPR for children: one hand or two? Resuscitation 2005;64:205—8.

27. Gurnett CA, Atkins DL. Successful use of a biphasic waveform automated external defibrillator in a high-risk child. Am J Cardiol 2000;86:1051—3.

28. Konig B, Benger J, Goldsworthy L. Automatic external defibrillation in a 6 year old. Arch Dis Child 2005;90:310—1.

29. Atkinson E, Mikysa B, Conway JA, et al. Specificity and sensitivity of automated external defibrillator rhythm analysis in infants and children. Ann Emerg Med 2003;42:185—96.

30. Cecchin F, Jorgenson DB, Berul CI, et al. Is arrhythmia detection by automatic external defibrillator accurate for children? Sensitivity and specificity of an automatic external defibrillator algorithm in 696 pediatric arrhythmias. Circulation 2001;103:2483—8.

31. Samson R, Berg R, Bingham R. Pediatric Advanced Life Support Task Force ILCoR. Use of automated external defibrillators for children: an update. An advisory statement from the Pediatric Advanced Life Support Task Force of the International Liaison Committee on Resuscitation. Resuscitation 2003;57:237—43.

32. Jorgenson D, Morgan C, Snyder D, et al. Energy attenuator for pediatric application of an automated external defibrillator. Crit Care Med 2002;30:S145—7.

33. Tang W, Weil MH, Jorgenson D, et al. Fixed-energy biphasic waveform defibrillation in a pediatric model of cardiac arrest and resuscitation. Crit Care Med 2002;30:2736—41.

34. Berg RA, Chapman FW, Berg MD, et al. Attenuated adult biphasic shocks compared with weight-based monophasic shocks in a swine model of prolonged pediatric ventricular fibrillation. Resuscitation 2004;61:189—97.

35. Berg RA, Samson RA, Berg MD, et al. Better outcome after pediatric defibrillation dosage than adult dosage in a swine model of pediatric ventricular fibrillation. J Am Coll Cardiol 2005;45:786—9.

36. Rossano JQ, Schiff L, Kenney MA, Atkins DL. Survival is not correlated with defibrillation dosing in pediatric out-of-hospital ventricular fibrillation. Circulation 2003;108:320–1.

37. Clark CB, Zhang Y, Davies LR, Karlsson G, Kerber RE. Pediatric transthoracic defibrillation: biphasic versus monophasic waveforms in an experimental model. Resuscitation 2001;51:159–63.

38. Schneider T, Martens PR, Paschen H, et al. Multicenter, randomized, controlled trial of 150-J biphasic shocks compared with 200- to 360-J monophasic shocks in the resuscitation of out-of-hospital cardiac arrest victims. Optimized Response to Cardiac Arrest (ORCA) Investigators. Circulation 2000;102:1780–7.

39. Faddy SC, Powell J, Craig JC. Biphasic and monophasic shocks for transthoracic defibrillation: a meta analysis of randomised controlled trials. Resuscitation 2003;58:9–16.

40. van Alem AP, Chapman FW, Lank P, Hart AA, Koster RW. A prospective, randomised and blinded comparison of first shock success of monophasic and biphasic waveforms in out-of-hospital cardiac arrest. Resuscitation 2003;58:17–24.

41. Redding JS. The choking controversy: critique of evidence on the Heimlich maneuver. Crit Care Med 1979;7:475–9.

42. International Liaison Committee on Resuscitation. Part 2. Adult Basic Life Support. 2005 International Consensus on Cardiopulmonary Resuscitation and Emergency Cardiovascular Care Science with Treatment Recommendations. Resuscitation 2005;67:187–200.

43. Sirbaugh PE, Pepe PE, Shook JE, et al. A prospective, population-based study of the demographics, epidemiology, management, and outcome of out-of-hospital pediatric cardiopulmonary arrest. Ann Emerg Med 1999;33:174–84.

44. Hickey RW, Cohen DM, Strausbaugh S, Dietrich AM. Pediatric patients requiring CPR in the prehospital setting. Ann Emerg Med 1995;25:495–501.

45. Reis AG, Nadkarni V, Perondi MB, Grisi S, Berg RA. A prospective investigation into the epidemiology of in-hospital pediatric cardiopulmonary resuscitation using the international Utstein reporting style. Pediatrics 2002;109:200–9.

46. Young KD, Gausche-Hill M, McClung CD, Lewis RJ. A prospective, population-based study of the epidemiology and outcome of out-of-hospital pediatric cardiopulmonary arrest. Pediatrics 2004;114:157–64.

47. Richman PB, Nashed AH. The etiology of cardiac arrest in children and young adults: special considerations for ED management. Am J Emerg Med 1999;17:264–70.

48. Engdahl J, Bang A, Karlson BW, Lindqvist J, Herlitz J. Characteristics and outcome among patients suffering from out of hospital cardiac arrest of non-cardiac aetiology. Resuscitation 2003;57:33–41.

49. Carcillo JA. Pediatric septic shock and multiple organ failure. Crit Care Clin 2003;19:413–40, viii.

50. Eberle B, Dick WF, Schneider T, Wisser G, Doetsch S, Tzanova I. Checking the carotid pulse check: diagnostic accuracy of first responders in patients with and without a pulse. Resuscitation 1996;33:107–16.

51. Moule P. Checking the carotid pulse: diagnostic accuracy in students of the healthcare professions. Resuscitation 2000;44:195–201.

52. Lapostolle F, Le Toumelin P, Agostinucci JM, Catineau J, Adnet F. Basic cardiac life support providers checking the carotid pulse: performance, degree of conviction, and influencing factors. Acad Emerg Med 2004;11:878–80.

53. Frederick K, Bixby E, Orzel MN, Stewart-Brown S, Willett K. Will changing the emphasis from 'pulseless' to 'no signs of circulation' improve the recall scores for effective life support skills in children? Resuscitation 2002;55:255–61.

54. Park C, Bahk JH, Ahn WS, Do SH, Lee KH. The laryngeal mask airway in infants and children. Can J Anaesth 2001;48:413–7.

55. Hedges JR, Dronen SC, Feero S, Hawkins S, Syverud SA, Shultz B. Succinylcholine-assisted intubations in prehospital care. Ann Emerg Med 1988;17:469–72.

56. Murphy-Macabobby M, Marshall WJ, Schneider C, Dries D. Neuromuscular blockade in aeromedical airway management. Ann Emerg Med 1992;21:664–8.

57. Sayre M, Weisgerber I. The use of neuromuscular blocking agents by air medical services. J Air Med Transp 1992;11:7–11.

58. Rose W, Anderson L, Edmond S. Analysis of intubations. Before and after establishment of a rapid sequence intubation protocol for air medical use. Air Med J 1994;13:475–8.

59. Sing RF, Reilly PM, Rotondo MF, Lynch MJ, McCans JP, Schwab CW. Out-of-hospital rapid-sequence induction for intubation of the pediatric patient. Acad Emerg Med 1996;3:41–5.

60. Ma OJ, Atchley RB, Hatley T, Green M, Young J, Brady W. Intubation success rates improve for an air medical program after implementing the use of neuromuscular blocking agents. Am J Emerg Med 1998;16:125–7.

61. Tayal V, Riggs R, Marx J, Tomaszewski C, Schneider R. Rapid-sequence intubation at an emergency medicine residency: success rate and adverse events during a two-year period. Acad Emerg Med 1999;6:31–7.

62. Wang HE, Sweeney TA, O'Connor RE, Rubinstein H. Failed prehospital intubations: an analysis of emergency department courses and outcomes. Prehosp Emerg Care 2001;5:134–41.

63. Sagarin MJ, Chiang V, Sakles JC, et al. Rapid sequence intubation for pediatric emergency airway management. Pediatr Emerg Care 2002;18:417–43.

64. Kaye K, Frascone RJ, Held T. Prehospital rapid-sequence intubation: a pilot training program. Prehosp Emerg Care 2003;7:235–40.

65. Wang HE, Kupas DF, Paris PM, Bates RR, Costantino JP, Yealy DM. Multivariate predictors of failed prehospital endotracheal intubation. Acad Emerg Med 2003;10:717–24.

66. Pepe P, Zachariah B, Chandra N. Invasive airway technique in resuscitation. Ann Emerg Med 1991;22:393–403.

67. Luten RC, Wears RL, Broselow J, et al. Length-based endotracheal tube and emergency equipment in pediatrics. Ann Emerg Med 1992;21:900–4.

68. Deakers TW, Reynolds G, Stretton M, Newth CJ. Cuffed endotracheal tubes in pediatric intensive care. J Pediatr 1994;125:57–62.

69. Khine HH, Corddry DH, Kettrick RG, et al. Comparison of cuffed and uncuffed endotracheal tubes in young children during general anesthesia. Anesthesiology 1997;86:627–31.

70. Newth CJ, Rachman B, Patel N, Hammer J. The use of cuffed versus uncuffed endotracheal tubes in pediatric intensive care. J Pediatr 2004;144:333–7.

71. Mhanna MJ, Zamel YB, Tichy CM, Super DM. The ''air leak'' test around the endotracheal tube, as a predictor of postextubation stridor, is age dependent in children. Crit Care Med 2002;30:2639–43.

72. Katz SH, Falk JL. Misplaced endotracheal tubes by paramedics in an urban emergency medical services system. Ann Emerg Med 2001;37:32–7.

73. Gausche M, Lewis RJ, Stratton SJ, et al. Effect of out-of-hospital pediatric endotracheal intubation on survival and neurological outcome: a controlled clinical trial. JAMA 2000;283:783—90.

74. Kelly JJ, Eynon CA, Kaplan JL, de Garavilla L, Dalsey WC. Use of tube condensation as an indicator of endotracheal tube placement. Ann Emerg Med 1998;31:575—8.

75. Andersen KH, Hald A. Assessing the position of the tracheal tube: the reliability of different methods. Anaesthesia 1989;44:984—5.

76. Andersen KH, Schultz-Lebahn T. Oesophageal intubation can be undetected by auscultation of the chest. Acta Anaesthesiol Scand 1994;38:580—2.

77. Hartrey R, Kestin IG. Movement of oral and nasal tracheal tubes as a result of changes in head and neck position. Anaesthesia 1995;50:682—7.

78. Van de Louw A, Cracco C, Cerf C, et al. Accuracy of pulse oximetry in the intensive care unit. Intensive Care Med 2001;27:1606—13.

79. Seguin P, Le Rouzo A, Tanguy M, Guillou YM, Feuillu A, Malledant Y. Evidence for the need of bedside accuracy of pulse oximetry in an intensive care unit. Crit Care Med 2000;28:703—6.

80. Tan A, Schulze A, O'Donnell CP, Davis PG. Air versus oxygen for resuscitation of infants at birth. Cochrane Database Syst Rev 2004:CD002273.

81. Ramji S, Rasaily R, Mishra PK, et al. Resuscitation of asphyxiated newborns with room air or 100% oxygen at birth: a multicentric clinical trial. Indian Pediatr 2003;40:510—7.

82. Vento M, Asensi M, Sastre J, Garcia-Sala F, Pallardo FV, Vina J. Resuscitation with room air instead of 100% oxygen prevents oxidative stress in moderately asphyxiated term neonates. Pediatrics 2001;107:642—7.

83. Saugstad OD. Resuscitation of newborn infants with room air or oxygen. Semin Neonatol 2001;6:233—9.

84. Aufderheide TP, Lurie KG. Death by hyperventilation: a common and life-threatening problem during cardiopulmonary resuscitation. Crit Care Med 2004;32:S345—51.

85. Aufderheide TP, Sigurdsson G, Pirrallo RG, et al. Hyperventilation-induced hypotension during cardiopulmonary resuscitation. Circulation 2004;109:1960—5.

86. Wik L, Kramer-Johansen J, Myklebust H, et al. Quality of cardiopulmonary resuscitation during out-of-hospital cardiac arrest. JAMA 2005;293:299—304.

87. Abella BS, Alvarado JP, Myklebust H, et al. Quality of cardiopulmonary resuscitation during in-hospital cardiac arrest. AMA 2005;293:305—10.

88. Abella BS, Sandbo N, Vassilatos P, et al. Chest compression rates during cardiopulmonary resuscitation are suboptimal: a prospective study during in-hospital cardiac arrest. Circulation 2005;111:428—34.

89. Borke WB, Munkeby BH, Morkrid L, Thaulow E, Saugstad OD. Resuscitation with 100% O(2) does not protect the myocardium in hypoxic newborn piglets. Arch Dis Child Fetal Neonatal Ed 2004;89:F156—60.

90. Stockinger ZT, McSwain Jr NE. Prehospital endotracheal intubation for trauma does not improve survival over bag-valve-mask ventilation. J Trauma 2004;56:531—6.

91. Pitetti R, Glustein JZ, Bhende MS. Prehospital care and outcome of pediatric out-of-hospital cardiac arrest. Prehosp Emerg Care 2002;6:283—90.

92. Cooper A, DiScala C, Foltin G, Tunik M, Markenson D, Welborn C. Prehospital endotracheal intubation for severe head injury in children: a reappraisal. Semin Pediatr Surg 2001;10:3—6.

93. Bhende MS, Thompson AE, Cook DR, Saville AL. Validity of a disposable end-tidal CO_2 detector in verifying endotracheal tube placement in infants and children. Ann Emerg Med 1992;21:142—5.

94. Bhende MS, Thompson AE, Orr RA. Utility of an end-tidal carbon dioxide detector during stabilization and transport of critically ill children. Pediatrics 1992;89(pt 1):1042—4.

95. Bhende MS, LaCovey DC. End-tidal carbon dioxide monitoring in the prehospital setting. Prehosp Emerg Care 2001;5:208—13.

96. Ornato JP, Shipley JB, Racht EM, et al. Multicenter study of a portable, hand-size, colorimetric end-tidal carbon dioxide detection device. Ann Emerg Med 1992;21:518—23.

97. Gonzalez del Rey JA, Poirier MP, Digiulio GA. Evaluation of an ambu-bag valve with a self-contained, colorimetric end-tidal CO_2 system in the detection of airway mishaps: an animal trial. Pediatr Emerg Care 2000;16:121—3.

98. Bhende MS, Thompson AE. Evaluation of an end-tidal CO_2 detector during pediatric cardiopulmonary resuscitation. Pediatrics 1995;95:395—9.

99. Bhende MS, Karasic DG, Karasic RB. End-tidal carbon dioxide changes during cardiopulmonary resuscitation after experimental asphyxial cardiac arrest. Am J Emerg Med 1996;14:349—50.

100. DeBehnke DJ, Hilander SJ, Dobler DW, Wickman LL, Swart GL. The hemodynamic and arterial blood gas response to asphyxiation: a canine model of pulseless electrical activity. Resuscitation 1995;30:169—75.

101. Ornato JP, Garnett AR, Glauser FL. Relationship between cardiac output and the end-tidal carbon dioxide tension. Ann Emerg Med 1990;19:1104—6.

102. Sharieff GQ, Rodarte A, Wilton N, Silva PD, Bleyle D. The self-inflating bulb as an esophageal detector device in children weighing more than twenty kilograms: a comparison of two techniques. Ann Emerg Med 2003;41:623—9.

103. Sharieff GQ, Rodarte A, Wilton N, Bleyle D. The self-inflating bulb as an airway adjunct: is it reliable in children weighing less than 20 kilograms? Acad Emerg Med 2003;10:303—8.

104. Poirier MP, Gonzalez Del-Rey JA, McAneney CM, DiGiulio GA. Utility of monitoring capnography, pulse oximetry, and vital signs in the detection of airway mishaps: a hyperoxemic animal model. Am J Emerg Med 1998;16:350—2.

105. Lillis KA, Jaffe DM. Prehospital intravenous access in children. Ann Emerg Med 1992;21:1430—4.

106. Kanter RK, Zimmerman JJ, Strauss RH, Stoeckel KA. Pediatric emergency intravenous access. Evaluation of a protocol. Am J Dis Child 1986;140:132—4.

107. Banerjee S, Singhi SC, Singh S, Singh M. The intraosseous route is a suitable alternative to intravenous route for fluid resuscitation in severely dehydrated children. Indian Pediatr 1994;31:1511—20.

108. Glaeser PW, Hellmich TR, Szewczuga D, Losek JD, Smith DS. Five-year experience in prehospital intraosseous infusions in children and adults. Ann Emerg Med 1993;22:1119—24.

109. Guy J, Haley K, Zuspan SJ. Use of intraosseous infusion in the pediatric trauma patient. J Pediatr Surg 1993;28:158—61.

110. Orlowski JP, Julius CJ, Petras RE, Porembka DT, Gallagher JM. The safety of intraosseous infusions: risks of fat and bone marrow emboli to the lungs. Ann Emerg Med 1989;18:1062—7.

111. Orlowski JP, Porembka DT, Gallagher JM, Lockrem JD, VanLente F. Comparison study of intraosseous, central intravenous, and peripheral intravenous infusions of emergency drugs. Am J Dis Child 1990;144:112—7.

112. Abe KK, Blum GT, Yamamoto LG. Intraosseous is faster and easier than umbilical venous catheterization in new-

born emergency vascular access models. Am J Emerg Med 2000;18:126—9.

113. Ellemunter H, Simma B, Trawoger R, Maurer H. Intraosseous lines in preterm and full term neonates. Arch Dis Child Fetal Neonatal Ed 1999;80:F74—5.

114. Cameron JL, Fontanarosa PB, Passalaqua AM. A comparative study of peripheral to central circulation delivery times between intraosseous and intravenous injection using a radionuclide technique in normovolemic and hypovolemic canines. J Emerg Med 1989;7:123—7.

115. Warren DW, Kissoon N, Sommerauer JF, Rieder MJ. Comparison of fluid infusion rates among peripheral intravenous and humerus, femur, malleolus, and tibial intraosseous sites in normovolemic and hypovolemic piglets. Ann Emerg Med 1993;22:183—6.

116. Brickman KR, Krupp K, Rega P, Alexander J, Guinness M. Typing and screening of blood from intraosseous access. Ann Emerg Med 1992;21:414—7.

117. Johnson L, Kissoon N, Fiallos M, Abdelmoneim T, Murphy S. Use of intraosseous blood to assess blood chemistries and hemoglobin during cardiopulmonary resuscitation with drug infusions. Crit Care Med 1999;27:1147—52.

118. Ummenhofer W, Frei FJ, Urwyler A, Drewe J. Are laboratory values in bone marrow aspirate predictable for venous blood in paediatric patients? Resuscitation 1994;27:123—8.

119. Kissoon N, Idris A, Wenzel V, Murphy S, Rush W. Intraosseous and central venous blood acid—base relationship during cardiopulmonary resuscitation. Pediatr Emerg Care 1997;13:250—3.

120. Abdelmoneim T, Kissoon N, Johnson L, Fiallos M, Murphy S. Acid-base status of blood from intraosseous and mixed venous sites during prolonged cardiopulmonary resuscitation and drug infusions. Crit Care Med 1999;27:1923—8.

121. Venkataraman ST, Orr RA, Thompson AE. Percutaneous infraclavicular subclavian vein catheterization in critically ill infants and children. J Pediatr 1988;113:480—5.

122. Fleisher G, Caputo G, Baskin M. Comparison of external jugular and peripheral venous administration of sodium bicarbonate in puppies. Crit Care Med 1989;17:251—4.

123. Hedges JR, Barsan WB, Doan LA, et al. Central versus peripheral intravenous routes in cardiopulmonary resuscitation. Am J Emerg Med 1984;2:385—90.

124. Neufeld JD, Marx JA, Moore EE, Light AI. Comparison of intraosseous, central, and peripheral routes of crystalloid infusion for resuscitation of hemorrhagic shock in a swine model. J Trauma 1993;34:422—8.

125. Stenzel JP, Green TP, Fuhrman BP, Carlson PE, Marchessault RP. Percutaneous femoral venous catheterizations: a prospective study of complications. J Pediatr 1989;114:411—5.

126. Kleinman ME, Oh W, Stonestreet BS. Comparison of intravenous and endotracheal epinephrine during cardiopulmonary resuscitation in newborn piglets. Crit Care Med 1999;27:2748—54.

127. Efrati O, Ben-Abraham R, Barak A, et al. Endobronchial adrenaline: should it be reconsidered? Dose response and haemodynamic effect in dogs. Resuscitation 2003;59:117—22.

128. Howard RF, Bingham RM. Endotracheal compared with intravenous administration of atropine. Arch Dis Child 1990;65:449—50.

129. Prengel AW, Lindner KH, Hahnel J, Ahnefeld FW. Endotracheal and endobronchial lidocaine administration: effects on plasma lidocaine concentration and blood gases. Crit Care Med 1991;19:911—5.

130. Crespo SG, Schoffstall JM, Fuhs LR, Spivey WH. Comparison of two doses of endotracheal epinephrine in a cardiac arrest model. Ann Emerg Med 1991;20:230—4.

131. Lee PL, Chung YT, Lee BY, Yeh CY, Lin SY, Chao CC. The optimal dose of atropine via the endotracheal route. Ma Zui Xue Za Zhi 1989;27:35—8.

132. Hahnel JH, Lindner KH, Schurmann C, Prengel A, Ahnefeld FW. Plasma lidocaine levels and PaO_2 with endobronchial administration: dilution with normal saline or distilled water? Ann Emerg Med 1990;19:1314—7.

133. Jasani MS, Nadkarni VM, Finkelstein MS, Mandell GA, Salzman SK, Norman ME. Effects of different techniques of endotracheal epinephrine administration in pediatric porcine hypoxic-hypercarbic cardiopulmonary arrest. Crit Care Med 1994;22:1174—80.

134. Steinfath M, Scholz J, Schulte am Esch J, Laer S, Reymann A, Scholz H. The technique of endobronchial lidocaine administration does not influence plasma concentration profiles and pharmacokinetic parameters in humans. Resuscitation 1995;29:55—62.

135. Carcillo JA, Fields AI. Clinical practice parameters for hemodynamic support of pediatric and neonatal patients in septic shock. Crit Care Med 2002;30:1365—78.

136. Simma B, Burger R, Falk M, Sacher P, Fanconi S. A prospective, randomized, and controlled study of fluid management in children with severe head injury: lactated Ringer's solution versus hypertonic saline. Crit Care Med 1998;26:1265—70.

137. Rocha e Silva M. Hypertonic saline resuscitation. Medicina (B Aries) 1998; 58:393-402.

138. Katz LM, Wang Y, Ebmeyer U, Radovsky A, Safar P. Glucose plus insulin infusion improves cerebral outcome after asphyxial cardiac arrest. Neuroreport 1998;9:3363—7.

139. Longstreth Jr WT, Copass MK, Dennis LK, Rauch-Matthews ME, Stark MS, Cobb LA. Intravenous glucose after out-of-hospital cardiopulmonary arrest: a community-based randomized trial. Neurology 1993;43:2534—41.

140. Chang YS, Park WS, Ko SY, et al. Effects of fasting and insulin-induced hypoglycemia on brain cell membrane function and energy metabolism during hypoxia-ischemia in newborn piglets. Brain Res 1999;844:135—42.

141. Cherian L, Goodman JC, Robertson CS. Hyperglycemia increases brain injury caused by secondary ischemia after cortical impact injury in rats. Crit Care Med 1997;25:1378—83.

142. Paul T, Bertram H, Bokenkamp R, Hausdorf G. Supraventricular tachycardia in infants, children and adolescents: diagnosis, and pharmacological and interventional therapy. Paediatr Drugs 2000;2:171—81.

143. Losek JD, Endom E, Dietrich A, Stewart G, Zempsky W, Smith K. Adenosine and pediatric supraventricular tachycardia in the emergency department: multicenter study and review. Ann Emerg Med 1999;33:185—91.

144. Roberts JR, Greenburg MI, Knaub M, Baskin SI. Comparison of the pharmacological effects of epinephrine administered by the intravenous and endotracheal routes. JACEP 1978;7:260—4.

145. Zaritsky A. Pediatric resuscitation pharmacology. Members of the Medications in Pediatric Resuscitation Panel. Ann Emerg Med 1993;22(pt 2):445—55.

146. Manisterski Y, Vaknin Z, Ben-Abraham R, et al. Endotracheal epinephrine: a call for larger doses. Anesth Analg 2002;95:1037—41 [table of contents].

147. Patterson MD, Boenning DA, Klein BL, et al. The use of high-dose epinephrine for patients with out-of-hospital cardiopulmonary arrest refractory to prehospital interventions. Pediatr Emerg Care 2005;21:227—37.

148. Perondi MB, Reis AG, Paiva EF, Nadkarni VM, Berg RA. A comparison of high-dose and standard-dose epinephrine in children with cardiac arrest. N Engl J Med 2004;350: 1722—30.

149. Carpenter TC, Stenmark KR. High-dose epinephrine is not superior to standard-dose epinephrine in pediatric in-hospital cardiopulmonary arrest. Pediatrics 1997;99:403—8.

150. Dieckmann R, Vardis R. High-dose epinephrine in pediatric out-of-hospital cardiopulmonary arrest. Pediatrics 1995;95:901—13.

151. Berg RA, Otto CW, Kern KB, et al. High-dose epinephrine results in greater early mortality after resuscitation from prolonged cardiac arrest in pigs: a prospective, randomized study. Crit Care Med 1994;22:282—90.

152. Rubertsson S, Wiklund L. Hemodynamic effects of epinephrine in combination with different alkaline buffers during experimental, open-chest, cardiopulmonary resuscitation. Crit Care Med 1993;21:1051—7.

153. Somberg JC, Timar S, Bailin SJ, et al. Lack of a hypotensive effect with rapid administration of a new aqueous formulation of intravenous amiodarone. Am J Cardiol 2004;93:576—81.

154. Yap S-C, Hoomtje T, Sreeram N. Polymorphic ventricular tachycardia after use of intravenous amiodarone for postoperative junctional ectopic tachycardia. Int J Cardiol 2000;76:245—7.

155. Dauchot P, Gravenstein JS. Effects of atropine on the electrocardiogram in different age groups. Clin Pharmacol Ther 1971;12:274—80.

156. Stulz PM, Scheidegger D, Drop LJ, Lowenstein E, Laver MB. Ventricular pump performance during hypocalcemia: clinical and experimental studies. J Thorac Cardiovasc Surg 1979;78:185—94.

157. van Walraven C, Stiell IG, Wells GA, Hebert PC, Vandemheen K, The OTAC Study Group. Do advanced cardiac life support drugs increase resuscitation rates from in-hospital cardiac arrest? Ann Emerg Med 1998;32:544—53.

158. Paraskos JA. Cardiovascular pharmacology III: atropine, calcium, calcium blockers, and (beta)-blockers. Circulation 1986;74:IV-86—9.

159. Stueven HA, Thompson B, Aprahamian C, Tonsfeldt DJ, Kastenson EH. The effectiveness of calcium chloride in refractory electromechanical dissociation. Ann Emerg Med 1985;14:626—9.

160. Stueven HA, Thompson B, Aprahamian C, Tonsfeldt DJ, Kastenson EH. Lack of effectiveness of calcium chloride in refractory asystole. Ann Emerg Med 1985;14:630—2.

161. Srinivasan V, Spinella PC, Drott HR, Roth CL, Helfaer MA, Nadkarni V. Association of timing, duration, and intensity of hyperglycemia with intensive care unit mortality in critically ill children. Pediatr Crit Care Med 2004;5:329—36.

162. Krinsley JS. Effect of an intensive glucose management protocol on the mortality of critically ill adult patients. Mayo Clin Proc 2004;79:992—1000.

163. Losek JD. Hypoglycemia and the ABC'S (sugar) of pediatric resuscitation. Ann Emerg Med 2000;35:43—6.

164. Finney SJ, Zekveld C, Elia A, Evans TW. Glucose control and mortality in critically ill patients. Jama 2003;290:2041—7.

165. Allegra J, Lavery R, Cody R, et al. Magnesium sulfate in the treatment of refractory ventricular fibrillation in the prehospital setting. Resuscitation 2001;49:245—9.

166. Tzivoni D, Banai S, Schuger C, et al. Treatment of torsade de pointes with magnesium sulfate. Circulation 1988;77:392—7.

167. Lokesh L, Kumar P, Murki S, Narang A. A randomized controlled trial of sodium bicarbonate in neonatal resuscitation-effect on immediate outcome. Resuscitation 2004;60:219—23.

168. Bar-Joseph G, Abramson NS, Kelsey SF, Mashiach T, Craig MT, Safar P. Improved resuscitation outcome in emergency medical systems with increased usage of sodium bicarbonate during cardiopulmonary resuscitation. Acta Anaesthesiol Scand 2005;49:6—15.

169. Dorian P, Cass D, Schwartz B, Cooper R, Gelaznikas R, Barr A. Amiodarone as compared with lidocaine for shock-resistant ventricular fibrillation. N Engl J Med 2002;346:884—90.

170. Walsh EP, Saul JP, Sholler GF, et al. Evaluation of a staged treatment protocol for rapid automatic junctional tachycardia after operation for congenital heart disease. J Am Coll Cardiol 1997;29:1046—53.

171. Wang L. Congenital long QT syndrome: 50 years of electrophysiological research from cell to bedside. Acta Cardiologica 2003;58:133—8.

172. Singh BN, Kehoe R, Woosley RL, Scheinman M, Quart B, Sotalol Multicenter Study Group. Multicenter trial of sotalol compared with procainamide in the suppression of inducible ventricular tachycardia: a double-blind, randomized parallel evaluation. Am Heart J 1995;129:87—97.

173. Luedtke SA, Kuhn RJ, McCaffrey FM. Pharmacologic management of supraventricular tachycardias in children, part 2: atrial flutter, atrial fibrillation, and junctional and atrial ectopic tachycardia. Ann Pharmacother 1997;31:1347—59.

174. Luedtke SA, Kuhn RJ, McCaffrey FM. Pharmacologic management of supraventricular tachycardias in children. Part 1: Wolff-Parkinson-White and atrioventricular nodal reentry. Ann Pharmacother 1997;31:1227—43.

175. Mandapati R, Byrum CJ, Kavey RE, et al. Procainamide for rate control of postsurgical junctional tachycardia. Pediatr Cardiol 2000;21:123—8.

176. Wang JN, Wu JM, Tsai YC, Lin CS. Ectopic atrial tachycardia in children. J Formos Med Assoc 2000;99:766—70.

177. Holmes CL, Landry DW, Granton JT. Science review: Vasopressin and the cardiovascular system part 1—receptor physiology. Crit Care 2003;7:427—34.

178. Voelckel WG, Lurie KG, McKnite S, et al. Effects of epinephrine and vasopressin in a piglet model of prolonged ventricular fibrillation and cardiopulmonary resuscitation. Crit Care Med 2002;30:957—62.

179. Voelckel WG, Lurie KG, McKnite S, et al. Comparison of epinephrine and vasopressin in a pediatric porcine model of asphyxial cardiac arrest. Crit Care Med 2000;28:3777—83.

180. Mann K, Berg RA, Nadkarni V. Beneficial effects of vasopressin in prolonged pediatric cardiac arrest: a case series. Resuscitation 2002;52:149—56.

181. Atkins DL, Kerber RE. Pediatric defibrillation: current flow is improved by using ''adult'' electrode paddles. Pediatrics 1994;94:90—3.

182. Atkins DL, Sirna S, Kieso R, Charbonnier F, Kerber RE. Pediatric defibrillation: importance of paddle size in determining transthoracic impedance. Pediatrics 1988;82:914—8.

183. Bennetts SH, Deakin CD, Petley GW, Clewlow F. Is optimal paddle force applied during paediatric external defibrillation? Resuscitation 2004;60:29—32.

184. Deakin C, Bennetts S, Petley G, Clewlow F. What is the optimal paddle force for paediatric defibrillation? Resuscitation 2002;55:59.

185. Atkins DL, Hartley LL, York DK. Accurate recognition and effective treatment of ventricular fibrillation by automated external defibrillators in adolescents. Pediatrics 1998;101(pt 1):393—7.

186. Pierpont GL, Kruse JA, Nelson DH. Intra-arterial monitoring during cardiopulmonary resuscitation. Cathet Cardiovasc Diagn 1985;11:513—20.

187. Zaritsky A, Nadkarni V, Getson P, Kuehl K. CPR in children. Ann Emerg Med 1987;16:1107—11.

188. Mogayzel C, Quan L, Graves JR, Tiedeman D, Fahrenbruch C, Herndon P. Out-of-hospital ventricular fibrillation in children and adolescents: causes and outcomes. Ann Emerg Med 1995;25:484—91.

189. Herlitz J, Engdahl J, Svensson L, Young M, Angquist KA, Holmberg S. Characteristics and outcome among children suffering from out of hospital cardiac arrest in Sweden. Resuscitation 2005;64:37—40.

190. Berg RA. Role of mouth-to-mouth rescue breathing in bystander cardiopulmonary resuscitation for asphyxial cardiac arrest. Crit Care Med 2000;28(Suppl.):N193—5.

191. Appleton GO, Cummins RO, Larson MP, Graves JR. CPR and the single rescuer: at what age should you ''call first'' rather than ''call fast''? Ann Emerg Med 1995;25:492—4.

192. Larsen MP, Eisenberg MS, Cummins RO, Hallstrom AP. Predicting survival from out-of-hospital cardiac arrest: a graphic model. Ann Emerg Med 1993;22:1652—8.

193. Cobb LA, Fahrenbruch CE, Walsh TR, et al. Influence of cardiopulmonary resuscitation prior to defibrillation in patients with out-of-hospital ventricular fibrillation. JAMA 1999;281:1182—8.

194. Wik L, Hansen TB, Fylling F, et al. Delaying defibrillation to give basic cardiopulmonary resuscitation to patients with out-of-hospital ventricular fibrillation: a randomized trial. JAMA 2003;289:1389—95.

195. Jacobs IG, Finn JC, Oxer HF, Jelinek GA. CPR before defibrillation in out-of-hospital cardiac arrest: a randomized trial. Emerg Med Australas 2005;17:39—45.

196. Somberg JC, Bailin SJ, Haffajee CI, et al. Intravenous lidocaine versus intravenous amiodarone (in a new aqueous formulation) for incessant ventricular tachycardia. Am J Cardiol 2002;90:853—9.

197. Kudenchuk PJ, Cobb LA, Copass MK, et al. Amiodarone for resuscitation after out-of-hospital cardiac arrest due to ventricular fibrillation. N Engl J Med 1999;341:871—8.

198. Perry JC, Fenrich AL, Hulse JE, Triedman JK, Friedman RA, Lamberti JJ. Pediatric use of intravenous amiodarone: efficacy and safety in critically ill patients from a multicenter protocol. J Am Coll Cardiol 1996;27:1246—50.

199. Cummins RO, Graves JR, Larsen MP, et al. Out-of-hospital transcutaneous pacing by emergency medical technicians in patients with asystolic cardiac arrest. N Engl J Med 1993;328:1377—82.

200. Sreeram N, Wren C. Supraventricular tachycardia in infants: response to initial treatment. Arch Dis Child 1990;65:127—9.

201. Bianconi L, Castro AMD, Dinelli M, et al. Comparison of intravenously administered dofetilide versus amiodarone in the acute termination of atrial fibrillation and flutter. A multicentre, randomized, double-blind, placebo-controlled study. Eur Heart J 2000;21:1265—73.

202. Burri S, Hug MI, Bauersfeld U. Efficacy and safety of intravenous amiodarone for incessant tachycardias in infants. Eur J Pediatr 2003;162:880—4.

203. Celiker A, Ceviz N, Ozme S. Effectiveness and safety of intravenous amiodarone in drug-resistant tachyarrhythmias of children. Acta Paediatrica Japonica 1998;40:567—72.

204. Dodge-Khatami A, Miller O, Anderson R, Gil-Jaurena J, Goldman A, de Leval M. Impact of junctional ectopic tachycardia on postoperative morbidity following repair of congenital heart defects. Eur J Cardio-Thoracic Surg 2002;21:255—9.

205. Figa FH, Gow RM, Hamilton RM, Freedom RM. Clinical efficacy and safety of intravenous Amiodarone in infants and children. Am J Cardiol 1994;74:573—7.

206. Hoffman TM, Bush DM, Wernovsky G, et al. Postoperative junctional ectopic tachycardia in children: incidence, risk factors, and treatment. Ann Thorac Surg 2002;74:1607—11.

207. Soult JA, Munoz M, Lopez JD, Romero A, Santos J, Tovaruela A. Efficacy and safety of intravenous amiodarone for short-term treatment of paroxysmal supraventricular tachycardia in children. Pediatr Cardiol 1995;16:16—9.

208. Benson Jr D, Smith W, Dunnigan A, Sterba R, Gallagher J. Mechanisms of regular wide QRS tachycardia in infants and children. Am J Cardiol 1982;49:1778—88.

209. Drago F, Mazza A, Guccione P, Mafrici A, Di Liso G, Ragonese P. Amiodarone used alone or in combination with propranolol: a very effective therapy for tachyarrhythmias in infants and children. Pediatr Cardiol 1998;19:445—9.

210. Benson DJ, Dunnigan A, Green T, Benditt D, Schneider S. Periodic procainamide for paroxysmal tachycardia. Circulation 1985;72:147—52.

211. Komatsu C, Ishinaga T, Tateishi O, Tokuhisa Y, Yoshimura S. Effects of four antiarrhythmic drugs on the induction and termination of paroxysmal supraventricular tachycardia. Jpn Circ J 1986;50:961—72.

212. Mandel WJ, Laks MM, Obayashi K, Hayakawa H, Daley W. The Wolff-Parkinson-White syndrome: pharmacologic effects of procaine amide. Am Heart J 1975;90:744—54.

213. Meldon SW, Brady WJ, Berger S, Mannenbach M. Pediatric ventricular tachycardia: a review with three illustrative cases. Pediatr Emerg Care 1994;10:294—300.

214. Shih JY, Gillette PC, Kugler JD, et al. The electrophysiologic effects of procainamide in the immature heart. Pediatr Pharmacol (New York) 1982;2:65—73.

215. Hildebrand CA, Hartmann AG, Arcinue EL, Gomez RJ, Bing RJ. Cardiac performance in pediatric near-drowning. Crit Care Med 1988;16:331—5.

216. Checchia PA, Sehra R, Moynihan J, Daher N, Tang W, Weil MH. Myocardial injury in children following resuscitation after cardiac arrest. Resuscitation 2003;57:131—7.

217. Hickey RW, Ferimer H, Alexander HL, et al. Delayed, spontaneous hypothermia reduces neuronal damage after asphyxial cardiac arrest in rats. Crit Care Med 2000;28:3511—6.

218. Hypothermia After Cardiac Arrest Study Aroup. Mild therapeutic hypothermia to improve the neurologic outcome after cardiac arrest. N Engl J Med 2002;346:549—56.

219. Bernard SA, Gray TW, Buist MD, et al. Treatment of comatose survivors of out-of-hospital cardiac arrest with induced hypothermia. N Engl J Med 2002;346:557—63.

220. Gluckman PD, Wyatt JS, Azzopardi D, et al. Selective head cooling with mild systemic hypothermia after neonatal encephalopathy: multicentre randomised trial. Lancet 2005;365:663—70.

221. Battin MR, Penrice J, Gunn TR, Gunn AJ. Treatment of term infants with head cooling and mild systemic hypothermia (35.0 degrees C and 34.5 degrees C) after perinatal asphyxia. Pediatrics 2003;111:244—51.

222. Compagnoni G, Pogliani L, Lista G, Castoldi F, Fontana P, Mosca F. Hypothermia reduces neurological damage in asphyxiated newborn infants. Biol Neonate 2002;82:222—7.

223. Gunn AJ, Gluckman PD, Gunn TR. Selective head cooling in newborn infants after perinatal asphyxia: a safety study. Pediatrics 1998;102:885—92.

224. Debillon T, Daoud P, Durand P, et al. Whole-body cooling after perinatal asphyxia: a pilot study in term neonates. Dev Med Child Neurol 2003;45:17—23.

225. Hachimi-Idrissi S, Corne L, Ebinger G, Michotte Y, Huyghens L. Mild hypothermia induced by a helmet device: a clinical feasibility study. Resuscitation 2001;51:275—81.

226. Bernard S, Buist M, Monteiro O, Smith K. Induced hypothermia using large volume, ice-cold intravenous fluid in comatose survivors of out-of-hospital cardiac arrest: a preliminary report. Resuscitation 2003;56:9—13.

227. Kliegel A, Losert H, Sterz F, et al. Cold simple intravenous infusions preceding special endovascular cooling for faster induction of mild hypothermia after cardiac arrest—a feasibility study. Resuscitation 2005;64:347—51.

228. Polderman KH, Peerdeman SM, Girbes AR. Hypophosphatemia and hypomagnesemia induced by cooling in patients with severe head injury. J Neurosurg 2001;94:697—705.

229. Polderman KH. Application of therapeutic hypothermia in the intensive care unit. Opportunities and pitfalls of a promising treatment modality—Part 2. Practical aspects and side effects. Intensive Care Med 2004;30:757—69.

230. Zeiner A, Holzer M, Sterz F, et al. Hyperthermia after cardiac arrest is associated with an unfavorable neurologic outcome. Arch Intern Med 2001;161:2007—12.

231. Takino M, Okada Y. Hyperthermia following cardiopulmonary resuscitation. Intensive Care Med 1991;17:419—20.

232. Takasu A, Saitoh D, Kaneko N, Sakamoto T, Okada Y. Hyperthermia: is it an ominous sign after cardiac arrest? Resuscitation 2001;49:273—7.

233. Coimbra C, Boris-Moller F, Drake M, Wieloch T. Diminished neuronal damage in the rat brain by late treatment with the antipyretic drug dipyrone or cooling following cerebral ischemia. Acta Neuropathol (Berl) 1996;92:447—53.

234. Coimbra C, Drake M, Boris-Moller F, Wieloch T. Long-lasting neuroprotective effect of postischemic hypothermia and treatment with an anti-inflammatory/antipyretic drug: evidence for chronic encephalopathic processes following ischemia. Stroke 1996;27:1578—85.

235. Gillis J, Dickson D, Rieder M, Steward D, Edmonds J. Results of inpatient pediatric resuscitation. Crit Care Med 1986;14:469—71.

236. Schindler MB, Bohn D, Cox PN, et al. Outcome of out-of-hospital cardiac or respiratory arrest in children. N Engl J Med 1996;335:1473—9.

237. Suominen P, Korpela R, Kuisma M, Silfvast T, Olkkola KT. Paediatric cardiac arrest and resuscitation provided by physician-staffed emergency care units. Acta Anaesthesiol Scand 1997;41:260—5.

238. Lopez-Herce J, Garcia C, Rodriguez-Nunez A, et al. Long-term outcome of paediatric cardiorespiratory arrest in Spain. Resuscitation 2005;64:79—85.

239. Lopez-Herce J, Garcia C, Dominguez P, et al. Characteristics and outcome of cardiorespiratory arrest in children. Resuscitation 2004;63:311—20.

240. Hazinski MF, Chahine AA, Holcomb III GW, Morris Jr JA. Outcome of cardiovascular collapse in pediatric blunt trauma. Ann Emerg Med 1994;23:1229—35.

241. Morris MC, Wernovsky G, Nadkarni VM. Survival outcomes after extracorporeal cardiopulmonary resuscitation instituted during active chest compressions following refractory in-hospital pediatric cardiac arrest. Pediatr Crit Care Med 2004;5:440—6.

242. Duncan BW, Ibrahim AE, Hraska V, et al. Use of rapid-deployment extracorporeal membrane oxygenation for the resuscitation of pediatric patients with heart disease after cardiac arrest. J Thorac Cardiovasc Surg 1998;116:305—11.

243. Parra DA, Totapally BR, Zahn E, et al. Outcome of cardiopulmonary resuscitation in a pediatric cardiac intensive care unit. Crit Care Med 2000;28:3296—300.

244. Idris AH, Berg RA, Bierens J, et al. Recommended guidelines for uniform reporting of data from drowning: the ''Utstein style''. Resuscitation 2003;59:45—57.

245. Bauchner H, Waring C, Vinci R. Parental presence during procedures in an emergency room: results from 50 observations. Pediatrics 1991;87:544—8.

246. Bauchner H, Vinci R, Waring C. Pediatric procedures: do parents want to watch? Pediatrics 1989;84:907—9 [comment].

247. Bauchner H, Zuckerman B. Cocaine, sudden infant death syndrome, and home monitoring. J Pediatr 1990;117:904—6.

248. Haimi-Cohen Y, Amir J, Harel L, Straussberg R, Varsano Y. Parental presence during lumbar puncture: anxiety and attitude toward the procedure. Clin Pediatr (Phila) 1996;35:2—4.

249. Sacchetti A, Lichenstein R, Carraccio CA, Harris RH. Family member presence during pediatric emergency department procedures. Pediatr Emerg Care 1996;12:268—71.

250. Boie ET, Moore GP, Brummett C, Nelson DR. Do parents want to be present during invasive procedures performed on their children in the emergency department? A survey of 400 parents. Ann Emerg Med 1999;34:70—4.

251. Taylor N, Bonilla L, Silver P, Sagy M. Pediatric procedure: do parents want to be present? Crit Care Med 1996;24:A131.

252. Powers KS, Rubenstein JS. Family presence during invasive procedures in the pediatric intensive care unit: a prospective study. Arch Pediatr Adolesc Med 1999;153:955—8.

253. Cameron JA, Bond MJ, Pointer SC. Reducing the anxiety of children undergoing surgery: parental presence during anaesthetic induction. J Paediatr Child Health 1996;32:51—6.

254. Merritt KA, Sargent JR, Osborn LM. Attitudes regarding parental presence during medical procedures. Am J Dis Child 1990;144:270—1.

255. Wolfram RW, Turner ED. Effects of parental presence during children's venipuncture. Acad Emerg Med 1996;3:58—64.

256. Jarvis AS. Parental presence during resuscitation: attitudes of staff on a paediatric intensive care unit. Intensive Crit Care Nurs 1998;14:3—7.

257. Meyers TA, Eichhorn DJ, Guzzetta CE. Do families want to be present during CPR? A retrospective survey. J Emerg Nurs 1998;24:400—5.

258. Doyle CJ, Post H, Burney RE, Maino J, Keefe M, Rhee KJ. Family participation during resuscitation: an option. Ann Emerg Med 1987;16:673—5.

259. Hanson C, Strawser D. Family presence during cardiopulmonary resuscitation: Foote Hospital emergency department's nine-year perspective. J Emerg Nurs 1992;18:104—6.

260. Robinson SM, Mackenzie-Ross S, Campbell Hewson GL, Egleston CV, Prevost AT. Psychological effect of witnessed resuscitation on bereaved relatives. Lancet 1998;352:614—7.

261. Meyers TA, Eichhorn DJ, Guzzetta CE, et al. Family presence during invasive procedures and resuscitation. Am J Nurs 2000;100:32—42 [quiz 3].

262. Beckman AW, Sloan BK, Moore GP, et al. Should parents be present during emergency department procedures on children, and who should make that decision? A survey of emergency physician and nurse attitudes. Acad Emerg Med 2002;9:154—8.

263. Eppich WJ, Arnold LD. Family member presence in the pediatric emergency department. Curr Opin Pediatr 2003;15:294—8.

264. Eichhorn DJ, Meyers TA, Mitchell TG, Guzzetta CE. Opening the doors: family presence during resuscitation. J Cardiovasc Nurs 1996;10:59—70.

265. International Liaison Committee on Resuscitation. Part 7. Neonatal Life Support. 2005 International Consensus on Cardiopulmonary Resuscitation and Emergency Cardiovascular Care Science with Treatment Recommendations. Resuscitation 2005;67:293—303.

266. Resuscitation Council (UK). Resuscitation at birth. Newborn life support course provider manual. London, Resuscitation Council (UK); 2001.

267. Niermeyer S, Kattwinkel J, Van Reempts P, et al. International Guidelines for Neonatal Resuscitation: an excerpt from the Guidelines 2000 for Cardiopulmonary Resuscitation and Emergency Cardiovascular Care: International Consensus on Science. Contributors and Reviewers for the Neonatal Resuscitation Guidelines. Pediatrics E2000;106:29.

268. Palme-Kilander C. Methods of resuscitation in low-Apgar-score newborn infants—a national survey. Acta Paediatr 1992;81:739—44.

269. British Paediatric Association Working Party. Neonatal Resuscitation. London: British Paediatric Association; 1993.

270. Dahm LS, James LS. Newborn temperature and calculated heat loss in the delivery room. Pediatrics 1972;49:504—13.

271. Stephenson J, Du J, Tk O. The effect if cooling on blood gas tensions in newborn infants. J Pediatr 1970;76:848—52.

272. Gandy GM, Adamsons Jr K, Cunningham N, Silverman WA, James LS. Thermal environment and acid—base homeostasis in human infants during the first few hours of life. J Clin Invest 1964;43:751—8.

273. Apgar V. A proposal for a new method of evaluation of the newborn infant. Curr Res Anesth Analg 1953:32.

274. Anonymous. Is the Apgar score outmoded? Lancet 1989;i:591—2.

275. Chamberlain G, Banks J. Assessment of the Apgar score. Lancet 1974;2:1225—8.

276. Owen CJ, Wyllie JP. Determination of heart rate in the baby at birth. Resuscitation 2004;60:213—7.

277. Cordero Jr L, Hon EH. Neonatal bradycardia following nasopharyngeal stimulation. J Pediatr 1971;78:441—7.

278. Thaler MM, Stobie GH. An improved technique of external caridac compression in infants and young children. N Engl J Med 1963;269:606—10.

279. Todres ID, Rogers MC. Methods of external cardiac massage in the newborn infant. J Pediatr 1975;86:781—2.

280. Dean JM, Koehler RC, Schleien CL, et al. Improved blood flow during prolonged cardiopulmonary resuscitation with 30% duty cycle in infant pigs. Circulation 1991;84:896—904.

281. Whyte SD, Sinha AK, Wyllie JP. Neonatal resuscitation: a practical assessment. Resuscitation 1999;40:21—5.

282. Costeloe K, Hennessy E, Gibson AT, Marlow N, Wilkinson AR. The EPICure study: outcomes to discharge from hospital for infants born at the threshold of viability. Pediatrics 2000;106:659—71.

283. Vohra S, Frent G, Campbell V, Abbott M, Whyte R. Effect of polyethylene occlusive skin wrapping on heat loss in very low birth weight infants at delivery: a randomized trial. J Pediatr 1999;134:547—51.

284. Lenclen R, Mazraani M, Jugie M, et al. Use of a polyethylene bag: a way to improve the thermal environment of the premature newborn at the delivery room. Arch Pediatr 2002;9:238—44.

285. Bjorklund LJ, Hellstrom-Westas L. Reducing heat loss at birth in very preterm infants. J Pediatr 2000;137:739—40.

286. Vohra S, Roberts RS, Zhang B, Janes M, Schmidt B. Heat loss prevention (HeLP) in the delivery room: a randomized controlled trial of polyethylene occlusive skin wrapping in very preterm infants. J Pediatr 2004;145:750—3.

287. Lieberman E, Eichenwald E, Mathur G, Richardson D, Heffner L, Cohen A. Intrapartum fever and unexplained seizures in term infants. Pediatrics 2000;106:983—8.

288. Grether JK, Nelson KB. Maternal infection and cerebral palsy in infants of normal birth weight. JAMA 1997;278:207—11.

289. Dietrich WD, Alonso O, Halley M, Busto R. Delayed posttraumatic brain hyperthermia worsens outcome after fluid percussion brain injury: a light and electron microscopic study in rats. Neurosurgery 1996;38:533—41 [discussion 41].

290. Wiswell TE, Gannon CM, Jacob J, et al. Delivery room management of the apparently vigorous meconium-stained neonate: results of the multicenter, international collaborative trial. Pediatrics 2000;105:1—7.

291. Vain NE, Szyld EG, Prudent LM, Wiswell TE, Aguilar AM, Vivas NI. Oropharyngeal and nasopharyngeal suctioning of meconium-stained neonates before delivery of their shoulders: multicentre, randomised controlled trial. Lancet 2004;364:597—602.

292. Solas AB, Kutzsche S, Vinje M, Saugstad OD. Cerebral hypoxemia-ischemia and reoxygenation with 21% or 100% oxygen in newborn piglets: effects on extracellular levels of excitatory amino acids and microcirculation. Pediatr Crit Care Med 2001;2:340—5.

293. Solas AB, Kalous P, Saugstad OD. Reoxygenation with 100 or 21% oxygen after cerebral hypoxemia-ischemia-hypercapnia in newborn piglets. Biol Neonate 2004;85:105—11.

294. Solas AB, Munkeby BH, Saugstad OD. Comparison of short- and long-duration oxygen treatment after cerebral asphyxia in newborn piglets. Pediatr Res 2004;56:125—31.

295. Huang CC, Yonetani M, Lajevardi N, Delivoria-Papadopoulos M, Wilson DF, Pastuszko A. Comparison of postasphyxial resuscitation with 100% and 21% oxygen on cortical oxygen pressure and striatal dopamine metabolism in newborn piglets. J Neurochem 1995;64:292—8.

296. Kutzsche S, Ilves P, Kirkeby OJ, Saugstad OD. Hydrogen peroxide production in leukocytes during cerebral hypoxia and reoxygenation with 100% or 21% oxygen in newborn piglets. Pediatr Res 2001;49:834—42.

297. Lundstrom KE, Pryds O, Greisen G. Oxygen at birth and prolonged cerebral vasoconstriction in preterm infants. Arch Dis Child Fetal Neonatal Ed 1995;73:F81—6.

298. Davis PG, Tan A, O'Donnell CP, Schulze A. Resuscitation of newborn infants with 100% oxygen or air: a systematic review and meta-analysis. Lancet 2004;364:1329—33.

299. Harris AP, Sendak MJ, Donham RT. Changes in arterial oxygen saturation immediately after birth in the human neonate. J Pediatr 1986;109:117—9.

300. Reddy VK, Holzman IR, Wedgwood JF. Pulse oximetry saturations in the first 6 hours of life in normal term infants. Clin Pediatr (Phila) 1999;38:87—92.

301. Toth B, Becker A, Seelbach-Gobel B. Oxygen saturation in healthy newborn infants immediately after birth measured by pulse oximetry. Arch Gynecol Obstet 2002;266:105—7.

302. Karlberg P, Koch G. Respiratory studies in newborn infants. III. Development of mechanics of breathing during the first week of life. A longitudinal study Acta Paediatr 1962;(Suppl. 135):121—9.

303. Vyas H, Milner AD, Hopkins IE. Intrathoracic pressure and volume changes during the spontaneous onset of respiration in babies born by cesarean section and by vaginal delivery. J Pediatr 1981;99:787—91.

304. Mortola JP, Fisher JT, Smith JB, Fox GS, Weeks S, Willis D. Onset of respiration in infants delivered by cesarean section. J Appl Physiol 1982;52:716—24.

305. Hull D. Lung expansion and ventilation during resuscitation of asphyxiated newborn infants. J Pediatr 1969;75:47—58.

306. Upton CJ, Milner AD. Endotracheal resuscitation of neonates using a rebreathing bag. Arch Dis Child 1991;66:39—42.

307. Vyas H, Milner AD, Hopkin IE, Boon AW. Physiologic responses to prolonged and slow-rise inflation in the resuscitation of the asphyxiated newborn infant. J Pediatr 1981;99:635—9.

308. Vyas H, Field D, Milner AD, Hopkin IE. Determinants of the first inspiratory volume and functional residual capacity at birth. Pediatr Pulmonol 1986;2:189—93.

309. Boon AW, Milner AD, Hopkin IE. Lung expansion, tidal exchange, and formation of the functional residual capacity during resuscitation of asphyxiated neonates. J Pediatr 1979;95:1031—6.

310. Ingimarsson J, Bjorklund LJ, Curstedt T, et al. Incomplete protection by prophylactic surfactant against the adverse effects of large lung inflations at birth in immature lambs. Intensive Care Med 2004;30:1446—53.

311. Nilsson R, Grossmann G, Robertson B. Bronchiolar epithelial lesions induced in the premature rabbit neonate by short periods of artificial ventilation. Acta Pathol Microbiol Scand [A] 1980;88:359—67.

312. Probyn ME, Hooper SB, Dargaville PA, et al. Positive end expiratory pressure during resuscitation of premature lambs rapidly improves blood gases without adversely affecting arterial pressure. Pediatr Res 2004;56:198—204.

313. Hird MF, Greenough A, Gamsu HR. Inflating pressures for effective resuscitation of preterm infants. Early Hum Dev 1991;26:69—72.

314. Lindner W, Vossbeck S, Hummler H, Pohlandt F. Delivery room management of extremely low birth weight infants: spontaneous breathing or intubation? Pediatrics 1999;103:961—7.

315. Allwood AC, Madar RJ, Baumer JH, Readdy L, Wright D. Changes in resuscitation practice at birth. Arch Dis Child Fetal Neonatal Ed 2003;88:F375—9.

316. Cole AF, Rolbin SH, Hew EM, Pynn S. An improved ventilator system for delivery-room management of the newborn. Anesthesiology 1979;51:356—8.

317. Hoskyns EW, Milner AD, Hopkin IE. A simple method of face mask resuscitation at birth. Arch Dis Child 1987;62:376—8.

318. Ganga-Zandzou PS, Diependaele JF, Storme L, et al. Is Ambu ventilation of newborn infants a simple question of finger-touch? Arch Pediatr 1996;3:1270—2.

319. Finer NN, Rich W, Craft A, Henderson C. Comparison of methods of bag and mask ventilation for neonatal resuscitation. Resuscitation 2001;49:299—305.

320. Kanter RK. Evaluation of mask-bag ventilation in resuscitation of infants. Am J Dis Child 1987;141:761—3.

321. Esmail N, Saleh M, et al. Laryngeal mask airway versus endotracheal intubation for Apgar score improvement in neonatal resuscitation. Egypt J Anesthesiol 2002;18:115—21.

322. Gandini D, Brimacombe JR. Neonatal resuscitation with the laryngeal mask airway in normal and low birth weight infants. Anesth Analg 1999;89:642—3.

323. Brimacombe J, Gandini D. Airway rescue and drug delivery in an 800 g neonate with the laryngeal mask airway. Paediatr Anaesth 1999;9:178.

324. Lonnqvist PA. Successful use of laryngeal mask airway in low-weight expremature infants with bronchopulmonary dysplasia undergoing cryotherapy for retinopathy of the premature. Anesthesiology 1995;83:422—4.

325. Paterson SJ, Byrne PJ, Molesky MG, Seal RF, Finucane BT. Neonatal resuscitation using the laryngeal mask airway. Anesthesiology 1994;80:1248—53.

326. Trevisanuto D, Ferrarese P, Zanardo V, Chiandetti L. Laryngeal mask airway in neonatal resuscitation: a survey of current practice and perceived role by anaesthesiologists and paediatricians. Resuscitation 2004;60:291—6.

327. Hansen TG, Joensen H, Henneberg SW, Hole P. Laryngeal mask airway guided tracheal intubation in a neonate with the Pierre Robin syndrome. Acta Anaesthesiol Scand 1995;39:129—31.

328. Osses H, Poblete M, Asenjo F. Laryngeal mask for difficult intubation in children. Paediatr Anaesth 1999;9:399—401.

329. Stocks RM, Egerman R, Thompson JW, Peery M. Airway management of the severely retrognathic child: use of the laryngeal mask airway. Ear Nose Throat J 2002;81:223—6.

330. Palme-Kilander C, Tunell R, Chiwei Y. Pulmonary gas exchange immediately after birth in spontaneously breathing infants. Arch Dis Child 1993;68:6—10.

331. Aziz HF, Martin JB, Moore JJ. The pediatric disposable end-tidal carbon dioxide detector role in endotracheal intubation in newborns. J Perinatol 1999;19:110—3.

332. Bhende MS, LaCovey D. A note of caution about the continuous use of colorimetric end-tidal CO_2 detectors in children. Pediatrics 1995;95:800—1.

333. Repetto JE, Donohue P-CP, Baker SF, Kelly L, Nogee LM. Use of capnography in the delivery room for assessment of endotracheal tube placement. J Perinatol 2001;21:284—7.

334. Roberts WA, Maniscalco WM, Cohen AR, Litman RS, Chhibber A. The use of capnography for recognition of esophageal intubation in the neonatal intensive care unit. Pediatr Pulmonol 1995;19:262—8.

335. Berg RA, Otto CW, Kern KB, et al. A randomized, blinded trial of high-dose epinephrine versus standard-dose epinephrine in a swine model of pediatric asphyxial cardiac arrest. Crit Care Med 1996;24:1695—700.

336. Burchfield DJ, Preziosi MP, Lucas VW, Fan J. Effects of graded doses of epinephrine during asphxia-induced bradycardia in newborn lambs. Resuscitation 1993;25:235—44.

337. Ralston SH, Voorhees WD, Babbs CF. Intrapulmonary epinephrine during prolonged cardiopulmonary resuscitation: improved regional blood flow and resuscitation in dogs. Ann Emerg Med 1984;13:79—86.

338. Ralston SH, Tacker WA, Showen L, Carter A, Babbs CF. Endotracheal versus intravenous epinephrine during electromechanical dissociation with CPR in dogs. Ann Emerg Med 1985;14:1044—8.

339. Redding JS, Asuncion JS, Pearson JW. Effective routes of drug administration during cardiac arrest. Anesth Analg 1967;46:253—8.

340. Schwab KO, von Stockhausen HB. Plasma catecholamines after endotracheal administration of adrenaline during postnatal resuscitation. Arch Dis Child Fetal Neonatal Ed 1994;70:F213—7.

341. Brambrink AM, Ichord RN, Martin LJ, Koehler RC, Traystman RJ. Poor outcome after hypoxia-ischemia in newborns is associated with physiological abnormalities during early recovery. Possible relevance to secondary brain injury after head trauma in infants. Exp Toxicol Pathol 1999;51:151—62.

342. Vannucci RC, Vannucci SJ. Cerebral carbohydrate metabolism during hypoglycemia and anoxia in newborn rats. Ann Neurol 1978;4:73—9.

343. Yager JY, Heitjan DF, Towfighi J, Vannucci RC. Effect of insulin-induced and fasting hypoglycemia on peri-

natal hypoxic-ischemic brain damage. Pediatr Res 1992;31:138—42.

344. Salhab WA, Wyckoff MH, Laptook AR, Perlman JM. Initial hypoglycemia and neonatal brain injury in term infants with severe fetal acidemia. Pediatrics 2004;114:361—6.

345. Kent TA, Soukup VM, Fabian RH. Heterogeneity affecting outcome from acute stroke therapy: making reperfusion worse. Stroke 2001;32:2318—27.

346. Eicher DJ, Wagner CL, Katikaneni LP, et al. Moderate hypothermia in neonatal encephalopathy: efficacy outcomes. Pediatr Neurol 2005;32:11—7.

347. Thoresen M, Whitelaw A. Cardiovascular changes during mild therapeutic hypothermia and rewarming in infants with hypoxic-ischemic encephalopathy. Pediatrics 2000;106:92—9.

348. Shankaran S, Laptook A, Wright LL, et al. Whole-body hypothermia for neonatal encephalopathy: animal observations as a basis for a randomized, controlled pilot study in term infants. Pediatrics 2002;110:377—85.

349. De Leeuw R, Cuttini M, Nadai M, et al. Treatment choices for extremely preterm infants: an international perspective. J Pediatr 2000;137:608—16.

350. Lee SK, Penner PL, Cox M. Comparison of the attitudes of health care professionals and parents toward active treatment of very low birth weight infants. Pediatrics 1991;88:110—4.

351. Kopelman LM, Irons TG, Kopelman AE. Neonatologists judge the ''Baby Doe'' regulations. N Engl J Med 1988;318:677—83.

352. Sanders MR, Donohue PK, Oberdorf MA, Rosenkrantz TS, Allen MC. Perceptions of the limit of viability: neonatologists' attitudes toward extremely preterm infants. J Perinatol 1995;15:494—502.

353. Draper ES, Manktelow B, Field DJ, James D. Tables for predicting survival for preterm births are updated. BMJ 2003;327:872.

354. Jain L, Ferre C, Vidyasagar D, Nath S, Sheftel D. Cardiopulmonary resuscitation of apparently stillborn infants: survival and long-term outcome. J Pediatr 1991;118:778—82.

355. Haddad B, Mercer BM, Livingston JC, Talati A, Sibai BM. Outcome after successful resuscitation of babies born with apgar scores of 0 at both 1 and 5 minutes. Am J Obstet Gynecol 2000;182:1210—4.

Resuscitation (2005) **67S1**, S135—S170

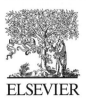

ELSEVIER

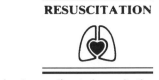

RESUSCITATION

www.elsevier.com/locate/resuscitation

European Resuscitation Council Guidelines for Resuscitation 2005
Section 7. Cardiac arrest in special circumstances

Jasmeet Soar, Charles D. Deakin, Jerry P. Nolan, Gamal Abbas, Annette Alfonzo, Anthony J. Handley, David Lockey, Gavin D. Perkins, Karl Thies

7a. Life-threatening electrolyte disorders

Overview

Electrolyte abnormalities can cause cardiac arrhythmias or cardiopulmonary arrest. Life-threatening arrhythmias are associated commonly with potassium disorders, particularly hyperkalaemia, and less commonly with disorders of serum calcium and magnesium. In some cases therapy for life-threatening electrolyte disorders should start before the laboratory results become available.

The electrolyte values for definitions have been chosen as a guide to clinical decision-making. The precise values that trigger treatment decisions will depend on the patient's clinical condition and the rate of change of the electrolyte values.

There is little or no evidence base for the treatment of electrolyte abnormalities during cardiac arrest. Guidance during cardiac arrest is based on the strategies used in the non-arrest patient. There are no major changes in the treatment of these disorders since the International Guidelines 2000.[1]

Prevention of electrolyte disorders

- Treat life-threatening electrolyte abnormalities before cardiac arrest occurs.
- After initial treatment, remove any precipitating factors (e.g., drugs) and monitor electrolyte levels to prevent recurrence of the abnormality.
- Monitor renal function in patients at risk of electrolyte disorders.
- In haemodialysis patients, review the dialysis prescription regularly to avoid inappropriate electrolyte shifts during treatment.

Potassium disorders

Potassium homeostasis

Extracellular potassium concentration is regulated tightly between $3.5-5.0 \, \text{mmol} \, l^{-1}$. A large concentration gradient normally exists between the intracellular and extracellular fluid compartments. This potassium gradient across the cell membranes contributes to the excitability of nerve and muscle cells, including the myocardium. Evaluation of serum potassium must take into consideration the effects of changes in serum pH. When serum pH decreases, serum potassium increases because

0300-9572/$ — see front matter © 2005 European Resuscitation Council. All Rights Reserved. Published by Elsevier Ireland Ltd.
doi:10.1016/j.resuscitation.2005.10.004

potassium shifts from the cellular to the vascular space. When serum pH increases, serum potassium decreases because potassium shifts intracellularly. We therefore anticipate the effects of pH changes on serum potassium during the therapy for hyperkalaemia or hypokalaemia.

Hyperkalaemia

This is the most common electrolyte disorder associated with cardiopulmonary arrest. It is usually caused by increased potassium release from the cells or impaired excretion by the kidneys.

Definition. There is no universal definition, although we have defined hyperkalaemia as a serum potassium concentration higher than $5.5\,mmol\,l^{-1}$; in practice, hyperkalaemia is a continuum. As the potassium concentration increases above this value, the risk of adverse events increases and the need for urgent treatment increases. Severe hyperkalaemia has been defined as a serum potassium concentration higher than $6.5\,mmol\,l^{-1}$.

Causes. There are several potential causes of hyperkalaemia, including renal failure, drugs (angiotensin converting enzyme inhibitors (ACEI), angiotensin II receptor blockers (ARB), potassium-sparing diuretics, non-steroidal anti-inflammatory drugs (NSAIDs), beta-blockers, trimethoprim, tissue breakdown (rhabdomyolysis, tumour lysis, haemolysis), metabolic acidosis, endocrine disorders (Addison's disease), hyperkalaemic periodic paralysis, or diet, which may be the sole cause in patients with established renal failure. Abnormal erythrocytes or thrombocytosis may cause a spuriously high potassium concentration. The risk of hyperkalaemia is even greater when there is a combination of factors, such as the concomitant use of ACEI and NSAIDs or potassium-sparing diuretics.

Recognition of hyperkalaemia. Exclude hyperkalaemia in patients with an arrhythmia or cardiac arrest.[2] Patients may present with weakness progressing to flaccid paralysis, paraesthesia or depressed deep tendon reflexes. The first indicator of hyperkalaemia may also be the presence of ECG abnormalities, arrhythmias, cardiopulmonary arrest or sudden death. The effect of hyperkalaemia on the ECG depends on the absolute serum potassium as well as the rate of increase. Most patients will have ECG abnormalities at a serum potassium concentration higher than $6.7\,mmol\,l^{-1}$.[3] The ECG manifestations of hyperkalaemia are usually progressive and include:

- first-degree heart block (prolonged PR interval) >0.2 s;
- flattened or absent P waves;
- tall, peaked (tented) T waves, larger than R wave in more than one lead;
- ST segment depression;
- S and T waves merging;
- widened QRS >0.12 s;
- ventricular tachycardia (VT);
- bradycardia;
- cardiac arrest, i.e., pulseless electrical activity (PEA), ventricular fibrillation (VF), asystole.

Treatment of hyperkalaemia. The five key steps in treating hyperkalaemia are:

1. cardiac protection by antagonising the effects of hyperkalaemia;
2. shifting potassium into cells;
3. removing potassium from the body;
4. monitoring serum potassium for rebound hyperkalaemia;
5. prevention of recurrence of hyperkalaemia.

When hyperkalaemia is strongly suspected, e.g., in the presence of ECG changes, start life-saving treatment even before laboratory results are available. The management of hyperkalaemia is the subject of a recent Cochrane review.[4]

Patient not in cardiac arrest. If the patient is not in cardiac arrest, assess fluid status; if hypovolaemic, give fluid to enhance urinary potassium excretion. The values for classification are an approximate guide. For mild elevation ($5.5-6\,mmol\,l^{-1}$), remove potassium from the body with:

- potassium exchange resins, i.e., calcium resonium 15—30 g or sodium polystyrene sulfonate (Kayexalate®) 15—30 g in 50—100 ml of 20% sorbitol, given either orally or by retention enema (onset in 1—3 h, maximal effect at 6 h);
- diuretics, i.e., furosemide $1\,mg\,kg^{-1}$ IV slowly (onset with the diuresis);
- dialysis; haemodialysis is more efficient than peritoneal dialysis at removing potassium (immediate onset, 25—30 mmol potassium h^{-1} removed with haemodialysis).

For moderate elevation ($6-6.5\,mmol\,l^{-1}$) without ECG changes, shift potassium into cells with:

- dextrose/insulin: 10 units short-acting insulin and 50 g glucose IV over 15—30 min (onset in 15—30 min, maximal effect at 30—60 min; monitor blood glucose). Use in addition to removal strategies above.

For severe elevation ($\geq$6.5 mmol l^{-1}) without ECG changes, shift potassium into cells with:

- salbutamol, 5 mg nebulised. Several doses may be required (onset in 15–30 min);
- sodium bicarbonate, 50 mmol IV over 5 min if metabolic acidosis present (onset in 15–30 min). Bicarbonate alone is less effective than glucose plus insulin or nebulised salbutamol; it is best used in conjunction with these medications;[5,6]
- use multiple shifting agents in addition to removal strategies above.

For severe elevation ($\geq$6.5 mmol l^{-1}) with toxic ECG changes, protect the heart *first* with:

- calcium chloride, i.e., 10 ml 10% calcium chloride IV over 2–5 min to antagonise the toxic effects of hyperkalaemia at the myocardial cell membrane. This protects the heart by reducing the risk of VF, but does not lower serum potassium (onset in 1–3 min). Use in addition to potassium removal and shifting strategies stated above.

Patient in cardiac arrest. If the patient is in cardiac arrest, there are no modifications to BLS in the presence of electrolyte abnormalities. For ALS, follow the universal algorithm. The general approach to treatment depends on the degree of hyperkalaemia, rate of rise of serum potassium and the patient's clinical condition.

In cardiopulmonary arrest, protect the heart first, then apply shifting and removal strategies using:

- calcium chloride: 10 ml of 10% calcium chloride IV by rapid bolus injection to antagonise the toxic effects of hyperkalaemia at the myocardial cell membrane;
- sodium bicarbonate: 50 mmol IV by rapid injection (if severe acidosis or renal failure);
- dextrose/insulin: 10 units short-acting insulin and 50 g glucose IV by rapid injection;
- haemodialysis: consider this for cardiac arrest induced by hyperkalaemia, which is resistant to medical treatment.

Indications for dialysis. Haemodialysis is the most effective method of removal of potassium from the body. The principal mechanism of action is the diffusion of potassium ions across the transmembrane potassium ion gradient. The typical decline in serum potassium is 1 mmol l^{-1} in the first 60 min, followed by 1 mmol l^{-1} over the next 2 h. Consider haemodialysis early for hyperkalaemia associated with established renal failure, oliguric acute renal failure (<400 ml day^{-1} urine output) or when there is marked tissue breakdown. Dialysis is also indicated when hyperkalaemia is resistant to medical management. Serum potassium frequently rebounds after initial treatment. In unstable patients, continuous veno-venous haemofiltration (CVVH) is less likely to compromise cardiac output than intermittent haemodialysis.

Hypokalaemia

Hypokalaemia is common in hospital patients.[7] Hypokalaemia increases the incidence of arrhythmias, particularly in patients with pre-existing heart disease and in those treated with digoxin.

Definition. Hypokalaemia is defined as a serum potassium <3.5 mmol l^{-1}. Severe hypokalaemia is defined as a K$^+$ < 2.5 mmol l^{-1} and may be associated with symptoms.

Causes. Causes of hypokalaemia include gastrointestinal loss (diarrhoea), drugs (diuretics, laxatives, steroids), renal losses (renal tubular disorders, diabetes insipidus, dialysis), endocrine disorders (Cushing's syndrome, hyperaldosteronism), metabolic alkalosis, magnesium depletion and poor dietary intake. Treatment strategies used for hyperkalaemia may also induce hypokalaemia.

Recognition of hypokalaemia. Exclude hypokalaemia in every patient with an arrhythmia or cardiac arrest. In dialysis patients, hypokalaemia occurs commonly at the end of a haemodialysis session or during treatment with continuous ambulatory peritoneal dialysis (CAPD).

As serum potassium concentration decreases, the nerves and muscles are predominantly affected, causing fatigue, weakness, leg cramps and constipation. In severe cases (K$^+$ < 2.5 mmol l^{-1}), rhabdomyolysis, ascending paralysis and respiratory difficulties may occur.

ECG features of hypokalaemia comprise:

- *U* waves;
- *T*-wave flattening;
- ST segment changes;
- arrhythmias, especially if patient is taking digoxin;
- cardiopulmonary arrest (PEA, VF, asystole).

Treatment. Treatment depends on the severity of hypokalaemia and the presence of symptoms and ECG abnormalities. Gradual replacement of potassium is preferable but in emergency intravenous potassium is required. The maximum recommended IV dose of potassium is 20 mmol h^{-1}, but more rapid infusion, e.g., 2 mmol min^{-1} for 10 min followed by 10 mmol over 5–10 min is indicated for unstable arrhythmias when cardiac arrest is imminent. Continuous ECG monitoring is essential during IV infusion, and the dose should be titrated after repeated sampling of serum potassium levels.

Many patients who are potassium deficient are also deficient in magnesium. Magnesium is important for potassium uptake and for the maintenance of intracellular potassium levels, particularly in the myocardium. Repletion of magnesium stores will facilitate more rapid correction of hypokalaemia and is recommended in severe cases of hypokalaemia.[8]

Calcium and magnesium disorders

The recognition and management of calcium and magnesium disorders is summarised in Table 7.1.

Summary

Electrolyte abnormalities are among the most common causes of cardiac arrhythmias. Of all the electrolyte abnormalities, hyperkalaemia is most rapidly fatal. A high degree of clinical suspicion and immediate treatment of the underlying electrolyte abnormalities can prevent many patients from progressing to cardiac arrest.

7b. Poisoning

General considerations

Poisoning is an infrequent cause of cardiac arrest, but remains a leading cause in victims younger than 40 years.[9–12] Most research on this topic consists primarily of small case series, animal studies and case reports.

Self-poisoning with therapeutic or recreational drugs is the main reason for hospital admission. Drug toxicity can also be caused by inappropriate dosing and drug interactions. Accidental poisoning is commonest in children. Homicidal poisoning is uncommon. Industrial accidents, warfare or terrorism may cause extensive chemical or radiation exposure. Decontamination and safe management for mass casualty incidents is not part of these guidelines.

Resuscitation

Treatment of the self-poisoning ('overdose') patient is based on an ABCDE approach to prevent cardiorespiratory arrest whilst awaiting drug elimination.[13] Airway obstruction and respiratory arrest secondary to a decreased conscious level is a common cause of death. Alcohol excess is often associated with self-poisoning.

- After opening and clearing the airway, check for breathing and a pulse. Avoid mouth-to-mouth resuscitation in the presence of toxins, such as cyanide, hydrogen sulphide, corrosives and organophosphates. Ventilate the patient's lungs using a pocket- or bag-mask and the highest possible concentration of oxygen. Be careful in paraquat poisoning as pulmonary injury may be exacerbated by high concentrations of oxygen.[14]
- There is a high incidence of pulmonary aspiration of gastric contents after poisoning. Intubate unconscious patients who cannot protect their airway early, using a rapid-sequence induction with cricoid pressure to decrease the risk of aspiration (see section 4d). This must be undertaken by persons trained in the technique.
- In the event of cardiac arrest, provide standard basic and advanced life support.
- With the exception of torsades de pointes (see below), cardioversion is indicated for life-threatening tachyarrhythmias (see section 4f).
- Drug-induced hypotension is common after self-poisoning. This usually responds to fluid therapy, but occasionally inotropic support is required.
- Once resuscitation is under way, try to identify the poison(s). Relatives, friends and ambulance crews can usually provide useful information. Examination of the patient may reveal diagnostic clues, such as odours, needle puncture marks, pinpoint pupils, tablet residues, signs of corrosion in the mouth or blisters associated with prolonged coma.
- Measure the patient's temperature; hypo- or hyperthermia may occur after drug overdose (see sections 7d and 7e).
- Consult regional or national poisons centres for information on treatment of the poisoned patient.[15,16] The World Health Organization lists poison centres on its website: http://www.who.int/ipcs/poisons/centre/en/.

Specific therapeutic measures

There are few specific therapeutic measures for poisons that are useful immediately. The emphasis is on intensive supportive therapy, with correction of hypoxia, hypotension and acid/base and electrolyte disorders.

Therapeutic measures include limiting absorption of ingested poisons, enhancing elimination, or the use of specific antidotes. For up-to-date guidance in severe or uncommon poisonings, seek

Table 7.1 Calcium (Ca^{2+}) and magnesium (Mg^{2+}) disorders with associated clinical presentation, ECG manifestations and recommended treatment

Disorder	Causes	Presentation	ECG	Treatment
Hypercalcaemia (Ca^{2+} >2.6 mmol l^{-1})	Primary or tertiary hyperparathyroidism Malignancy Sarcoidosis Drugs	Confusion Weakness Abdominal pain Hypotension Arrhythmias Cardiac arrest	Short QT interval Prolonged QRS interval Flat T waves AV-block Cardiac arrest	Fluid replacement IV Furosemide, 1 mg kg^{-1} IV Hydrocortisone, 200–300 mg IV Pamidronate, 60–90 mg IV Calcitonin, 4–8 units kg^{-1} 8 h^{-1} IM Review medication Haemodialysis
Hypocalcaemia (Ca^{2+} <2.1 mmol l^{-1})	Chronic renal failure Acute pancreatitis Calcium channel blocker overdose Toxic shock syndrome Rhabdomyolysis Tumour lysis syndrome	Paraesthesia Tetany Seizures AV-block Cardiac arrest	Prolonged QT interval T-wave inversion Heart block Cardiac arrest	Calcium chloride 10%, 10–40 ml Magnesium sulphate 50%, 4–8 mmol (if necessary)
Hypermagnesaemia (Mg^{2+} > 1.1 mmol l^{-1})	Renal failure Iatrogenic	Confusion Weakness Respiratory depression AV-block Cardiac arrest	Prolonged PR and QT intervals T-wave peaking AV-block Cardiac arrest	Calcium chloride 10%, 5–10 ml, repeated if necessary Ventilatory support if necessary Saline diuresis: 0.9% saline with furosemide 1 mg kg^{-1} IV Haemodialysis
Hypomagnesaemia (Mg^{2+} <0.6 mmol l^{-1})	Gastrointestinal loss Polyuria Starvation Alcoholism Malabsorption	Tremor Ataxia Nystagmus Seizures Arrhythmias: torsades de pointes Cardiac arrest	Prolonged PR and QT Intervals ST-segment depression Torsades de pointes T-wave inversion Flattened P waves Increased QRS duration	Severe or symptomatic: 2 g 50% magnesium sulphate (4 ml = 8 mmol) IV over 15 min Torsade de pointes: 2 g 50% magnesium sulphate (4 ml = 8 mmol) IV over 1–2 min Seizure: 2 g 50% magnesium sulphate (4 ml = 8 mmol) IV over 10 min

advice from a poisons centre.

- Activated charcoal is known to adsorb certain drugs. Its value decreases over time after ingestion. There is no evidence that ingestion of charcoal improves clinical outcome. According to evidence from volunteer studies, consider giving a single dose of activated charcoal to patients who have ingested a potentially toxic amount of poison (known to be adsorbed by activated charcoal) up to 1 h previously.[17] Give it only to patients with an intact or protected airway. Multiple doses of activated charcoal can be beneficial in life-threatening poisoning with carbemazepine, dapsone, phenobarbital, quinine and theophylline.
- Gastric lavage followed by activated charcoal therapy is useful only within 1 h of ingesting the poison.[17] Generally this should be carried out after tracheal intubation. Delayed gastric lavage has very little effect on drug absorption and may propel drugs further along the gastrointestinal tract.[18] Do not give ipecacuanha syrup to induce vomiting; there is little evidence of benefit.[19]
- There is little evidence for the use of laxatives, e.g., lactulose or magnesium citrate, to enhance drug elimination from the gut.[20]
- Whole-bowel irrigation by enteral administration of a polyethylene glycol solution can reduce drug absorption by cleansing the gastrointestinal tract. It can be useful in cases of potentially toxic ingestion of sustained release or enteric-coated drugs, oral iron poisoning and the removal of ingested packets of illicit drugs.[21]
- Urine alkalinisation (pH 7.5) by giving IV sodium bicarbonate can be useful in moderate-to-severe salicylate poisoning in patients who do not need haemodialysis.[22] Urine alkalinisation can also be useful in tricyclic overdose (see below).
- Haemodialysis or haemoperfusion can be useful for elimination of specific life-threatening toxins. Haemodialysis removes drugs or metabolites that are water soluble, have a low volume of distribution and low plasma protein binding.[23] It may be considered for poisoning with methanol, ethylene glycol, salicylates and lithium. Haemoperfusion involves passing blood through an absorptive-containing cartridge (usually charcoal). This technique removes substances that have a high degree of plasma protein binding. Charcoal haemoperfusion may be indicated for intoxications with carbamazepine, phenobarbital, phenytoin and theophylline.
- Specific antidotes (see below) which may be effective include: N-acetylcysteine for paracetamol; high-dose atropine for organophosphate insecticides; sodium nitrite, sodium thiosulphate or dicobalt edetate for cyanides; digoxin-specific Fab antibodies for digoxin; flumazenil for benzodiazepines; and naloxone for opioids. Reversal of benzodiazepine intoxication with flumazenil is associated with significant toxicity in patients with benzodiazepine dependence or co-ingestion of proconvulsant medications, such as tricyclic antidepressants.[24] The routine use of flumazenil in the comatose patient with an overdose is not recommended.

Specific antidotes

These guidelines will address only some causes of cardiorespiratory arrest due to poisoning.

Opioid poisoning

Opioid poisoning commonly causes respiratory depression followed by respiratory insufficiency or respiratory arrest. The respiratory effects of opioids are reversed rapidly by the opiate antagonist naloxone. In severe respiratory depression, the evidence shows fewer adverse events when airway opening, oxygen administration and ventilation are carried out before giving naloxone in cases of opioid-induced respiratory depression;[25–30] however, the use of naloxone can prevent the need for intubation. The preferred route for giving naloxone depends on the skills of the rescuer: IV, intramuscular (IM), subcutaneous (SC), endotracheal (ET) and intranasal (IN) routes can be used. The non-IV routes can be quicker because time is saved in not having to establish IV access, which can be extremely difficult in an IV drug abuser. The initial doses of naloxone are 400 mcg IV,[27] 800 mcg IM, 800 mcg SC,[27] 2 mg IN[31] or 1–2 mg ET. Large opioid overdoses may require titration to a total naloxone dose of 6–10 mg. The duration of action of naloxone is approximately 45–70 min, but respiratory depression can persist for 4–5 h after opioid overdose. Thus, the clinical effects of naloxone may not last as long as those of a significant opioid overdose. Titrate the dose until the victim is breathing adequately and has protective airway reflexes.

Acute withdrawal from opioids produces a state of sympathetic excess and may cause complications, such as pulmonary oedema, ventricular arrhythmia and severe agitation. Use naloxone reversal of opiate intoxication with caution in patients suspected of opioid dependence.

There is no good evidence that naloxone improves outcome once cardiac arrest associated with opioid toxicity has occurred. Cardiac arrest is usually secondary to a respiratory arrest and associated with severe brain hypoxia. Prognosis is poor.[26]

Giving naloxone is unlikely to be harmful. Once cardiac arrest has occurred, follow the standard resuscitation protocols.

Tricyclic antidepressants

Self-poisoning with tricyclic antidepressants is common and can cause hypotension, seizures and arrhythmias. Anticholinergic effects include mydriasis, fever, dry skin, delirium, tachycardia, ileus and urinary retention. Most life-threatening problems occur within the first 6 h after ingestion. A widening QRS complex indicates a greater risk of arrhythmias. There is evidence to support the use of sodium bicarbonate to treat arrhythmias induced by tricyclic antidepressants and/or hypotension.[32–47] The exact threshold for starting treatment based on QRS duration has not been established. No study has investigated the optimal target arterial or urinary pH with bicarbonate therapy, but an arterial pH of 7.45–7.55 has been commonly accepted and seems reasonable. Hypertonic saline may also be effective in treating cardiac toxicity.[48]

Cocaine toxicity

Sympathetic overstimulation associated with cocaine toxicity may cause agitation, symptomatic tachycardia, hypertensive crisis, hyperthermia and myocardial ischaemia with angina. Glyceryl trinitrate and phentolamine reverse cocaine-induced coronary vasoconstriction, labetalol has no significant effect, and propranolol makes it worse.[49–52] Small doses of IV benzodiazepines (midazolam, diazepam, lorazepam) are effective first-line drugs. Use nitrates only as second-line therapy for myocardial ischaemia. Labetalol (alpha- and beta-blocker) is useful for the treatment of tachycardia and hypertensive emergencies due to cocaine toxicity.

Drug-induced severe bradycardia

Severe bradycardia from poisoning or drug overdose may be refractory to standard ALS protocols because of prolonged receptor binding or direct cellular toxicity. Atropine may be life saving in organophosphate, carbamate or nerve agent poisoning. Give atropine for bradycardia caused by acetylcholinesterase-inhibiting substances. Large (2–4 mg) and repeated doses may be required to achieve a clinical effect. Isoprenaline may be useful at high doses in refractory bradycardia induced by beta-antagonist receptor blockade. Heart block and ventricular arrhythmias associated with digoxin or digitalis glycoside poisoning may be treated effec-tively with digoxin-specific antibody fragments.[53] Antibody-specific therapy may also be effective in poisoning from plants as well as Chinese herbal medications containing digitalis glycosides.[53–55]

Vasopressors, inotropes, calcium, glucagon, phosphodiesterase inhibitors and insulin-glucose may all be useful in beta-blocker and calcium channel blocker overdose.[56–58] Transcutaneous pacing may be effective for severe bradycardia caused by poisoning and overdose (see section 3).

Further treatment and prognosis

A long period of coma in a single position can cause pressure sores and rhabdomyolysis. Measure electrolytes (particularly potassium), blood glucose and arterial blood gases. Monitor temperature because thermoregulation is impaired. Both hypothermia and hyperthermia (hyperpyrexia) can occur after the overdose of some drugs. Retain samples of blood and urine for analysis.

Be prepared to continue resuscitation for a prolonged period, particularly in young patients as the poison may be metabolised or excreted during extended life support measures.

Alternative approaches which may be effective in severely poisoned patients include:

- higher doses of medication than in standard protocols;
- non-standard drug therapies;
- prolonged CPR.

7c. Drowning

Overview

Drowning is a common cause of accidental death in Europe. The most important and detrimental consequence of drowning is hypoxia. The duration of hypoxia is the critical factor in determining the victim's outcome. Therefore, oxygenation, ventilation and perfusion should be restored as rapidly as possible. Immediate resuscitation at the scene is essential for survival and neurological recovery after drowning. This will require bystander provision of CPR plus immediate activation of the EMS system. Victims who have spontaneous circulation and breathing when they reach hospital usually recover with good outcomes.

Epidemiology

The World Health Organization (WHO) estimates that, worldwide, drowning accounts for approximately 450,000 deaths each year. A further 1.3 million disability-adjusted life-years are lost each year as a result of premature death or disability from drowning;[59] 97% of deaths from drowning occur in low- and middle-income countries.[59] In 2002, there were 427 deaths from drowning in the United Kingdom (Royal Society for the Prevention of Accidents 2002) and 4073 in the United States (National Center for Injury Prevention 2002), yielding an annual incidence of drowning of 0.8 and 1.45 per 100,000 population, respectively. Death from drowning is more common in young males and is the leading cause of accidental death in Europe in this group.[59] Alcohol consumption is a contributory factor in up to 70% of drownings.[60]

The guidelines in this chapter focus on the treatment of the individual drowning victim rather than the management of mass casualty aquatic incidents.

Definitions, classifications and reporting

Over 30 different terms have been used to describe the process and outcome from submersion- and immersion-related incidents.[61] To improve clarity and to help comparability of future scientific and epidemiological reports, the International Liaison Committee on Resuscitation (ILCOR) has proposed new definitions related to drowning.[62] Drowning itself is defined as a process resulting in primary respiratory impairment from submersion/immersion in a liquid medium. Implicit in this definition is that a liquid/air interface is present at the entrance of the victim's airway, preventing the victim from breathing air. The victim may live or die after this process, but whatever the outcome, he or she has been involved in a drowning incident. Immersion means to be covered in water or other fluid. For drowning to occur, usually at least the face and airway must be immersed. Submersion implies that the entire body, including the airway, is under the water or other fluid.

ILCOR recommends that the following terms, previously used, should no longer be used: dry and wet drowning, active and passive drowning, silent drowning, secondary drowning and drowned versus near-drowned.[62]

Basic life support

Aquatic rescue and recovery from the water

Always be aware of personal safety and minimise the danger to yourself and the victim at all times. Whenever possible, attempt to save the drowning victim without entry into water. Talking to the victim, reaching with a rescue aid (e.g., stick or clothing), or throwing a rope or buoyant rescue aid may be effective if the victim is close to dry land. Alternatively, use a boat or other water vehicle to assist with the rescue. Avoid entry into the water whenever possible. If entry into the water is essential, take a buoyant rescue aid or flotation device.

Remove all the drowning victims from the water by the fastest and safest means available and resuscitate as quickly as possible. The incidence of cervical spine injury in drowning victims is low (approximately 0.5%).[63] Spinal immobilisation can be difficult to perform in the water and can delay removal from the water and adequate resuscitation of the victim. Poorly applied cervical collars can also cause airway obstruction in unconscious patients.[64] Despite potential spinal injury, victims who are pulseless and apnoeic should be removed from water as quickly as possible (even if a back support device is not available), while attempting to limit neck flexion and extension. Cervical spine immobilisation is not indicated unless signs of severe injury are apparent or the history is consistent with the possibility of severe injury.[65] These circumstances include a history of diving, water-slide use, signs of trauma or signs of alcohol intoxication. Whenever possible, remove the victim from the water in a horizontal position to minimise the risks of post-immersion hypotension and cardiovascular collapse.[66]

Rescue breathing

The first and most important treatment for the drowning victim is alleviation of hypoxaemia. Prompt initiation of rescue breathing or positive pressure ventilation increases the survival.[67,68] In the apnoeic victim, start rescue breathing as soon as the victim's airway is opened and the rescuer's safety ensured. This can sometimes be achieved when the victim is still in shallow water. It is likely to be difficult to pinch the victim's nose, so mouth-to-nose ventilation may be used as an alternative to mouth-to-mouth ventilation. If the victim is in deep water, start in-water rescue breathing if trained to do so, ideally with the support of a buoyant rescue aid,[69] although in-water, unsupported resuscitation may also be possible.[70] Untrained rescuers should not attempt to perform any form of resuscitation with a victim in deep water.

If there is no spontaneous breathing after opening the airway, give rescue breaths for approximately 1 min.[69] If the victim does not start breathing spontaneously, further management depends on the distance from land. If the victim can be brought to land in <5 min of rescue time, continue rescue breaths while towing. If more than an estimated 5 min from land, give further rescue breaths over 1 min, then bring the victim to land as quickly as possible without further attempts at ventilation.[69]

There is no need to clear the airway of aspirated water. The majority of drowning victims aspirate only a modest amount of water, and this is absorbed rapidly into the central circulation. An attempt to remove water from the air passages by any means other than suction is unnecessary and dangerous. Abdominal thrusts cause regurgitation of gastric contents and subsequent aspiration. They have been associated with other life-threatening injuries and should not be performed unless there are clear signs of foreign-body airway obstruction.[71]

Chest compression

As soon as the victim is removed from water, check for breathing. A healthcare professional who is trained in pulse checking may also check for pulse, but this may be even more difficult to find in a drowning victim, particularly if cold. If the victim is not breathing, start chest compressions immediately. Chest compression is ineffective in water.[72,73]

Defibrillation

If the victim is unresponsive and not breathing and an AED is available, attach it to the victim and turn it on. Before attaching the AED pads, dry the victim's chest to enable adherence. Deliver shocks according to the AED prompts. If the victim is hypothermic with a core body temperature ≤30 °C (86 °F), limit defibrillation to a total of three attempts until the core body temperature rises above 30 °C (86 °F).[74]

Regurgitation during resuscitation

Regurgitation of stomach contents is common following resuscitation from drowning and will complicate efforts to maintain a patent airway. In one study, regurgitation occurred in two-thirds of victims who received rescue breathing and 86% of victims who required compression and ventilation.[75] If regurgitation occurs, turn the victim's mouth to the side and remove the regurgitated material using directed suction if possible. If spinal cord injury is suspected, log-roll the victim, keeping the head, neck and torso aligned, before aspirating the regurgitated material. Log-rolling will require several rescuers.

Advanced life support

Airway and breathing

Give high-flow oxygen during the initial assessment of the spontaneously breathing drowning victim. Consider non-invasive ventilation or continuous positive airway pressure if the victim fails to respond to treatment with high-flow oxygen.[76] Use pulse oximetry and arterial blood gas analysis to titrate the concentration of inspired oxygen and to provide an indicator of the adequacy of ventilation. Consider early intubation and controlled ventilation for victims who fail to respond to these initial measures or who have a reduced level of consciousness. Take care to ensure optimal preoxygenation before intubation. Use a rapid-sequence induction with cricoid pressure to reduce the high risk of aspiration.[77] Protect the airway of the victim in cardiopulmonary arrest early in the resuscitation attempt, ideally with a tracheal tube. Reduced pulmonary compliance requiring high inflation pressures may limit the use of adjuncts, such as the laryngeal mask airway. Initiate ventilation with a high-inspired oxygen concentration as soon as possible, to treat the severe hypoxaemia that is likely to be present.

Circulation and defibrillation

Follow standard advanced life support protocols. If severe hypothermia is present (core body temperature ≤30 °C or 86 °F), limit defibrillation attempts to three, and withhold IV drugs until the core body temperature increases above these levels. If moderate hypothermia is present, give IV drugs at longer than standard intervals (see section 7d).

During prolonged immersion, victims may become hypovolaemic from the hydrostatic pressure of water on the body. Give IV fluid to correct the hypovolaemia but avoid excessive volumes, which may cause pulmonary oedema. After return of spontaneous circulation, use haemodynamic monitoring to guide fluid resuscitation.

Discontinuing resuscitation efforts

Making a decision to discontinue resuscitation efforts on a victim of drowning is notoriously difficult. No single factor can accurately predict good or poor survival with 100% certainty. Decisions made in the field frequently prove later to have been incorrect.[78] Continue resuscitation unless there is clear evidence that resuscitation attempts are futile (e.g., massive traumatic injuries, *rigor mortis*, putrefaction etc.), or timely evacuation to a medical facility is not possible. Neurologically intact survival has been reported in several victims submerged for greater than 60 min.[79,80]

Post-resuscitation care

Salt versus fresh water

Much attention has been focused in the past on differences between salt- and fresh-water drowning. Extensive data from animal studies and human case series have shown that, irrespective of the tonicity of the inhaled fluid, the predominant pathophysiological process is hypoxaemia, driven by surfactant wash-out and dysfunction, alveolar collapse, atelectasis and intrapulmonary shunting. Small differences in electrolyte disturbance are rarely of any clinical relevance and do not usually require treatment.

Lung injury

Victims of drowning are at high risk of developing acute respiratory distress syndrome (ARDS) for upto 72 h after submersion. Protective ventilation strategies improve survival in patients with ARDS.[81] The propensity towards alveolar collapse may require the use of PEEP or other alveolar recruitment manoeuvres to reverse severe hypoxaemia.[82] Extracorporeal membrane oxygenation and nitric oxide administration have been used in some centres for refractory hypoxaemia in drowning victims but the efficacy of these treatments is unproven.[65]

Pneumonia is common after drowning. Prophylactic antibiotics have not been shown to be of benefit, although they may be considered after submersion in grossly contaminated water such as sewage. Give broad-spectrum antibiotics if signs of infection develop subsequently.[65]

Hypothermia

Victims of submersion may develop primary or secondary hypothermia. If the submersion occurs in icy water (<5 °C or 41 °F), hypothermia may develop rapidly and provide some protection against hypoxia. Such effects, however, have typically been reported after submersion of children in icy water.[59] Hypothermia may also develop as a secondary complication of the submersion, and subsequent heat loss through evaporation during attempted resuscitation. In these victims the hypothermia is not protective (see section 7d).

Several small clinical studies in patients with accidental hypothermia have shown that survival may be improved by either passive or active warming out of hospital or in the emergency room.[65]

In contrast, there is evidence of benefit from induced hypothermia for comatose victims resuscitated from prehospital cardiac arrests.[83] To date, there is no convincing evidence to guide therapy in this patient group. A pragmatic approach might be to consider instituting active rewarming until a core temperature of 32—34 °C is achieved, and then actively to avoid hyperthermia (>37 °C) during the subsequent period of intensive care (International Life Saving Federation, 2003).

Other supportive care

Attempts have been made to improve neurological outcome following drowning with the use of barbiturates, intracranial pressure (ICP) monitoring and steroids. None of these interventions has been shown to alter the outcome. In fact, signs of high ICP serve as a symptom of significant neurological hypoxic injury, and no evidence that attempts to alter the ICP will affect the outcome.[65]

7d. Hypothermia

Definition

Hypothermia exists when the body core temperature is below 35 °C and is classified arbitrarily as mild (35—32 °C), moderate (32—30 °C) or severe (less than 30 °C). Hypothermia can occur in people with normal thermoregulation who are exposed to cold environments, particularly wet or windy conditions, or following immersion in cold water. When thermoregulation is impaired, for example, in the elderly and very young, hypothermia may follow a mild cold insult. The risk of hypothermia is also increased by drug or alcohol ingestion, illness, injury or neglect. Hypothermia may be suspected from the clinical history or a brief external examination of a collapsed patient. A low-reading thermometer is needed to measure the core temperature and confirm diagnosis.

In some cases, hypothermia may exert a protective effect on the brain after cardiac arrest.[84,85] Intact neurological recovery may be possible after hypothermic cardiac arrest, although those with non-asphyxial arrest have a better prognosis than those with asphyxial hypothermic arrest.[86—88] Lifesaving procedures should not be withheld on the basis of clinical presentation alone.[87]

Decision to resuscitate

Beware of pronouncing death in a hypothermic patient, as cold alone may produce a very slow, small-volume, irregular pulse and an unrecordable blood pressure. Hypothermia protects the brain and vital organs, and associated arrhythmias are potentially reversible either before or during rewarming. At 18 °C the brain can tolerate periods of circulatory arrest for 10 times longer than at 37 °C. Dilated pupils can be caused by a variety of insults and must not be taken as a sign of death.

On discovering a hypothermic cardiac arrest victim in cold environment, it is not always easy to distinguish between primary and secondary hypothermia. Cardiac arrest could be caused primarily by hypothermia, or hypothermia could follow a normothermic cardiac arrest (e.g., cardiac arrest caused by myocardial ischaemia in a person in cold environment).

Do not confirm death until the patient has been rewarmed or until attempts to raise the core temperature have failed; prolonged resuscitation may be necessary. In the prehospital setting, resuscitation should be withheld only if the patient has obvious lethal injuries or if the body is completely frozen making resuscitation attempts impossible.[89] In the hospital setting, use clinical judgment to determine when to stop resuscitating a hypothermic arrest victim.

Resuscitation

All the principles of prevention, basic and advanced life support apply to the hypothermic patient. Do not delay the urgent procedures, such as intubation and insertion of vascular catheters. Intubation can provoke VF in a patient with severe hypothermia.[87,90]

- Clear the airway and, if there is no spontaneous respiratory effort, ventilate the patient's lungs with high concentrations of oxygen. If possible, use warmed (40—46 °C) and humidified oxygen. Consider careful tracheal intubation when indicated according to the ALS algorithm.
- Palpate a major artery and, if available, look at the ECG for up to 1 min and look for signs of life before concluding that there is no cardiac output. If a Doppler ultrasound probe is available, use it to establish whether there is peripheral blood flow. If the victim is pulseless, start chest compressions immediately. If there is any doubt about whether a pulse is present, start CPR.
- Once resuscitation is under way, confirm hypothermia with a low-reading thermometer. The method of temperature measurement should be the same throughout resuscitation and rewarming. Use oesophageal, bladder, rectal or tympanic temperature measurements.[91,92]

Use the same ventilation and chest compression rates as for a normothermic patient. Hypothermia can cause stiffness of the chest wall, making ventilation and chest compression difficult.

The hypothermic heart may be unresponsive to cardioactive drugs, attempted electrical pacing and attempted defibrillation. Drug metabolism is slowed, leading to potentially toxic plasma concentrations of any drug given repeatedly.[90] The evidence for the efficacy of drugs in severe hypothermia is limited and based mainly on animal studies. Adrenaline may be effective in increasing coronary perfusion pressure, but not survival, in severe hypothermic cardiac arrest.[93,94] The efficacy of amiodarone is also reduced.[95] For these reasons, withhold adrenaline and other drugs until the patient has been warmed to a temperature greater than 30 °C. Once 30 °C has been reached, the intervals between doses should be doubled. As the patient's temperature returns towards normal, the standard drug protocols should be used.

Remember to rule out other primary causes of cardiorespiratory arrest using the four Hs and four Ts approach (e.g., drug overdose, hypothyroidism, trauma).

Arrhythmias

As the body core temperature decreases, sinus bradycardia tends to give way to atrial fibrillation (AF) followed by ventricular fibrillation (VF) and finally asystole.[96] Follow the standard treatment protocols.

Severely hypothermic victims (core temperature <30 °C) in cardiac arrest in hospital must be rapidly rewarmed using internal methods. Arrhythmias other than VF tend to revert spontaneously as the core temperature increases, and usually do not require immediate treatment. Bradycardia may be physiological in severe hypothermia, and cardiac pacing is not indicated unless bradycardia persists after rewarming.

The temperature at which defibrillation should first be attempted and how often it should be tried in the severely hypothermic patient has not been established. AEDs may be used on these patients. If VF is detected, give a shock; if VF/VT persists after three shocks, delay further defibrillation attempts until the core temperature is above 30 °C.[97,98] If an AED is used, follow the AED prompts while rewarming the patient.

Rewarming

General measures for all casualties include removal from the cold environment, prevention of further heat loss and rapid transfer to the hospital. Remove cold or wet clothing as soon as possible. Cover the dry casualties with blankets and keep them out of the wind.

Rewarming may be passive external, active external, or active internal. Passive warming is achieved with blankets and a warm room, and is suitable for conscious victims with mild hypothermia. In severe hypothermia or cardiac arrest, active warming is required, but this must not delay transport to a hospital where more advanced rewarming techniques are available. Several techniques have been described, although there are no clinical trials of outcome to determine the best rewarming method. Studies show that forced air rewarming and warm IV fluids are effective in patients with severe hypothermia and a perfusing rhythm.[99,100] Other warming techniques include the use of warm humidified gases, gastric, peritoneal, pleural or bladder lavage with warm fluids (at 40 °C), and extracorporeal blood warming with partial bypass.[87,90,101–103]

In the patient with cardiac arrest and hypothermia, cardiopulmonary bypass is the preferred method of active internal rewarming because it also provides circulation, oxygenation and ventilation, while the core body temperature is increased gradually.[104,105] Survivors in one case series had an average of 65 min of conventional CPR before cardiopulmonary bypass.[105] Unfortunately, facilities for cardiopulmonary bypass are not always available and a combination of methods may have to be used.

During rewarming, patients will require large volumes of fluids as their vascular space expands with vasodilation. Warm all the IV fluids. Use continuous haemodynamic monitoring and, if possible, treat the patient in a critical care unit. Avoid hyperthermia during and after the warming period. Although there are no formal studies, once ROSC has been achieved use standard strategies for postresuscitation care, including mild hypothermia if appropriate (section 4g). There is no evidence for the routine use of steroids, barbiturates or antibiotics.[106,107]

7e. Hyperthermia

Definition

Hyperthermia occurs when the body's ability to thermoregulate fails, and core temperature exceeds the one that is normally maintained by homeostatic mechanisms. Hyperthermia may be exogenous, caused by environmental conditions, or secondary to endogenous heat production.

Environment-related hyperthermia occurs where heat, usually in the form of radiant energy, is absorbed by the body at a rate faster than that can be lost by thermoregulatory mechanisms. Hyperthermia occurs along a continuum of heat-related conditions, starting with heat stress, progressing to heat exhaustion, to heat stroke (HS) and finally multiorgan dysfunction and cardiac arrest in some instances.[108]

Malignant hyperthermia (MH) is a rare disorder of skeletal muscle calcium homeostasis characterised by muscle contracture and life-threatening hypermetabolic crisis following exposure of genetically predisposed individuals to halogenated anaesthetics and depolarising muscle relaxants.[109,110]

The key features and treatment of heat stress and heat exhaustion are included in Table 7.2.

Heat stroke (HS)

HS is a systemic inflammatory response with a core temperature above 40.6 °C, accompanied by mental state change and varying levels of organ dysfunction. There are two forms of HS: classic non-exertion heat stroke (CHS) occuring during high environmental temperatures and often effecting the elderly during heat waves;[111] exertion heat stroke (EHS) occuring during strenuous physical exercise in high environmental temperatures and/or high humidity usually effecting healthy young adults.[112] Mortality from HS ranges between 10 and 50%.[113]

Predisposing factors

The elderly are at an increased risk for heat-related illness because of underlying illness, medication use, declining thermoregulatory mechanisms and limited social support. There are several risk factors: lack of acclimatisation, dehydration, obesity, alcohol, cardiovascular disease, skin conditions (psoriasis, eczema, scleroderma, burn, cystic fibrosis), hyperthyroidism, phaeochromocytoma and drugs (anticholinergics, diamorphine, cocaine, amphetamine, phenothiazines, sympathomimetics, calcium channel blockers, beta-blockers).

Clinical presentation

Heat stroke can resemble septic shock and may be caused by similar mechanisms.[114] Features include:

- core temperature 40.6 °C or more;
- hot, dry skin (sweating is present in about 50% of cases of exertional heat stroke);

Table 7.2   Heat stress and heat exhaustion

Condition	Features	Treatment
Heat stress	Normal or mild temperature elevation	Rest
	Heat oedema: swelling of feet and ankles	Elevation of oedematous limbs
	Heat syncope: vasodilation causing hypotension	Cooling
	Heat cramps: sodium depletion causing cramps	Oral rehydration
		Salt replacement
Heat exhaustion	Systemic reaction to prolonged heat exposure (hours to days)	As above
	Temperature >37 °C and <40 °C	Consider IV fluids and ice packs for severe cases
	Headache, dizziness, nausea, vomiting, tachycardia, hypotension, sweating muscle pain, weakness and cramps	
	Haemoconcentration	
	Hyponatraemia or hypernatraemia	
	May progress rapidly to heat stroke	

- early signs and symptoms, e.g., extreme fatigue, headache, fainting, facial flushing, vomiting and diarrhoea;
- cardiovascular dysfunction including arrhythmias[115] and hypotension;
- respiratory dysfunction including ARDS;[116]
- central nervous system dysfunction including seizures and coma;[117]
- liver and renal failure;[118]
- coagulopathy;[116]
- rhabdomyolysis.[119]

Other clinical conditions need to be considered, including:

- drug toxicity;[120,121]
- drug withdrawal syndrome;
- serotonin syndrome;[122]
- neuroleptic malignant syndrome[123]
- sepsis;[124]
- central nervous system infection;
- endocrine disorders, e.g., thyroid storm, phaeochromocytoma.[125]

Management

The mainstay of treatment is supportive therapy based on optimising the ABCDEs and cooling the patient.[126,127] Start cooling before the patient reaches the hospital. Aim to reduce the core temperature to approximately 39 °C. Patients with severe heat stroke need to be managed in a critical care setting. Use haemodynamic monitoring to guide fluid therapy. Large volumes of fluid may be required. Correct the electrolyte abnormalities as described in Section 7a.

Cooling techniques

Several cooling methods have been described, but there are few formal trials to determine which method is best. Simple cooling techniques include drinking cool fluids, fanning the completely undressed patient and spraying tepid water on the patient. Ice packs over areas where there are large superficial blood vessels (axillae, groins, neck) may also be useful. Surface cooling methods may cause shivering. In cooperative stable patients, immersion in cold water can be effective;[128] however, this may cause peripheral vasoconstriction, shunt blood away from the periphery and reduce heat dissipation. Immersion is also not practical in the most sick patients.

Further techniques to cool patients with hyperthermia are similar to those used for therapeutic hypothermia after cardiac arrest (see section 4g). Gastric, peritoneal,[129] pleural or bladder lavage with cold water lowers the core temperature. Intravascular cooling techniques include the use of cold IV fluids,[130] intravascular cooling catheters[131,132] and extracorporeal circuits,[133] e.g., continuous veno-venous haemofiltration or cardiopulmonary bypass.

Drug therapy in heat stroke

There are no specific drug therapies in heat stroke to lower the core temperature. There is no good evidence that antipyretics (e.g., non-steroidal anti-inflammatory drugs or paracetamol) are effective in heat stroke. Dantrolene (see below) has not been shown to be beneficial.[134]

Malignant hyperthermia (MH)

MH is a life-threatening genetic sensitivity of skeletal muscles to volatile anaesthetics and depolarising neuromuscular blocking drugs, occurring during or after anaesthesia. Stop triggering agents immediately; give oxygen, correct acidosis and electrolyte abnormalities. Start active cooling and give dantrolene.[135]

Modifications to cardiopulmonary resuscitation and post-resuscitation care

There are no specific studies on cardiac arrest in hyperthermia. If cardiac arrest occurs, follow standard procedures for basic and advanced life support and cool the patient. There are no data on the effects of hyperthermia on defibrillation threshold; therefore, attempt defibrillation according to current guidelines, while continuing to cool the patient. Animal studies suggest that the prognosis is poor compared with normothermic cardiac arrest.[136,137] The risk of unfavourable neurological outcome increases for each degree of body temperature >37 °C.[138] Provide post-resuscitation care according to the normal guidelines.

7f. Asthma

Introduction

Approximately 300 million people of all ages and ethnic backgrounds suffer from asthma worldwide.[139] Asthma still causes many deaths in young adults, mostly among those with chronic severe asthma, adverse psychosocial circumstances and poor medical management. National and international guidance for the management of asthma already exists.[139,140] The following guidelines focus on the treatment of patients with near-fatal asthma and cardiac arrest.

Causes of cardiac arrest

Cardiac arrest in the asthmatic person is often a terminal event after a period of hypoxaemia; occasionally, it may be sudden. Cardiac arrest in asthmatics has been linked to:

- severe bronchospasm and mucous plugging leading to asphyxia (this condition causes the vast majority of asthma-related deaths);
- cardiac arrhythmias caused by hypoxia, which is the common cause of asthma-related arrhythmia. Arrhythmias can be caused by stimulant drugs

(e.g., beta-adrenergic agonists, aminophylline) or electrolyte abnormalities;
- dynamic hyperinflation, i.e., autopositive end-expiratory pressure (auto-PEEP), can occur in mechanically ventilated asthmatics. Auto-PEEP is caused by air trapping and 'breath stacking' (breathed air entering and being unable to escape). Gradual build-up of pressure occurs and reduces blood flow and blood pressure;
- tension pneumothorax (often bilateral).

The four Hs and four Ts approach to reversible causes helps identify these causes in cardiac arrest.

Diagnosis

Wheezing is a common physical finding, but severity does not correlate with the degree of airway obstruction. The absence of wheezing may indicate critical airway obstruction, whereas increased wheezing may indicate a positive response to bronchodilator therapy. SaO_2 may not reflect progressive alveolar hypoventilation, particularly if oxygen is being given. The SaO_2 may initially decrease during the therapy because beta-agonists cause both bronchodilation and vasodilation and may increase intrapulmonary shunting initially.

Other causes of wheezing include: pulmonary oedema, chronic obstructive pulmonary disease (COPD), pneumonia, anaphylaxis,[141] pneumonia, foreign bodies, pulmonary embolism, bronchiectasis and subglottic mass.[142]

The severity of an asthma attack is defined in Table 7.3.

Key interventions to prevent arrest

The patient with severe asthma requires aggressive medical management to prevent deterioration. Base assessment and treatment on an ABCDE approach. Experienced clinicians should treat these high-risk patients in a critical care area. The specific drugs and the treatment sequence will vary according to local practice.

Oxygen

Use a concentration of inspired oxygen that will achieve an SaO_2 ≥92%. High-flow oxygen by mask is sometimes necessary. Consider rapid-sequence induction and tracheal intubation if, despite efforts to optimise drug therapy, the patient has:

- decreased conscious level, coma;
- profuse sweating;
- reduced muscle tone (clinical signs of hypercarbia);

Table 7.3 The severity of asthma[140]

Asthma	Features
Near-fatal	Raised $PaCO_2$ and/or requiring mechanical ventilation with raised inflation pressures
Life-threatening	Any one of: PEF <33% best or predicted Bradycardia SpO_2 <92%, dysrhythmia PaO_2 <8 kPa, hypotension Normal $PaCO_2$ (4.6—6.0 kPa (35—45 mmHg)), exhaustion Silent chest, confusion Cyanosis, coma Feeble respiratory effort
Acute severe	Any one of: PEF 33-50% best or predicted Respiratory rate >25/min Heart rate >110/min Inability to complete sentences in one breath
Moderate exacerbation	Increasing symptoms PEF >50—75% best or predicted No features of acute severe asthma
Brittle	Type 1: wide PEF variability (>40% diurnal variation for >50% of the time over a period >150 days) despite intense therapy Type 2: sudden severe attacks on a background of apparently well controlled asthma

PEF, peak expiratory flow.

- findings of severe agitation, confusion and fighting against the oxygen mask (clinical signs of hypoxemia).

Elevation of the $PaCO_2$ alone does not indicate the need for tracheal intubation. Treat the patient, not the numbers.

Nebulised beta$_2$-agonists

Salbutamol, 5 mg nebulised, is the cornerstone of therapy for acute asthma in most of the world. Repeated doses every 15—20 min are often needed. Severe asthma may necessitate continuous nebulised salbutamol. Nebuliser units that can be driven by high-flow oxygen should be available. The hypoventilation associated with severe or near-fatal asthma may prevent effective delivery of nebulised drugs.

Intravenous corticosteroids

Oxygen and beta-agonists are the most important therapies initially, but give corticosteroids (hydrocortisone, 200 mg IV,) early. Although there is no difference in clinical effects between oral and IV formulations of corticosteroids,[143] the IV route is preferable because patients with near-fatal asthma may vomit or be unable to swallow.

Nebulised anticholinergics

Nebulised anticholinergics (ipratropium, 0.5 mg 4—6 h) may produce additional bronchodilation in severe asthma or in those who do not respond to beta-agonists.[144,145]

Intravenous salbutamol

Several studies have shown intravenous salbutamol (250 mcg IV slowly) to provide additional benefit in severe asthmatics who are already receiving nebulised salbutamol.[146] Give an infusion of 3—20 mcg min^{-1}.

Intravenous magnesium sulphate

Magnesium sulphate (2 g, IV slowly) may be useful as a bronchodilator in severe or near-fatal asthma. A Cochrane meta-analysis of seven studies concluded that magnesium is beneficial, particularly for those with the most severe exacerbations.[147] Magnesium causes bronchial smooth muscle relaxation independent of the serum magnesium level and has only minor side effects (flushing, light-headedness).

Intravenous theophylline

Theophylline is given IV as aminophylline, a mixture of theophylline with ethylenediamine, which is 20 times more soluble than theophylline alone. Aminophylline should only be considered in severe or near-fatal asthma. A loading dose of $5 \, mg \, kg^{-1}$ is given over 20—30 min (unless on maintenance therapy), followed by an infusion of $500-700 \, mcg \, kg^{-1} \, h^{-1}$. Addition of this drug to high doses of beta-agonists increases side effects more than it increases bronchodilation. Check levels to avoid toxicity.

Subcutaneous or intramuscular adrenaline and terbutaline

Adrenaline and terbutaline are adrenergic agents that may be given subcutaneously to patients with acute severe asthma. The dose of subcutaneous adrenaline is 300 mcg up to a total of three doses at 20-min intervals. Adrenaline may cause an increase in heart rate, myocardial irritability and increased oxygen demand; however, its use (even in patients over 35 years old) is well tolerated.[148] Terbutaline is given in a dose of 250 mcg subcutaneously, which can be repeated in 30—60 min. These drugs are more commonly given to children with acute asthma and, although most studies have shown them to be equally effective,[149] one study concluded that terbutaline was superior.[150] These alternative routes may need to be considered when IV access is impossible.

Intravenous fluids

Severe or near-fatal asthma is associated with dehydration and hypovolaemia, and this will further compromise the circulation in patients with dynamic hyperinflation of the lungs. If there is evidence of hypovolaemia or dehydration, give IV fluids.

Heliox

Heliox is a mixture of helium and oxygen (usually 80:20 or 70:30). A recent meta-analysis of four clinical trials did not support the use of heliox in the initial treatment of patients with acute asthma.[151]

Ketamine

Ketamine is a parenteral dissociative anaesthetic with bronchodilatory properties. One case series suggested substantial effectiveness,[152] but the single randomised trial published to date showed no benefit to ketamine compared with standard care.[153]

Non-invasive ventilation

Non-invasive ventilation decreases the intubation rate and mortality in COPD;[154] however, its role in patients with severe acute asthma is uncertain. Although promising, a recent Cochrane review suggests that more studies are needed.[155]

Management of cardiac arrest

Basic life support

Give basic life support according to the standard guidelines. Ventilation will be difficult because of increased airway resistance; try to prevent gastric inflation.

Advanced life support

Modifications to standard ALS guidelines. Consider the need for intubation early. The peak airway pressures recorded during the ventilation of patients with severe asthma (mean $67.8 \pm 11.1 \, cmH_2O$ in 12 patients) are significantly higher than the normal lower oesophageal sphincter pressure (approximately $20 \, cmH_2O$).[156] There is a significant risk of gastric inflation and hypoventilation of the lungs when attempting to ventilate a severe asthmatic without a tracheal tube. During cardiac arrest this risk is even higher because the lower oesophageal sphincter pressure is substantially less than normal.[157]

The new recommended respiratory rate ($10 \, breaths \, min^{-1}$) and tidal volume required for a normal chest rise during CPR should not cause dynamic hyperinflation of the lungs (gas trapping). Tidal volume depends on the inspiratory time and inspiratory flow, while lung emptying depends on the expiratory time and expiratory flow. In mechanically ventilated severe asthmatics, increasing the expiratory time (achieved by reducing the respiratory rate) provides only moderate gains in terms of reduced gas trapping when a minute volume of less than $10 \, l \, min^{-1}$ is used.[156]

There is limited evidence from the case reports of unexpected ROSC in patients with suspected gas trapping when the tracheal tube is disconnected.[158—161] If dynamic hyperinflation of the lungs is suspected during CPR, compression of the chest wall and/or a period of apnoea (disconnection of tracheal tube) may relieve gas trapping if dynamic hyperinflation occurs. Although this procedure is supported by limited evidence, it is unlikely to be harmful in an otherwise desperate situation.

Dynamic hyperinflation increases transthoracic impedance.[162] Consider the higher shock energies for defibrillation if initial defibrillation attempts fail.

There is no good evidence for the use of open-chest cardiac compressions in patients with asthma-associated cardiac arrest. Working through the four Hs and four Ts will identify potentially reversible courses of asthma related cardiac arrest. Tension pneumothorax can be difficult to diagnose in cardiac arrest; it may be indicated by unilateral expansion of the chest wall, shifting of the trachea and subcutaneous emphysema. Release air from the pleural space with needle decompression. Insert a large-gauge cannula in the second intercostal space in the mid clavicular line, being careful to avoid direct puncture of the lung. If air is emitted, insert a chest tube. Always consider bilateral pneumothoraces in asthma-related cardiac arrest.

Post-resuscitation care

The following should be added to usual management after ROSC:

- Optimise the medical management of bronchospasm.
- Use permissive hypercapnia; it may not be possible to achieve normal oxygenation and ventilation in a patient with severe bronchospasm. Efforts to achieve normal arterial blood gas values may worsen lung injury. Mild hypoventilation reduces the risk of barotraumas, and hypercapnoea is typically well-tolerated.[163] Target lower arterial blood oxygen saturations (e.g., 90%).
- Provide sedation (neuromuscular paralysis if needed) and controlled ventilation. Despite the absence of formal studies, ketamine and inhalational anaesthetics have bronchodilator properties that may be useful in the asthmatic patient who is difficult to ventilate.
- Involve a senior critical care doctor early.

7g. Anaphylaxis

Introduction

Anaphylaxis is a rare, but potentially reversible, cause of cardiac arrest. Although the management of cardiac arrest secondary to anaphylaxis follows the general principles described elsewhere in these guidelines, the pathophysiological processes occurring during anaphylaxis may require additional specific therapy.

Anaphylaxis is a severe life-threatening, generalised or systemic hypersensitivity reaction. Investigations will show whether the reaction is allergic (immunoglobulin E (IgE) or non IgE mediated) or non-allergic anaphylaxis. The term anaphylactoid reaction is no longer used. An anaphylactic reaction is generally defined as a severe, systemic allergic reaction characterized by multisystem involvement, including the airway, vascular system, gastrointestinal tract and skin. Severe cases may cause complete airway obstruction secondary to laryngeal oedema, bronchospasm, hypotension, cardiovascular collapse and death. Other symptoms include rhinitis, conjunctivitis, abdominal pain, vomiting, diarrhoea and a sense of impending doom. There is also usually a colour change; the patient may appear either flushed or pale. Anaphylactic reactions vary in severity, and progress may be rapid, slow or (unusually) biphasic. Rarely, manifestations may be delayed (this may occur with latex allergy), or persist for more than 24 h.

Pathophysiology

Initial exposure to an allergen may trigger an immune response that sensitises the body to subsequent exposure. This sensitisation results in antigen-specific IgE bound to the cell membrane of basophils and mast cells. On repeat exposure, the antigen is bound by the IgE, triggering release of a series of inflammatory mediators including histamines, leukotrienes, prostaglandins, thromboxanes and bradykinins. These mediators act systemically to cause increased mucous membrane secretion, increased capillary permeability and markedly reduced vascular smooth muscle tone. This causes the clinical symptoms of angioedema and airway swelling, bronchospasm, hypotension and cardiovascular collapse.

Anaphylaxis is caused by a hypersensitivity reaction in which histamine, serotonin and other vasoactive substances are released from basophils and mast cells in response to an IgE-mediated reaction. Antigen-specific immunoglobulins are produced after initial exposure to an allergen. Subsequent re-exposure to this allergen provokes an anaphylactic reaction, although many anaphylactic reactions occur without known previous exposure.

Aetiology

Although anaphylaxis is relatively common, progression to a severe life-threatening reaction is rare. Any antigen capable of activating IgE can theoretically be a trigger for anaphylaxis. The commonest causes of life-threatening reactions are drugs, stinging insects and food. In as many as 5% of the cases, the antigen triggering the anaphylaxis cannot be identified.

Drugs

Neuromuscular blocking drugs (particularly suxamethonium) and antibiotics are the most common triggers for drug-induced anaphylaxis.[164] Aspirin, non-steroidal anti-inflammatory drugs and IV contrast agents are also common causes of life-threatening anaphylaxis.

Latex

Latex, or natural rubber, is a significant trigger of anaphylaxis among hospitalised patients because of frequent instrumentation and operations in which latex products are used. Avoidance is the only effective therapy, and the availability of latex-free clinic and hospital environments, including patient and operating rooms, is now a priority.[165] Life-threatening anaphylactic reactions to latex are very rare[166,167] with a decade-long registry of anaphylactic deaths in England not registering any latex-associated deaths.[168,169]

Stinging insects

The prevalence of IgE-mediated systemic reactions to insect stings is 2.8% in temperate climates, although higher in countries, such as Australia where exposure to insect stings is more common.[170] The stinging insects belong to the *Hymenoptera* order and include hornets, wasps, honeybees and fire ants. Most stings cause local reactions with pain and swelling at the site but progress to anaphylaxis in susceptible persons. Fatal anaphylaxis occurs in people who are re-stung after a previous sting has induced IgE antibodies. Fatal reactions occur within 10—15 min, with cardiovascular collapse being the commonest cause of death.[168,169,171]

Foods

Life-threatening allergic reactions to food are increasing. Peanuts, seafood (in particular prawns and shellfish) and wheat are the foods associated most frequently with life-threatening anaphylaxis.[172] Bronchospasm, angioedema, airway obstruction and asphyxia comprise the most common fatal mechanism.[168,169,171]

Signs and symptoms

Anaphylaxis should be considered when two or more body systems are affected (cutaneous, respiratory, cardiovascular, neurological or gastrointestinal), with or without cardiovascular or airway involvement. Symptoms may be particularly severe in patients with asthma, those taking beta-adrenoceptor blockers and during neuraxial anaesthesia: states associated with reduced endogenous catecholamine response. The speed of the onset of signs and symptoms is related to the likely severity of the ensuing anaphylaxis.

Early signs and symptoms include urticaria, rhinitis, conjunctivitis, abdominal pain, vomiting and diarrhoea. Flushing is common but pallor may also occur. Marked upper airway (laryngeal) oedema and bronchospasm may develop, causing stridor and wheezing (or high airway pressures in ventilated patients). In asthmatics, this may be particularly severe and difficult to treat. Cardiovascular collapse is the most common peri-arrest manifestation. Vasodilation causes relative hypovolaemia, exacerbated by true volume loss as increased capillary permeability results in extravasation of intravascular fluid. Additional cardiac dysfunction may follow from underlying disease or from the development of myocardial ischaemia from adrenaline administration.[168,169,171]

Differential diagnosis

The lack of any consistent clinical manifestation and a wide range of possible presentations may cause diagnostic difficulty. In each case, take as full a history and examination as possible. The history of previous allergic reactions, as well as that of the recent incident is important. Pay particular attention to the condition of the skin, the pulse rate, the blood pressure and the upper airways, and auscultate the chest. Measure and record the peak flow where possible. Consider the diagnosis of other conditions only after anaphylaxis has been excluded; failure to identify and treat anaphylaxis can be fatal:[173,174]

- ACE inhibitors may cause angioedema with marked swelling of the upper airway. This reaction may occur at any time and is not related to an initial exposure to the drug. The best treatment for this form of angioedema is unclear, but early recognition and appropriate airway management are critical.[175]
- Hereditary angioedema is familial and indistinguishable from the early angioedema of anaphylaxis or drug-related angioedema. An important

distinguishing feature is the absence of urticaria with hereditary angioedema. This is treated with C1 esterase inhibitor, either as a specific concentrate or contained within fresh frozen plasma.

- Severe asthma may present with bronchospasm and stridor, which are also common features of severe anaphylaxis. However, asthma attacks do not usually present with urticaria or angioedema.
- Rarely, panic attacks may be associated with functional stridor as a result of forced adduction of the vocal cords. As with asthma, there is no urticaria, angioedema, hypoxia or hypotension.
- Vasovagal reactions cause sudden collapse and extreme bradycardia that may be mistaken for absence of a pulse. Recovery is usually relatively rapid, and is not associated with urticaria, angioedema or bronchospasm.

Considerations in relation to treatment

Wide variations in aetiology, severity and organ involvement preclude standardised treatment recommendations. The lack of clinical trials necessitates guidelines based on consensus opinion.

Adrenaline is generally agreed to be the most important drug for any severe anaphylactic reaction. As an alpha-agonist, it reverses peripheral vasodilation and reduces oedema. Its beta-agonist properties dilate the airways, increase the force of myocardial contraction and suppress histamine and leukotriene release.

Adrenaline is most effective when given early after the onset of the reaction, but it is not without risk, particularly when given IV. When given intramuscularly, adrenaline is very safe. Adverse effects are extremely rare, and the only patient reported to have had a myocardial infarction after intramuscular injection had numerous risk factors for coronary disease. Sometimes there has been uncertainty as to whether complications (e.g., myocardial ischaemia) have been due to the effects of the allergen itself or to adrenaline given as treatment for it.[168,176]

Rarely, adrenaline may fail to reverse the clinical manifestations of anaphylaxis, particularly in late reactions or in patients treated with beta-blockers. Other measures then assume greater importance, particularly volume replacement.

General resuscitation measures

All victims should recline in a position of comfort. Remove the likely allergen (i.e., stop drug infusion or blood transfusion). Lying flat, with or without leg elevation, may be helpful for hypotension but not helpful for breathing difficulties. Airway obstruction can develop rapidly due to soft tissue swelling. Consider early tracheal intubation; delay may make intubation extremely difficult.

Oxygen

Give high-flow oxygen (10—15 l min^{-1}).

Adrenaline

Give adrenaline intramuscularly to all patients with clinical signs of shock, airway swelling or definite breathing difficulty; adrenaline will be absorbed rapidly. Inspiratory stridor, wheeze, cyanosis, pronounced tachycardia and decreased capillary filling indicate a severe reaction. For adults, give an IM dose of adrenaline, 0.5 ml of 1:1000 solution (500 mcg). If the patient's condition fails to improve, repeat the dose after about 5 min. In some cases several doses may be needed, particularly if improvement is transient. The IM route is preferable to SC administration because absorption is more rapid in shock.[177,178]

IV adrenaline (in a dilution of at least 1:10,000; never 1:1000) is hazardous and must be reserved for patients with profound shock that is immediately life threatening and for special indications, for example during anaesthesia. A further 10-fold dilution to 1:100,000 adrenaline enables finer titration of the dose and increases its safety by reducing the risk of unwanted adverse effects. This should be carried out with a minimum of electrocardiographic monitoring. Doctors experienced in the use of IV adrenaline may prefer to use the IV route in any patient with signs of severe anaphylaxis.

Antihistamine

Give an H$_1$-antihistamine (e.g., chlorphenamine 10—20 mg) by slow IV injection. Consider also an H$_2$-blocker, e.g., ranitidine, 50 mg IV.[179]

Hydrocortisone

Give hydrocortisone by slow IV injection after severe attacks to help avert late sequelae. This is particularly important for asthmatics (who are at an increased risk of severe or fatal anaphylaxis) if they have been treated with corticosteroids previously. Corticosteroids are considered as slow-acting drugs and may take up to 4—6 h to have an effect, even if given IV. However, they may help in the emergency treatment of an acute attack, and they also have a role in preventing or shortening the protracted reactions.

Inhaled bronchodilators

An inhaled beta$_2$ agonist, such as salbutamol (5 mg, repeated if necessary), may help reverse the refractory bronchospasm. Inhaled ipratropium (500 mcg, repeated as necessary) may be particularly useful for the treatment of bronchospasm in patients on beta-blockers. Some cases of near-fatal asthma may really be anaphylaxis, resulting in mistaken overtreatment with conventional bronchodilators rather than more specific treatment with adrenaline.[141]

Intravenous fluids

If severe hypotension does not respond rapidly to drug treatment, give fluid; a rapid infusion of 1–2 l may be required. Further fluid is likely to be necessary.

Potential therapies

Vasopressin. There are case reports that vasopressin may benefit severely hypotensive patients.[180,181]

Atropine. Case reports also suggest that, when relative or severe bradycardia is present, there may be a role for atropine.[174]

Glucagon. For patients unresponsive to adrenaline, especially those receiving beta-blockers, glucagon may be effective. This agent is short-acting (1–2 mg every 5 min IM, or IV). Nausea, vomiting and hyperglycaemia are common side effects.

Envenomation

Rarely, insect envenomation by bees, but not wasps, leaves a venom sac. Immediately scrape away any insect parts at the site of the sting.[182] Squeezing may increase envenomation.

Cardiac arrest

In addition to the ALS drugs, consider the following therapies.

Rapid fluid resuscitation

Near-fatal anaphylaxis produces profound vasodilation and a relative hypovolaemia. Massive volume replacement is essential. Use at least two large-bore cannulae with pressure bags to give large volumes (as much as 4–8 l IV fluid may be necessary in the immediate resuscitation period).

Antihistamines

Give an antihistamine IV if antihistamine has not already been given before the arrest.[179]

Steroids

Steroids given during a cardiac arrest will have little immediate effect but, if ROSC is restored, they may be effective in the post-resuscitation period.

Prolonged CPR

Patients with anaphylaxis are often young, with healthy hearts and cardiovascular systems. Effective CPR may maintain sufficient oxygen delivery until the catastrophic effects of the anaphylactic reaction resolve.

Airway obstruction

Airway obstruction may occur rapidly in severe anaphylaxis, particularly in patients with angioedema. Warning signs are lingual and labial swelling, hoarseness and oropharyngeal swelling. Consider early, elective intubation. As airway obstruction progresses, both LMAs and Combitubes are likely to be difficult to insert. Tracheal intubation and cricothyroidotomy will also become increasingly difficult. Attempts at tracheal intubation may exacerbate laryngeal oedema. Early involvement of a senior anaesthetist is mandatory when managing these patients.

Observation

Warn patients with even moderate attacks of the possibility of an early recurrence of symptoms and, in some circumstances, keep them under observation for 8–24 h. This caution is particularly applicable to:

- severe reactions with slow onset due to idiopathic anaphylaxis;
- reactions in severe asthmatics or with a severe asthmatic component;
- reactions with the possibility of continuing absorption of allergen;
- patients with a previous history of biphasic reactions.[179,183–187]

A patient who remains symptom-free for 4 h after treatment may be discharged.[188]

Investigations and further management

Measurement of mast cell tryptase may help with retrospective diagnosis of anaphylaxis.[189,190] Take three 10-ml clotted blood samples:

- immediately after the reaction has been treated;
- about 1 h after reaction;
- about 6 h and up to 24 h after reaction.

It is important to identify the allergen after successful resuscitation from anaphylaxis, to prevent recurrence. Refer the patient to a specialist clinic. Patients at very high risk of anaphylaxis may carry their own adrenaline syringe for self-administration and wear a 'MedicAlert' type bracelet. Report reactions to drugs to the appropriate monitoring agency.

7h. Cardiac arrest following cardiac surgery

Cardiac arrest following major cardiac surgery (both on and off bypass) is relatively common in the immediate postoperative phase, with a reported incidence of 0.7% in the first 24 h[191] and 1.4% within the first 8 days.[192] Cardiac arrest is usually caused by specific pathology that is reversible if treated promptly and appropriately, and therefore, has a relatively high survival rate. Cardiac arrest is usually preceded by physiological deterioration,[193] although it may occur suddenly in stable patients.[191] Continuous monitoring on the intensive care unit (ICU) enables immediate intervention at the time of arrest. Survival to hospital discharge of patients suffering from cardiac arrest during the first 24 h after adult cardiac surgery is reported as 54%[192]–79%[191,194] and 41% in children.[193]

Aetiology

Perioperative myocardial infarction is the commonest cause of sudden cardiac arrest and is often secondary to graft occlusion.[191,192]

The main causes of cardiac arrest in the initial postoperative period include:

- myocardial ischaemia;
- tension pneumothorax;
- haemorrhage causing hypovolaemic shock;
- cardiac tamponade;
- disconnection of pacing system in pacing-dependent patient;
- electrolyte disturbances (particularly hypo/hyperkalaemia).

Diagnosis

An immediate decision on the likely cause of cardiac arrest must be made to enable rapid intervention and successful resuscitation. Auscultation of the chest, examination of the ECG and chest radiograph, transoesophageal/transthoracic echocardiography and measurement of blood loss from chest drains will aid in identifying the cause of the arrest. Actively seek and exclude reversible causes of cardiac arrest: the four Hs and four Ts. Myocardial ischaemia often causes myocardial irritability and progressive hypotension before an arrest. A tension pneumothorax and cardiac tamponade will cause progressive hypotension and an increasing central venous pressure. Increasing airway pressures and poor air entry in the affected lung will differentiate between the two conditions. Lack of drainage of blood from the chest drains does not exclude haemorrhage or tamponade, because drains may block with clot.

Treatment

Treatment of cardiac arrest following cardiac surgery follows the same principles of BLS and ALS that have already been described in these guidelines. Seek assistance from experienced clinicians without delay. Exclude immediately correctable causes, such as pacing-lead disconnection and tension pneumothorax. Extreme bradycardia or asystole may respond to pacing via internal pacing-wires (if present) connected to an external pacemaker. Ensure correction of hypo/hyperkalaemia and hypomagnesaemia. Rapid restoration of an adequate blood volume is important, ensuring that haemoglobin levels are maintained no lower than $8.0\,g\,dl^{-1}$. Be careful when giving IV adrenaline, as the resulting hypertension may cause catastrophic failure of anastomoses.

External chest compressions

External chest compressions may be necessary but may cause sternal subluxation, fractured ribs and damage to grafts. Continuous observation of the invasive blood pressure will enable the force of compression to be optimised. Effective external chest compressions should take precedence over the concerns of damage to grafts.

Internal cardiac massage

Mechanical factors (e.g., haemorrhage, tamponade, graft occlusion) account for a substantial proportion of causes of sudden cardiac arrest occurring in haemodynamically stable patients during the immediate postoperative period.[191] Correction of this pathology may require chest reopening and therefore internal cardiac massage. Up to 10% of patients may need chest reopening following cardiac surgery.[195] Overall survival to discharge the following internal cardiac massage is 17%[196]–25%.[195] Cardiac arrest on the ICU, arrest within 24 h of surgery, and reopening within 10 min of arrest are independent predictors of survival.[195]

The high incidence of potentially correctable mechanical causes of arrest, in conjunction with the high survival rate achieved by open CPR, supports an early approach to open-chest CPR in these patients.[191,197] Reopen the patient's chest immediately if there is no output with external chest compressions or if there is a shockable rhythm refractory to cardioversion. Management of asystole usually requires prompt chest opening. Opening of the chest is relatively straightforward and, if indicated, should be undertaken within 10 min of cardiac arrest. Consider training the non-surgical medical staff to open the wound and remove sternal wires, while a surgeon is summoned. Make sure that a chest opening kit is immediately available on the ICU. The invasive blood pressure will guide the effectiveness of internal cardiac massage Remove the blood clot carefully, either manually or by suctioning, to avoid damaging the grafts. Early identification and treatment of underlying pathology is challenging under these circumstances and requires an experienced surgeon.

Reinstitution of emergency cardiopulmonary bypass

The need for emergency cardiopulmonary bypass (CPB) may occur in approximately 0.8% patients, occurring at a mean of 7 h postoperatively,[198] and is usually indicated to correct surgical bleeding or graft occlusion and rest an exhausted myocardium. Emergency institution of CPB should be available on all units undertaking cardiac surgery. Survival to discharge the rates of 32%,[195] 42%[198] and 56.3%[199] have been reported when CPB is reinstituted on the ICU. Survival rates decline rapidly when this procedure is undertaken more than 24 h after surgery and when performed on the ward rather than the ICU. Emergency CPB should probably be restricted to patients who arrest within 72 h of surgery, as surgically remediable problems are unlikely after this time.[195] Ensuring adequate re-anticoagulation before commencing CPB, or the use of a heparin-bonded CPB circuit, is important. The need for a further period of aortic cross-clamping does not preclude a favourable outcome.[198]

Internal defibrillation

Internal defibrillation using paddles applied directly across the ventricles requires considerably less energy than that used for external defibrillation. Biphasic shocks are substantially more effective than the monophasic shocks for direct defibrillation. For biphasic shocks, starting at 5 J creates the optimum conditions for lowest threshold and cumulative energy, whereas 10 or 20 J offers optimum conditions for more rapid defibrillation and fewer shocks.[200] Monophasic shocks require approximately double these energy levels.[200]

7i. Traumatic cardiorespiratory arrest

Introduction

Cardiac arrest secondary to traumatic injury has a very high mortality, with an overall survival of just 2.2% (range, 0–3.7%) (Table 7.4).[201–207] In those who survive, neurological disability is common, being absent in only 0.8% of those suffering from traumatic cardiorespiratory arrest (TCRA).

Diagnosis of traumatic cardiorespiratory arrest

The diagnosis of TCRA is made clinically: the trauma patient is unresponsive, apnoeic and pulseless. Both asystole and organised cardiac activity without cardiac output are regarded as TCRA.

Commotio cordis

Commotio cordis is actual or near cardiac arrest caused by a blunt impact to the chest wall over the heart.[208–211] A blow on the chest during the vulnerable phase of the cardiac cycle may cause malignant arrhythmias (usually VF). Syncope after chest wall impact may be caused by non-sustained arrhythmic events. Commotio cordis occurs mostly during sports (most commonly baseball) and recreational activities, and victims are usually young males (mean age 14 years). The Commotio Cordis Registry in Minneapolis is accruing 5–15 cases of commotio cordis each year. The overall survival rate from commotio cordis is 15%, but reaches 25% if resuscitation is started within 3 min.[211]

Trauma secondary to medical events

A cardiorespiratory arrest caused by a medical pathology (e.g., cardiac arrhythmia, hypoglycaemia, seizure) may precipitate a secondary traumatic event (e.g., fall, road traffic accident, etc.). Traumatic injuries may not be the primary cause of a cardiorespiratory arrest.

Mechanism of injury

Blunt trauma

Of 1242 patients with cardiac arrest after blunt trauma, 19 (1.5%) survived, but only 2 (0.16%) had a good neurological outcome (Table 7.4).

Penetrating trauma

Of 839 patients with cardiac arrest after penetrating injury, there were 16 (1.9%) survivors, of whom 12 (1.4%) had a good neurological outcome (Table 7.4).

Signs of life and initial ECG activity

There are no reliable predictors of survival for TCRA. One study reported that the presence of reactive pupils and sinus rhythm correlated significantly with survival.[217] In a study of penetrating trauma, pupil reactivity, respiratory activity and sinus rhythm were correlated with survival but were unreliable.[207] Three studies reported no survivors among patients presenting with asystole or agonal rhythms.[202,207,218] Another reported no survivors in PEA after blunt trauma.[219] Based on these studies, the American College of Surgeons and the National Association of EMS Physicians produced prehospital guidelines on withholding resuscitation.[220] They recommend withholding resuscitation in:

- blunt trauma victims presenting apnoeic and pulseless, and without organised ECG activity;
- penetrating trauma victims found apnoeic and pulseless after rapid assessment for signs of life, such as pupillary reflexes, spontaneous movement or organised ECG activity.

A recent retrospective study questions these recommendations: in a series of 184 TCRA victims, several survivors met the criteria for non-resuscitation.[221]

Treatment

Survival from TCRA is correlated with duration of CPR and prehospital time.[205,222–226] Prolonged CPR is associated with a poor outcome; the maximum CPR time associated with a favourable outcome is 16 min.[205,222–224] The level of prehospital intervention will depend on the skills of local EMS providers,

but treatment on scene should focus on good quality BLS and ALS and exclusion of reversible causes. Look for and treat any medical condition that may have precipitated the trauma event. Undertake only the essential lifesaving interventions on scene and, if the patient has signs of life, transfer rapidly to the nearest appropriate hospital. Consider on-scene thoracostomy for appropriate patients.[227,228] Do not delay for unproven interventions, such as spinal immobilisation.[229]

Resuscitative thoracotomy

Prehospital. Resuscitative thoracotomy has been reported as futile if out-of-hospital time has exceeded 30 min;[225] others consider thoracotomy to be futile in patients with blunt trauma requiring more than 5 min of prehospital CPR and in patients with penetrating trauma requiring more than 15 min of CPR.[226] With these time limits in mind, one UK service recommends that, if surgical intervention cannot be accomplished within 10 min after loss of pulse in patients with penetrating chest injury, on-scene thoracotomy should be considered.[227] Following this approach, of 39 patients who underwent thoracotomy at scene, 4 patients survived and 3 of these made a good neurological recovery.

Hospital. A relatively simple technique for resuscitative thoracotomy has been described recently.[228,230] The American College of Surgeons has published practice guidelines for emergency department thoracotomy (EDT) based on a meta-analysis of 42 outcome studies including 7035 EDTs.[231] The overall survival rate was 7.8%, and of 226 survivors (5%), only 34 (15%) exhibited a neurological deficit. The investigators concluded the following:

- After blunt trauma, EDT should be limited to those with vital signs on arrival and a witnessed cardiac arrest (estimated survival rate 1.6%).
- Emergency department thoracotomy is best applied to patients with penetrating cardiac injuries, who arrive at the trauma centre after short on-scene and transport times, with witnessed signs of life or ECG activity (estimated survival rate 31%).
- Emergency department thoracotomy should be undertaken in penetrating non-cardiac thoracic injuries even though survival rates are low.
- Emergency department thoracotomy should be undertaken in patients with exsanguinating abdominal vascular injury even though survival rates are low. This procedure should be used as

Table 7.4 Survival after traumatic cardiac arrest

Source	Entry criteria	Number of survivors neurologically intact	Number of survivors of penetrating trauma neurologically intact	Number of survivors of blunt trauma neurologically intact
Bouillon[212]	Pulseless, requiring CPR at scene	224 4 3		
Battistella[202]	Pulseless, requiring CPR at scene, en route or in ED	604 16 9	300 12 9	304 4 0
Pasquale[206]	CPR before or on hospital admission	106 3	21 1	85 2
Fisher[213]	Children requiring CPR before or on admission after blunt trauma	65 1 0		38 1 0
Hazinski[214]	Children requiring CPR or being severely hypotensive on admission after blunt trauma	38 1 0		65 1 0
Shimazu[203]	TCRA on admission	267 7 4		
Calkins[215]	Children requiring CPR after blunt trauma	25 2 2		25 2 2
Yanagawa[216]	OHCA in blunt trauma	332 6 0		332 6 0
Rosemurgy[201]	CPR before admission	138 0 0	42 0 0	96 0 0
Stratton[207]	Unconscious, pulseless at scene	879 9 3	497 4 3	382 5 0
Cera[217]	CPR on admission	161 15 ?		

For each study, the first number indicates the number of patients in cardiac arrest, the second indicates the numbers of survivors and the third indicates the number of survivors with a good neurological outcome. CPR = cardiopulmonary resuscitation; ED = emergency department; TCRA = traumatic cardiorespiratory arrest; OHCA = out-of-hospital cardiac arrest.

an adjunct to definitive repair of abdominal vascular injury.

Airway management

Effective airway management is essential to maintain oxygenation of the severely compromised trauma victim. In one study, tracheal intubation on-scene of patients with TCRA doubled the tolerated period of CPR, i.e., the mean time of CPR for survivors who were intubated in the field was 9.1 min versus 4.2 min for those who were not intubated.[224]

Tracheal intubation of trauma victims is a difficult procedure with a high failure rate if carried out by less experienced care providers.[232–235] Use the basic airway management manoeuvres and alternative airways to maintain oxygenation if tracheal intubation cannot be accomplished immediately. If these measures fail, a surgical airway is indicated.

Ventilation

In low cardiac output states positive pressure ventilation causes further circulatory depression, or even cardiac arrest, by impeding venous return to the heart.[236] Monitor ventilation with capnometry and adjust to achieve normocapnia. This may enable slow respiratory rates and low tidal volumes, and the corresponding decrease in transpulmonary pressure may increase venous return and cardiac output.

Chest decompression

Effective decompression of a tension pneumothorax can be achieved quickly by lateral thoracostomy, which is likely to be more effective than needle thoracostomy and quicker than inserting a chest tube.[237]

Effectiveness of chest compressions in TCRA

In hypovolaemic cardiac arrest or cardiac tamponade, chest compressions are unlikely to be as effective as in cardiac arrest from other causes;[238] nonetheless, return of spontaneous circulation with ALS in patients with TCRA is well described. Chest compressions are still the standard of care in patients with cardiac arrest, irrespective of aetiology.

Haemorrhage control

Early haemorrhage control is vital. Handle the patient gently at all times, to prevent clot disruption. Apply external compression and pelvic and limb splints when appropriate. Delays in surgical haemostasis are disastrous for patients with exsanguinating trauma.

Pericardiocentesis

In patients with suspected trauma-related cardiac tamponade, needle pericardiocentesis is probably not a useful procedure.[239] There is no evidence of benefit in the literature. It may increase scene time, cause myocardial injury and delay effective therapeutic measures, such as emergency thoracotomy.

Fluids and blood transfusion on scene

Fluid resuscitation of trauma victims before haemorrhage is controlled is controversial, and there is no clear consensus on when it should be started and what fluids should be given.[240] Limited evidence and general consensus support a more conservative approach to IV fluid infusion, with permissive hypotension until surgical haemostasis is achieved.[241,242] In the UK, the National Institute for Clinical Excellence (NICE) has published guidelines on prehospital fluid replacement in trauma.[243] The recommendations include giving 250 ml boluses of crystalloid solution until a radial pulse is achieved, and not delaying rapid transport of trauma victims for fluid infusion in the field. Prehospital fluid therapy may have a role in prolonged entrapments, but there is no reliable evidence for this.[244,245]

Ultrasound

Ultrasound is a valuable tool in the evaluation of the compromised trauma victim. Haemoperitoneum, haemo- or pneumothorax and cardiac tamponade can be diagnosed reliably in minutes even in the prehospital phase.[246] Diagnostic peritoneal lavage and needle pericardiocentesis have virtually disappeared from clinical practice since the introduction of sonography in trauma care. Prehospital ultrasound is now available, although its benefits are yet to be proven.

Vasopressors

The possible role of vasopressors (e.g., vasopressin) in trauma resuscitation is unclear and is based mainly on case reports.[247]

7j. Cardiac arrest associated with pregnancy

Overview

Mortality related to pregnancy in developed countries is rare, occurring in an estimated 1:30,000 deliveries.[248] The fetus must always be considered when an adverse cardiovascular event occurs in a pregnant woman. Resuscitation guidelines for pregnancy are based largely on case series and scientific rationale. Most reports address the causes in developed countries, whereas the majority of pregnancy-related deaths occur in the developing world.

Significant physiological changes occur during pregnancy, e.g., cardiac output, blood volume, minute ventilation and oxygen consumption all increase. Furthermore, the gravid uterus may cause significant compression of iliac and abdominal vessels when the mother is in the supine position, resulting in reduced cardiac output and hypotension.

Causes

There are many causes of cardiac arrest in pregnant women. A review of nearly 2 million pregnancies in the UK[248] showed that maternal death was associated with:

- pre-existing cardiac disease;
- thromboembolism;
- suicide;
- hypertensive disorders of pregnancy;
- sepsis;
- ectopic pregnancy;
- haemorrhage;
- amniotic fluid embolism;

Pregnant women can also suffer the same causes of cardiac arrest as women of the same age group.

Key interventions to prevent cardiac arrest

In an emergency, use an ABCDE approach. Many cardiovascular problems associated with pregnancy are caused by caval compression. Treat a distressed or compromised pregnant patient as follows:

- Place the patient in the left lateral position or manually and gently displace the uterus to the left.
- Give 100% oxygen.
- Give a fluid bolus.
- Immediately re-evaluate the need for any drugs being given.
- Seek expert help early.

Modifications to BLS guidelines for cardiac arrest

After 20 weeks' gestation, the pregnant woman's uterus can press down against the inferior vena cava and the aorta, impeding venous return and cardiac output. Uterine obstruction of venous return can cause pre-arrest hypotension or shock and, in the critically ill patient, may precipitate arrest.[249,250] After cardiac arrest, the compromise in venous return and cardiac output by the gravid uterus limit the effectiveness of chest compressions. Non-cardiac arrest data show that the gravid uterus can be shifted away from the cava in most cases by placing the patient in 15 degrees of left lateral decubitus position.[251] Tilt may be accomplished by manual or mechanical means. There is no evidence to guide the hand position for optimum chest compressions in the pregnant patient. A hand position higher than the normal position for chest compression may be needed to adjust for the elevation

of the diaphragm and abdominal contents caused by the gravid uterus. Attempt defibrillation using standard energy doses.[252] There is no evidence that shocks from a direct current defibrillator have adverse effects on the fetal heart. Left lateral tilt and large breasts will make it difficult to place an apical defibrillator paddle. Adhesive defibrillator pads are preferable to paddles in pregnancy.

Modifications to advanced life support

There is a greater potential for gastro-oesophageal sphincter insufficiency and risk of pulmonary aspiration of gastric contents. Early tracheal intubation with correctly applied cricoid pressure decreases this risk. Tracheal intubation will make ventilation of the lungs easier in the presence of increased intra-abdominal pressure.

A tracheal tube 0.5–1 mm internal diameter (ID) smaller than that used for a non-pregnant woman of similar size may be necessary because of maternal airway narrowing from oedema and swelling.[253] Tracheal intubation may be more difficult in the pregnant patient.[254] Expert help, a failed intubation drill and the use of alternative airway devices may be needed (see section 4d).[255]

Reversible causes

Rescuers should attempt to identify common and reversible causes of cardiac arrest in pregnancy during resuscitation attempts. The 4 Hs and 4 Ts approach helps to identify all the common causes of cardiac arrest in pregnancy. Pregnant patients are at risk of all the other causes of cardiac arrest for their age group (e.g., anaphylaxis, drug overdose, trauma). Consider the use of abdominal ultrasound by a skilled operator to detect pregnancy and possible causes during cardiac arrest in pregnancy; however, do not delay other treatments. Specific causes of cardiac arrest in pregnancy include the following:

Haemorrhage

Life-threatening haemorrhage can occur both antenatally and postnatally. Associations include ectopic pregnancy, placental abruption, placenta praevia and uterine rupture.[248] A massive haemorrhage protocol must be available in all units and should be updated and rehearsed regularly in conjunction with the blood bank. Women at high risk of bleeding should be delivered in centres with facilities for blood transfusion, intensive care and other interventions, and plans should be made in advance for their management. Treatment is based on an

ABCDE approach. The key step is to stop the bleeding. Consider the following:

- fluid resuscitation including use of rapid transfusion system and cell salvage;[256]
- correction of coagulopathy. There may be a role for recombinant Factor VIIa;[257]
- oxytocin and prostaglandins to correct uterine atony;[258]
- uterine compression sutures;[259]
- radiological embolisation;[260]
- hysterectomy;
- aortic cross-clamping in catastrophic haemorrhage.[261]

Drugs

Iatrogenic overdose is possible in eclamptic women receiving magnesium sulphate, particularly if the woman becomes oliguric. Give calcium to treat magnesium toxicity (see life-threatening electrolyte abnormalities).

Central neural blockade for analgesia or anaesthesia may cause problems due to sympathetic blockade (hypotension, bradycardia) or local anaesthetic toxicity.[262]

Cardiovascular disease

Pulmonary hypertension causes most deaths from congenital heart disease. Peripartum cardiomyopathy, myocardial infarction and aneurysm or dissection of the aorta or its branches cause most deaths from acquired cardiac disease.[263,264] Patients with known cardiac disease need to be managed in a specialist unit. Pregnant women with coronary artery disease may suffer an acute coronary syndrome. Percutaneous coronary intervention is the reperfusion strategy of choice for ST-elevation myocardial infarction in pregnancy because fibrinolytics are relatively contraindicated.[265]

Pre-eclampsia and eclampsia

Eclampsia is defined as the development of convulsions and/or unexplained coma during pregnancy or postpartum in patients with signs and symptoms of pre-eclampsia.[266,267] Magnesium sulphate is effective in preventing approximately half of the cases of eclampsia developing in labour or immediately postpartum in women with pre-eclampsia.

Life-threatening pulmonary embolism

Successful use of fibrinolytics for massive, life-threatening pulmonary embolism in pregnant women has been reported.[268–271]

Amniotic fluid embolism

Amniotic fluid embolism may present with breathlessness, cyanosis, arrhythmias, hypotension and haemorrhage associated with disseminated intravascular coagulopathy.[272] Presentation is variable and may be similar to anaphylaxis. Treatment is supportive, as there is no specific therapy. Successful use of cardiopulmonary bypass for women suffering life-threatening amniotic fluid embolism during labour and delivery is reported.[273]

If immediate resuscitation attempts fail

Consider the need for an emergency hysterotomy or Caesarean section as soon as a pregnant woman goes into cardiac arrest. In some circumstances immediate resuscitation attempts will restore a perfusing rhythm; in early pregnancy this may enable the pregnancy to proceed to term. When initial resuscitation attempts fail, delivery of the fetus may improve the chances of successful resuscitation of the mother and fetus.[274–276] The best survival rate for infants over 24–25 weeks' gestation occurs when delivery of the infant is achieved within 5 min after the mother's cardiac arrest.[274,277–279] This requires that the provider commence the hysterotomy at about 4 min after cardiac arrest. Delivery will relieve caval compression and improve chances of maternal resuscitation. The Caesarean delivery also enables access to the infant so that newborn resuscitation can begin.

Decision-making for emergency hysterotomy

Consider gestational age. The gravid uterus reaches a size that will begin to compromise aorto-caval blood flow at approximately 20 weeks' gestation; however, fetal viability begins at approximately 24–25 weeks. Portable ultrasounds are available in some emergency departments and may aid in determination of gestational age (in experienced hands) and positioning, provided their use does not delay the decision to perform emergency hysterotomy.[280]

- At gestational age <20 weeks, urgent Caesarean delivery need not be considered, because a gravid uterus of this size is unlikely to significantly compromise maternal cardiac output.
- At gestational age approximately 20–23 weeks, initiate emergency hysterotomy to enable successful resuscitation of the mother, not survival

of the delivered infant, which is unlikely at this gestational age.

- At gestational age approximately ≥24−25 weeks, initiate emergency hysterotomy to save the life of both the mother and the infant.

Planning for emergencies. Advanced life support in pregnancy requires coordination of maternal resuscitation, Caesarean delivery of the fetus and newborn resuscitation within 5 min. To achieve this, units likely to deal with cardiac arrest in pregnancy should:

- have plans and equipment for resuscitation of both the pregnant woman and newborn in place;
- ensure early involvement of obstetric and neonatal teams;
- ensure regular training in obstetric emergencies.

7k. Electrocution

Introduction

Electrical injury is a relatively infrequent but potentially devastating multisystem injury with high morbidity and mortality, causing 0.54 deaths per 100,000 people each year. Most electrical injuries in adults occur in the workplace and are associated generally with high voltage, whereas children are at risk primarily at home, where the voltage is lower (220 V in Europe, Australia and Asia; 110 V in the USA and Canada).[281] Electrocution from lightning strikes is rare, but worldwide it causes 1000 deaths each year.[282]

Electric shock injuries are caused by the direct effects of current on cell membranes and vascular smooth muscle. The thermal energy associated with high-voltage electrocution will also cause burns. Factors influencing the severity of electrical injury include whether the current is alternating (AC) or direct (DC), voltage, magnitude of energy delivered, resistance to current flow, pathway of current through the patient, and the area and duration of contact. Skin resistance is decreased by moisture, which increases the likelihood of injury. Electric current follows the path of least resistance; conductive neurovascular bundles within limbs are particularly prone to damage.

Contact with AC may cause tetanic contraction of skeletal muscle, which may prevent release from the source of electricity. Myocardial or respiratory failure may cause immediate death.

- Respiratory arrest may be caused by paralysis of the central respiratory control system or the respiratory muscles.

- Current may precipitate ventricular fibrillation (VF) if it traverses the myocardium during the vulnerable period (analogous to an R-on-T phenomenon).[283] Electrical current may also cause myocardial ischaemia because of coronary artery spasm. Asystole may be primary, or secondary to asphyxia following respiratory arrest.

Current that traverses the myocardium is more likely to be fatal. A transthoracic (hand-to-hand) pathway is more likely to be fatal than a vertical (hand-to-foot) or straddle (foot-to-foot) pathway. There may be extensive tissue destruction along the current pathway.

Lightning strike

Lightning strikes deliver as much as 300 kilovolts over a few ms. Most of the current from a lightning strike passes over the surface of the body in a process called 'external flashover'. Both industrial shocks and lightning strikes cause deep burns at the point of contact. For industry the points of contact are usually on the upper limbs, hands and wrists, whereas for lightning they are mostly on the head, neck and shoulders. Injury may also occur indirectly through ground current or current 'splashing' from a tree or other object that is hit by lightning.[284] Explosive force may cause blunt trauma.[285] The pattern and severity of injury from a lightning strike varies considerably, even among affected individuals from a single group.[286−288] As with industrial and domestic electric shock, death is caused by cardiac[287−291] or respiratory arrest.[284,292] In those who survive the initial shock, extensive catecholamine release or autonomic stimulation may occur, causing hypertension, tachycardia, non-specific ECG changes (including prolongation of the QT interval and transient T-wave inversion), and myocardial necrosis. Creatine kinase may be released from myocardial and skeletal muscle. Lightning can also cause central and peripheral nerve damage; brain haemorrhage and oedema, and peripheral nerve injury are common. Mortality from lightning injuries is as high as 30%, with up to 70% of survivors sustaining significant morbidity.[293−295]

Diagnosis

The circumstances surrounding the incident are not always known. Unconscious patients with linear or punctuate burns or feathering should be treated as a victims of lightning strike.[284]

Rescue

Ensure that any power source is switched off and do not approach the casualty until it is safe. High voltage (above domestic mains) electricity can arc and conduct through the ground for up to a few metres around the casualty. It is safe to approach and handle casualties after lightning strike, although it would be wise to move to a safer environment, particularly if lightning has been seen within 30 min.[284]

Resuscitation

Start standard basic and advanced life support without delay.

- Airway management may be difficult if there are electrical burns around the face and neck. Early tracheal intubation is needed in these cases, as extensive soft-tissue oedema may develop causing airway obstruction. Head and spine trauma can occur after electrocution. Immobilise the spine until evaluation can be performed.
- Muscular paralysis, especially after high voltage, may persist for several hours;[294] ventilatory support is required during this period.
- VF is the commonest initial arrhythmia after high-voltage AC shock; treat with prompt attempted defibrillation. Asystole is more common after DC shock; use standard protocols for this and other arrhythmias.
- Remove smouldering clothing and shoes to prevent further thermal injury.
- Vigorous fluid therapy is required if there is significant tissue destruction. Maintain a good urine output to enhance the excretion of myoglobin, potassium and other products of tissue damage.[291]
- Consider early surgical intervention in patients with severe thermal injuries.
- Maintain spinal immobilisation if there is a likelihood of head or neck trauma.[296,297]
- Conduct a thorough secondary survey to exclude traumatic injuries caused by tetanic muscular contraction or by the person being thrown.[297,298]
- Electrocution can cause severe, deep soft-tissue injury with relatively minor skin wounds, because current tends to follow neurovascular bundles; look carefully for features of compartment syndrome, which will necessitate fasciotomy.

Patients struck by lightning are most likely to die if they suffer immediate cardiac or respiratory arrest and are not treated rapidly. When multiple victims are struck simultaneously by lightning, rescuers should give highest priority to patients in respiratory or cardiac arrest. Victims with respiratory arrest may require only ventilation to avoid secondary hypoxic cardiac arrest. Resuscitative attempts may have higher success rates in lightning victims than in patients with cardiac arrest from other causes, and efforts may be effective even when the interval before the resuscitative attempt is prolonged.[292] Dilated or non-reactive pupils should never be used as a prognostic sign, particularly in patients suffering a lightning strike.[284]

There are conflicting reports on the vulnerability of the fetus to electric shock. The clinical spectrum of electrical injury ranges from a transient unpleasant sensation for the mother with no effect on her fetus, to fetal death either immediately or a few days later. Several factors, such as the magnitude of the current and the duration of contact, are thought to affect outcome.[299]

Further treatment and prognosis

Immediate resuscitation in young victims of cardiac arrest due to electrocution can result in survival. Successful resuscitation has been reported after prolonged life support. All those who survive electrical injury should be monitored in hospital if they have a history of cardiorespiratory problems or have suffered:

- loss of consciousness;
- cardiac arrest;
- electrocardiographic abnormalities;
- soft-tissue damage and burns.

Severe burns (thermal or electrical), myocardial necrosis, the extent of central nervous system injury, and secondary multisystem organ failure determine the morbidity and long-term prognosis. There is no specific therapy for electrical injury, and the management is symptomatic. Prevention remains the best way to minimise the prevalence and severity of electrical injury.

References

1. Guidelines 2000 for Cardiopulmonary Resuscitation and Emergency Cardiovascular Care: International Consensus on Science. Part 8: Advanced challenges in resuscitation. Section 1. Life-threatening electrolyte abnormalities. Circulation 2000;102:I-122—217.
2. Niemann JT, Cairns CB. Hyperkalemia and ionized hypocalcemia during cardiac arrest and resuscitation: possible culprits for postcountershock arrhythmias? Ann Emerg Med 1999;34:1—7.
3. Ahmed J, Weisberg LS. Hyperkalemia in dialysis patients. Semin Dial 2001;14:348—56.

4. Mahoney B, Smith W, Lo D, Tsoi K, Tonelli M, Clase C. Emergency interventions for hyperkalaemia. Cochrane Database Syst Rev 2005. CD003235.

5. Ngugi NN, McLigeyo SO, Kayima JK. Treatment of hyperkalaemia by altering the transcellular gradient in patients with renal failure: effect of various therapeutic approaches. East Afr Med J 1997;74:503—9.

6. Allon M, Shanklin N. Effect of bicarbonate administration on plasma potassium in dialysis patients: interactions with insulin and albuterol. Am J Kidney Dis 1996;28:508—14.

7. Rastegar A, Soleimani M. Hypokalaemia and hyperkalaemia. Postgrad Med J 2001;77:759—64.

8. Cohn JN, Kowey PR, Whelton PK, Prisant LM. New guidelines for potassium replacement in clinical practice: a contemporary review by the National Council on Potassium in Clinical Practice. Arch Intern Med 2000;160:2429—36.

9. Litovitz TL, Felberg L, White S, Klein-Schwartz W. 1995 annual report of the American Association of Poison Control Centers Toxic Exposure Surveillance System. Am J Emerg Med 1996;14:487—537.

10. McCaig LF, Burt CW. Poisoning-related visits to emergency departments in the United States, 1993—1996. J Toxicol Clin Toxicol 1999;37:817—26.

11. Fingerhut LA, Cox CS. Poisoning mortality, 1985—1995. Public Health Rep 1998;113:218—33.

12. Watson WA, Litovitz TL, Klein-Schwartz W, et al. 2003 annual report of the American Association of Poison Control Centers Toxic Exposure Surveillance System. Am J Emerg Med 2004;22:335—404.

13. Zimmerman JL. Poisonings and overdoses in the intensive care unit: general and specific management issues. Crit Care Med 2003;31:2794—801.

14. Suntres ZE. Role of antioxidants in paraquat toxicity. Toxicology 2002;180:65—77.

15. Facility assessment guidelines for regional toxicology treatment centers. American Academy of Clinical Toxicology. J Toxicol Clin Toxicol 1993;31:211—7.

16. Poison information and treatment systems. American College of Emergency Physicians. Ann Emerg Med 1996;28:384.

17. Chyka PA, Seger D, Krenzelok EP, Vale JA. Position paper: single-dose activated charcoal. Clin Toxicol (Phila) 2005;43:61—87.

18. Vale JA, Kulig K. Position paper: gastric lavage. J Toxicol Clin Toxicol 2004;42:933—43.

19. Krenzelok EP. Ipecac syrup-induced emesis.. no evidence of benefit. Clin Toxicol (Phila) 2005;43:11—2.

20. Position paper: cathartics. J Toxicol Clin Toxicol 2004;42:243—53.

21. Position paper: whole bowel irrigation. J Toxicol Clin Toxicol 2004;42:843—54.

22. Proudfoot AT, Krenzelok EP, Vale JA. Position Paper on urine alkalinization. J Toxicol Clin Toxicol 2004;42:1—26.

23. Golper TA, Bennett WM. Drug removal by continuous arteriovenous haemofiltration. A review of the evidence in poisoned patients. Med Toxicol Adverse Drug Exp 1988;3:341—9.

24. Pitetti RD, Singh S, Pierce MC. Safe and efficacious use of procedural sedation and analgesia by nonanesthesiologists in a pediatric emergency department. Arch Pediatr Adolesc Med 2003;157:1090—6.

25. Osterwalder JJ. Naloxone — for intoxications with intravenous heroin and heroin mixtures — harmless or hazardous? A prospective clinical study. J Toxicol Clin Toxicol 1996;34:409—16.

26. Sporer KA, Firestone J, Isaacs SM. Out-of-hospital treatment of opioid overdoses in an urban setting. Acad Emerg Med 1996;3:660—7.

27. Wanger K, Brough L, Macmillan I, Goulding J, MacPhail I, Christenson JM. Intravenous vs. subcutaneous naloxone for out-of-hospital management of presumed opioid overdose. Acad Emerg Med 1998;5:293—9.

28. Hasan RA, Benko AS, Nolan BM, Campe J, Duff J, Zureikat GY. Cardiorespiratory effects of naloxone in children. Ann Pharmacother 2003;37:1587—92.

29. Sporer KA. Acute heroin overdose. Ann Intern Med 1999;130:584—90.

30. Schneir AB, Vadeboncoeur TF, Offerman SR, et al. Massive oxycontin ingestion refractory to naloxone therapy. Ann Emerg Med 2002;40:425—8.

31. Kelly AM, Kerr D, Dietze P, Patrick I, Walker T, Koutsogiannis Z. Randomised trial of intranasal versus intramuscular naloxone in prehospital treatment for suspected opioid overdose. Med J Aust 2005;182:24—7.

32. Brown TC. Sodium bicarbonate treatment for tricyclic antidepressant arrhythmias in children. Med J Aust 1976;2:380—2.

33. Hoffman JR, Votey SR, Bayer M, Silver L. Effect of hypertonic sodium bicarbonate in the treatment of moderate-to-severe cyclic antidepressant overdose. Am J Emerg Med 1993;11:336—41.

34. Knudsen K, Abrahamsson J. Epinephrine and sodium bicarbonate independently and additively increase survival in experimental amitriptyline poisoning. Crit Care Med 1997;25:669—74.

35. Nattel S, Mittleman M. Treatment of ventricular tachyarrhythmias resulting from amitriptyline toxicity in dogs. J Pharmacol Exp Ther 1984;231:430—5.

36. Nattel S, Keable H, Sasyniuk BI. Experimental amitriptyline intoxication: electrophysiologic manifestations and management. J Cardiovasc Pharmacol 1984;6:83—9.

37. Pentel P, Benowitz N. Efficacy and mechanism of action of sodium bicarbonate in the treatment of desipramine toxicity in rats. J Pharmacol Exp Ther 1984;230:12—9.

38. Brown TC, Barker GA, Dunlop ME, Loughnan PM. The use of sodium bicarbonate in the treatment of tricyclic antidepressant-induced arrhythmias. Anaesth Intensive Care 1973;1:203—10.

39. Brown TC. Tricyclic antidepressant overdosage: experimental studies on the management of circulatory complications. Clin Toxicol 1976;9:255—72.

40. Hedges JR, Baker PB, Tasset JJ, Otten EJ, Dalsey WC, Syverud SA. Bicarbonate therapy for the cardiovascular toxicity of amitriptyline in an animal model. J Emerg Med 1985;3:253—60.

41. Sasyniuk BI, Jhamandas V, Valois M. Experimental amitriptyline intoxication: treatment of cardiac toxicity with sodium bicarbonate. Ann Emerg Med 1986;15:1052—9.

42. Stone CK, Kraemer CM, Carroll R, Low R. Does a sodium-free buffer affect QRS width in experimental amitriptyline overdose? Ann Emerg Med 1995;26:58—64.

43. McCabe JL, Cobaugh DJ, Menegazzi JJ, Fata J. Experimental tricyclic antidepressant toxicity: a randomized, controlled comparison of hypertonic saline solution, sodium bicarbonate, and hyperventilation. Ann Emerg Med 1998;32:329—33.

44. Sasyniuk BI, Jhamandas V. Mechanism of reversal of toxic effects of amitriptyline on cardiac Purkinje fibers by sodium bicarbonate. J Pharmacol Exp Ther 1984;231:387—94.

45. Sasyniuk BI, Jhamandas V. Frequency-dependent effects of amitriptyline on V_{max} in canine Purkinje fibers and its alteration by alkalosis. Proc West Pharmacol Soc 1986;29:73—5.

46. Bou-Abboud E, Nattel S. Molecular mechanisms of the reversal of imipramine-induced sodium channel blockade

by alkalinization in human cardiac myocytes. Cardiovasc Res 1998;38:395—404.

47. Levitt MA, Sullivan Jr JB, Owens SM, Burnham L, Finley PR. Amitriptyline plasma protein binding: effect of plasma pH and relevance to clinical overdose. Am J Emerg Med 1986;4:121—5.

48. McKinney PE, Rasmussen R. Reversal of severe tricyclic antidepressant-induced cardiotoxicity with intravenous hypertonic saline solution. Ann Emerg Med 2003;42:20—4.

49. Brogan WCI, Lange RA, Kim AS, Moliterno DJ, Hillis LD. Alleviation of cocaine-induced coronary vasoconstriction by nitroglycerin. J Am Coll Cardiol 1991;18:581—6.

50. Lange RA, Cigarroa RG, Yancy Jr CW, et al. Cocaine-induced coronary-artery vasoconstriction. N Engl J Med 1989;321:1557—62.

51. Lange RA, Cigarroa RG, Flores ED, et al. Potentiation of cocaine-induced coronary vasoconstriction by beta-adrenergic blockade. Ann Intern Med 1990;112:897—903.

52. Boehrer JD, Moliterno DJ, Willard JE, Hillis LD, Lange RA. Influence of labetalol on cocaine-induced coronary vasoconstriction in humans. Am J Med 1993;94:608—10.

53. Bosse GM, Pope TM. Recurrent digoxin overdose and treatment with digoxin-specific Fab antibody fragments. J Emerg Med 1994;12:179—85.

54. Eddleston M, Rajapakse S, Rajakanthan, et al. Anti-digoxin Fab fragments in cardiotoxicity induced by ingestion of yellow oleander: a randomised controlled trial. Lancet 2000;355:967—72.

55. Dasgupta A, Szelei-Stevens KA. Neutralization of free digoxin-like immunoreactive components of oriental medicines Dan Shen and Lu-Shen-Wan by the Fab fragment of antidigoxin antibody (Digibind). Am J Clin Pathol 2004;121:276—81.

56. Bailey B. Glucagon in beta-blocker and calcium channel blocker overdoses: a systematic review. J Toxicol Clin Toxicol 2003;41:595—602.

57. Dewitt CR, Waksman JC. Pharmacology, pathophysiology and management of calcium channel blocker and beta-blocker toxicity. Toxicol Rev 2004;23:223—38.

58. Wax PM, Erdman AR, Chyka PA, et al. beta-blocker ingestion: an evidence-based consensus guideline for out-of-hospital management. Clin Toxicol (Phila) 2005;43:131—46.

59. Peden MM, McGee K. The epidemiology of drowning worldwide. Inj Control Saf Promot 2003;10:195—9.

60. Driscoll TR, Harrison JA, Steenkamp M. Review of the role of alcohol in drowning associated with recreational aquatic activity. Inj Prev 2004;10:107—13.

61. Papa L, Hoelle R, Idris A. Systematic review of definitions for drowning incidents. Resuscitation 2005;65:255—64.

62. Idris AH, Berg RA, Bierens J, et al. Recommended guidelines for uniform reporting of data from drowning: The ''Utstein style''. Resuscitation 2003;59:45—57.

63. Watson RS, Cummings P, Quan L, Bratton S, Weiss NS. Cervical spine injuries among submersion victims. J Trauma 2001;51:658—62.

64. Dodd FM, Simon E, McKeown D, Patrick MR. The effect of a cervical collar on the tidal volume of anaesthetised adult patients. Anaesthesia 1995;50:961—3.

65. International Liaison Committee on Resuscitation 2005. International Consensus on Cardiopulmonary Resuscitation and Emergency Cardiovascular Care Science with Treatment Recommendations. Resuscitation 2005;67:157—341.

66. Golden FS, Hervey GR, Tipton MJ. Circum-rescue collapse: collapse, sometimes fatal, associated with rescue of immersion victims. J R Nav Med Serv 1991;77:139—49.

67. Goh SH, Low BY. Drowning and near-drowning—some lessons learnt. Ann Acad Med Singapore 1999;28:183—8.

68. Quan L, Wentz KR, Gore EJ, Copass MK. Outcome and predictors of outcome in pediatric submersion victims receiving prehospital care in King County. Wash Pediatr 1990;86:586—93.

69. Szpilman D, Soares M. In-water resuscitation—is it worthwhile? Resuscitation 2004;63:25—31.

70. Perkins GD. In-water resuscitation: a pilot evaluation. Resuscitation 2005;65:321—4.

71. Rosen P, Stoto M, Harley J. The use of the Heimlich maneuver in near-drowning: Institute of Medicine report. J Emerg Med 1995;13:397—405.

72. March NF, Matthews RC. New techniques in external cardiac compressions. Aquatic cardiopulmonary resuscitation. JAMA 1980;244:1229—32.

73. March NF, Matthews RC. Feasibility study of CPR in the water. Undersea Biomed Res 1980;7:141—8.

74. Thomas R, Cahill CJ. Successful defibrillation in profound hypothermia (core body temperature 25.6 degrees C). Resuscitation 2000;47:317—20.

75. Manolios N, Mackie I. Drowning and near-drowning on Australian beaches patrolled by life-savers: a 10-year study, 1973—1983. Med J Aust 1988;148:165—7, 70—71.

76. Modell JH, Calderwood HW, Ruiz BC, Downs JB, Chapman Jr R. Effects of ventilatory patterns on arterial oxygenation after near-drowning in sea water. Anesthesiology 1974;40:376—84.

77. Golden FS, Tipton MJ, Scott RC. Immersion, near-drowning and drowning. Br J Anaesth 1997;79:214—25.

78. Wyatt JP, Tomlinson GS, Busuttil A. Resuscitation of drowning victims in south-east Scotland. Resuscitation 1999;41:101—4.

79. Schmidt U, Fritz KW, Kasperczyk W, Tscherne H. Successful resuscitation of a child with severe hypothermia after cardiac arrest of 88 min. Prehosp Disaster Med 1995;10:60—2.

80. Bolte RG, Black PG, Bowers RS, Thorne JK, Corneli HM. The use of extracorporeal rewarming in a child submerged for 66 min. JAMA 1988;260:377—9.

81. The acute respiratory distress syndrome network. Ventilation with lower tidal volumes as compared with traditional tidal volumes for acute lung injury and the acute respiratory distress syndrome. N Engl J Med 2000;342:1301—8.

82. Moran I, Zavala E, Fernandez R, Blanch L, Mancebo J. Recruitment manoeuvres in acute lung injury/acute respiratory distress syndrome. Eur Respir J Suppl 2003;42:37s—42s.

83. Nolan JP, Morley PT, Vanden Hoek TL, Hickey RW. Therapeutic hypothermia after cardiac arrest. An advisory statement by the Advancement Life support Task Force of the International Liaison committee on Resuscitation. Resuscitation 2003;57:231—5.

84. Holzer M, Behringer W, Schorkhuber W, et al. Mild hypothermia and outcome after CPR. Hypothermia for Cardiac Arrest (HACA) Study Group. Acta Anaesthesiol Scand Suppl 1997;111:55—8.

85. Sterz F, Safar P, Tisherman S, Radovsky A, Kuboyama K, Oku K. Mild hypothermic cardiopulmonary resuscitation improves outcome after prolonged cardiac arrest in dogs. Crit Care Med 1991;19:379—89.

86. Farstad M, Andersen KS, Koller ME, Grong K, Segadal L, Husby P. Rewarming from accidental hypothermia by extracorporeal circulation. A retrospective study. Eur J Cardiothorac Surg 2001;20:58—64.

87. Schneider SM. Hypothermia: from recognition to rewarming. Emerg Med Rep 1992;13:1—20.

88. Gilbert M, Busund R, Skagseth A, Nilsen PÅ, Solbø JP. Resuscitation from accidental hypothermia of 13.7 °C with circulatory arrest. Lancet 2000;355:375–6.

89. Danzl DF, Pozos RS, Auerbach PS, et al. Multicenter hypothermia survey. Ann Emerg Med 1987;16:1042–55.

90. Reuler JB. Hypothermia: pathophysiology, clinical settings, and management. Ann Intern Med 1978;89:519–27.

91. Lefrant JY, Muller L, de La Coussaye JE, et al. Temperature measurement in intensive care patients: comparison of urinary bladder, oesophageal, rectal, axillary, and inguinal methods versus pulmonary artery core method. Intensive Care Med 2003;29:414–8.

92. Robinson J, Charlton J, Seal R, Spady D, Joffres MR. Oesophageal, rectal, axillary, tympanic and pulmonary artery temperatures during cardiac surgery. Can J Anaesth 1998;45:317–23.

93. Krismer AC, Lindner KH, Kornberger R, et al. Cardiopulmonary resuscitation during severe hypothermia in pigs: does epinephrine or vasopressin increase coronary perfusion pressure? Anesth Analg 2000;90:69–73.

94. Kornberger E, Lindner KH, Mayr VD, et al. Effects of epinephrine in a pig model of hypothermic cardiac arrest and closed-chest cardiopulmonary resuscitation combined with active rewarming. Resuscitation 2001;50:301–8.

95. Stoner J, Martin G, O'Mara K, Ehlers J, Tomlanovich M. Amiodarone and bretylium in the treatment of hypothermic ventricular fibrillation in a canine model. Acad Emerg Med 2003;10:187–91.

96. Mattu A, Brady WJ, Perron AD. Electrocardiographic manifestations of hypothermia. Am J Emerg Med 2002;20:314–26.

97. Southwick FS, Dalglish S P.H. Jr. Recovery after prolonged asystolic cardiac arrest in profound hypothermia: a case report and literature review. JAMA 1980;243:1250–3.

98. Ujhelyi MR, Sims JJ, Dubin SA, Vender J, Miller AW. Defibrillation energy requirements and electrical heterogeneity during total body hypothermia. Crit Care Med 2001;29:1006–11.

99. Kornberger E, Schwarz B, Lindner KH, Mair P. Forced air surface rewarming in patients with severe accidental hypothermia. Resuscitation 1999;41:105–11.

100. Roggla M, Frossard M, Wagner A, Holzer M, Bur A, Roggla G. Severe accidental hypothermia with or without hemodynamic instability: rewarming without the use of extracorporeal circulation. Wien Klin Wochenschr 2002;114:315–20.

101. Weinberg AD, Hamlet MP, Paturas JL, White RD, McAninch GW. Cold weather emergencies: principles of patient management. Branford, CN: American Medical Publishing Co.; 1990.

102. Zell SC, Kurtz KJ. Severe exposure hypothermia: a resuscitation protocol. Ann Emerg Med 1985;14:339–45.

103. Althaus U, Aeberhard P, Schupbach P, Nachbur BH, Muhlemann W. Management of profound accidental hypothermia with cardiorespiratory arrest. Ann Surg 1982;195:492–5.

104. Walpoth BH, Walpoth-Aslan BN, Mattle HP, et al. Outcome of survivors of accidental deep hypothermia and circulatory arrest treated with extracorporeal blood warming. N Engl J Med 1997;337:1500–5.

105. Silfvast T, Pettila V. Outcome from severe accidental hypothermia in Southern Finland—a 10-year review. Resuscitation 2003;59:285–90.

106. Moss J. Accidental severe hypothermia. Surg Gynecol Obstet 1986;162:501–13.

107. Safar P. Cerebral resuscitation after cardiac arrest: research initiatives and future directions [published correction appears in Ann Emerg Med. 1993;22:759]. Ann Emerg Med 1993;22(pt 2):324–49.

108. Bouchama A, Knochel JP. Heat stroke. N Engl J Med 2002;346:1978–88.

109. Wappler F. Malignant hyperthermia. Eur J Anaesthesiol 2001;18:632–52.

110. Ali SZ, Taguchi A, Rosenberg H. Malignant hyperthermia. Best Pract Res Clin Anaesthesiol 2003;17:519–33.

111. Bouchama A. The 2003 European heat wave. Intensive Care Med 2004;30:1–3.

112. Coris EE, Ramirez AM, Van Durme DJ. Heat illness in athletes: the dangerous combination of heat, humidity and exercise. Sports Med 2004;34:9–16.

113. Grogan H, Hopkins PM. Heat stroke: implications for critical care and anaesthesia. Br J Anaesth 2002;88:700–7.

114. Bouchama A, De Vol EB. Acid-base alterations in heatstroke. Intensive Care Med 2001;27:680–5.

115. Akhtar MJ, al-Nozha M, al-Harthi S, Nouh MS. Electrocardiographic abnormalities in patients with heat stroke. Chest 1993;104:411–4.

116. el-Kassimi FA, Al-Mashhadani S, Abdullah AK, Akhtar J. Adult respiratory distress syndrome and disseminated intravascular coagulation complicating heat stroke. Chest 1986;90:571–4.

117. Waruiru C, Appleton R. Febrile seizures: an update. Arch Dis Child 2004;89:751–6.

118. Berger J, Hart J, Millis M, Baker AL. Fulminant hepatic failure from heat stroke requiring liver transplantation. J Clin Gastroenterol 2000;30:429–31.

119. Huerta-Alardin AL, Varon J, Marik PE. Bench-to-bedside review: Rhabdomyolysis—an overview for clinicians. Crit Care 2005;9:158–69.

120. Wolff ED, Driessen OMJ. Theophylline intoxication in a child. Ned Tijdschr Geneeskd 1977;121:896–901.

121. Sidor K, Mikolajczyk W, Horwath-Stolarczyk A. Acute poisoning in children hospitalized at the Medical University Hospital No 3 in Warsaw, between 1996 and 2000. Pediatr Polska 2002;77:509–16.

122. Boyer EW, Shannon M. The serotonin syndrome. N Engl J Med 2005;352:1112–20.

123. Bhanushali MJ, Tuite PJ. The evaluation and management of patients with neuroleptic malignant syndrome. Neurol Clin 2004;22:389–411.

124. Abraham E, Matthay MA, Dinarello CA, et al. Consensus conference definitions for sepsis, septic shock, acute lung injury, and acute respiratory distress syndrome: time for a re-evaluation. Crit Care Med 2000;28:232–5.

125. Savage MW, Mah PM, Weetman AP, Newell-Price J. Endocrine emergencies. Postgrad Med J 2004;80:506–15.

126. Hadad E, Weinbroum AA, Ben-Abraham R. Drug-induced hyperthermia and muscle rigidity: a practical approach. Eur J Emerg Med 2003;10:149–54.

127. Halloran LL, Bernard DW. Management of drug-induced hyperthermia. Curr Opin Pediatr 2004;16:211–5.

128. Armstrong LE, Crago AE, Adams R, Roberts WO, Maresh CM. Whole-body cooling of hyperthermic runners: comparison of two field therapies. Am J Emerg Med 1996;14:355–8.

129. Horowitz BZ. The golden hour in heat stroke: use of iced peritoneal lavage. Am J Emerg Med 1989;7:616–9.

130. Bernard S, Buist M, Monteiro O, Smith K. Induced hypothermia using large volume, ice-cold intravenous fluid in comatose survivors of out-of-hospital cardiac arrest: a preliminary report. Resuscitation 2003;56:9–13.

131. Schmutzhard E, Engelhardt K, Beer R, et al. Safety and efficacy of a novel intravascular cooling device to control body temperature in neurologic intensive care patients: a prospective pilot study. Crit Care Med 2002;30: 2481—8.

132. Al-Senani FM, Graffagnino C, Grotta JC, et al. A prospective, multicenter pilot study to evaluate the feasibility and safety of using the CoolGard system and icy catheter following cardiac arrest. Resuscitation 2004;62:143—50.

133. Behringer W, Safar P, Wu X, et al. Veno-venous extracorporeal blood shunt cooling to induce mild hypothermia in dog experiments and review of cooling methods. Resuscitation 2002;54:89—98.

134. Hadad E, Cohen-Sivan Y, Heled Y, Epstein Y. Clinical review: treatment of heat stroke—should dantrolene be considered? Crit Care 2005;9:86—91.

135. Krause T, Gerbershagen MU, Fiege M, Weisshorn R, Wappler F. Dantrolene—a review of its pharmacology, therapeutic use and new developments. Anaesthesia 2004;59:364—73.

136. Eshel G, Safar P, Sassano J, Stezoski W. Hyperthermia-induced cardiac arrest in dogs and monkeys. Resuscitation 1990;20:129—43.

137. Eshel G, Safar P, Radovsky A, Stezoski SW. Hyperthermia-induced cardiac arrest in monkeys: limited efficacy of standard CPR. Aviat Space Environ Med 1997;68:415—20.

138. Zeiner A, Holzer M, Sterz F, et al. Hyperthermia after cardiac arrest is associated with an unfavorable neurologic outcome. Arch Intern Med 2001;161:2007—12.

139. Masoli M, Fabian D, Holt S, Beasley R. The global burden of asthma: executive summary of the GINA Dissemination Committee report. Allergy 2004;59:469—78.

140. BTS/SIGN. British Thoracic Society, Scottish Intercollegiate Guidelines Network (SIGN). British guideline on the management of asthma. Thorax 2003;58(Suppl. I):i1—94.

141. Rainbow J, Browne GJ. Fatal asthma or anaphylaxis? Emerg Med J 2002;19:415—7.

142. Kokturk N, Demir N, Kervan F, Dinc E, Koybasioglu A, Turktas H. A subglottic mass mimicking near-fatal asthma: a challenge of diagnosis. J Emerg Med 2004;26:57—60.

143. Ratto D, Alfaro C, Sipsey J, Glovsky MM, Sharma OP. Are intravenous corticosteroids required in status asthmaticus? JAMA 1988;260:527—9.

144. Aaron SD. The use of ipratropium bromide for the management of acute asthma exacerbation in adults and children: a systematic review. J Asthma 2001;38:521—30.

145. Rodrigo G, Rodrigo C, Burschtin O. A meta-analysis of the effects of ipratropium bromide in adults with acute asthma. Am J Med 1999;107:363—70.

146. Munro A, Jacobs M. Best evidence topic reports. Is intravenous aminophylline better than intravenous salbutamol in the treatment of moderate to severe asthma? Emerg Med J 2004;21:78—80.

147. Rowe BH, Bretzlaff JA, Bourdon C, Bota GW, Camargo Jr CA. Magnesium sulfate for treating exacerbations of acute asthma in the emergency department. Cochrane Database Syst Rev 2000:CD001490.

148. Cydulka R, Davison R, Grammer L, Parker M, Mathews IV J. The use of epinephrine in the treatment of older adult asthmatics. Ann Emerg Med 1988;17:322—6.

149. Victoria MS, Battista CJ, Nangia BS. Comparison of subcutaneous terbutaline with epinephrine in the treatment of asthma in children. J Allergy Clin Immunol 1977;59:128—35.

150. Victoria MS, Battista CJ, Nangia BS. Comparison between epinephrine and terbutaline injections in the acute management of asthma. J Asthma 1989;26:287—90.

151. Rodrigo GJ, Rodrigo C, Pollack CV, Rowe B. Use of helium-oxygen mixtures in the treatment of acute asthma: a systematic review. Chest 2003;123:891—6.

152. Petrillo TM, Fortenberry JD, Linzer JF, Simon HK. Emergency department use of ketamine in pediatric status asthmaticus. J Asthma 2001;38:657—64.

153. Howton JC, Rose J, Duffy S, Zoltanski T, Levitt MA. Randomized, double-blind, placebo-controlled trial of intravenous ketamine in acute asthma. Ann Emerg Med 1996;27:170—5.

154. Antonelli M, Pennisi MA, Montini L. Clinical review: noninvasive ventilation in the clinical setting—experience from the past 10 years. Crit Care 2005;9:98—103.

155. Ram FS, Wellington S, Rowe BH, Wedzicha JA. Non-invasive positive pressure ventilation for treatment of respiratory failure due to severe acute exacerbations of asthma. Cochrane Database Syst Rev 2005:CD004360.

156. Leatherman JW, McArthur C, Shapiro RS. Effect of prolongation of expiratory time on dynamic hyperinflation in mechanically ventilated patients with severe asthma. Crit Care Med 2004;32:1542—5.

157. Bowman FP, Menegazzi JJ, Check BD, Duckett TM. Lower esophageal sphincter pressure during prolonged cardiac arrest and resuscitation. Ann Emerg Med 1995;26:216—9.

158. Lapinsky SE, Leung RS. Auto-PEEP and electromechanical dissociation. N Engl J Med 1996;335:674.

159. Rogers PL, Schlichtig R, Miro A, Pinsky M. Auto-PEEP during CPR. An "occult" cause of electromechanical dissociation? Chest 1991;99:492—3.

160. Rosengarten PL, Tuxen DV, Dziukas L, Scheinkestel C, Merrett K, Bowes G. Circulatory arrest induced by intermittent positive pressure ventilation in a patient with severe asthma. Anaesth Intensive Care 1991;19:118—21.

161. Sprung J, Hunter K, Barnas GM, Bourke DL. Abdominal distention is not always a sign of esophageal intubation: cardiac arrest due to "auto-PEEP". Anesth Analg 1994;78:801—4.

162. Deakin CD, McLaren RM, Petley GW, Clewlow F, Dalrymple-Hay MJ. Effects of positive end-expiratory pressure on transthoracic impedance—implications for defibrillation. Resuscitation 1998;37:9—12.

163. Mazzeo AT, Spada A, Pratico C, Lucanto T, Santamaria LB. Hypercapnia: what is the limit in paediatric patients? A case of near-fatal asthma successfully treated by multipharmacological approach. Paediatr Anaesth 2004;14:596—603.

164. Mertes PM, Laxenaire MC, Alla F. Anaphylactic and anaphylactoid reactions occurring during anesthesia in France in 1999—2000. Anesthesiology 2003;99:536—45.

165. Yunginger JW. Latex allergy in the workplace: an overview of where we are. Ann Allergy Asthma Immunol 1999;83:630—3.

166. Dreyfus DH, Fraser B, Randolph CC. Anaphylaxis to latex in patients without identified risk factors for latex allergy. Conn Med 2004;68:217—22.

167. Ownby DR. A history of latex allergy. J Allergy Clin Immunol 2002;110:S27—32.

168. Pumphrey RS. Lessons for management of anaphylaxis from a study of fatal reactions. Clin Exp Allergy 2000;30:1144—50.

169. Pumphrey RS. Fatal anaphylaxis in the UK, 1992—2001. Novartis Found Symp 2004;257:116—28, discussion 28—32, 57—60, 276—285.

170. Incorvaia C, Senna G, Mauro M, et al. Prevalence of allergic reactions to Hymenoptera stings in northern Italy. Allerg Immunol (Paris) 2004;36:372—4.

171. Pumphrey RS, Roberts IS. Postmortem findings after fatal anaphylactic reactions. J Clin Pathol 2000;53:273—6.

172. Mullins RJ. Anaphylaxis: risk factors for recurrence. Clin Exp Allergy 2003;33:1033—40.

173. Brown AF. Anaphylaxis: quintessence, quarrels, and quandaries. Emerg Med J 2001;18:328.

174. Brown AF. Anaphylaxis gets the adrenaline going. Emerg Med J 2004;21:128—9.

175. Ishoo E, Shah UK, Grillone GA, Stram JR, Fuleihan NS. Predicting airway risk in angioedema: staging system based on presentation. Otolaryngol Head Neck Surg 1999;121:263—8.

176. Pumphrey R. Anaphylaxis: can we tell who is at risk of a fatal reaction? Curr Opin Allergy Clin Immunol 2004;4:285—90.

177. Simons FE, Gu X, Simons KJ. Epinephrine absorption in adults: intramuscular versus subcutaneous injection. J Allergy Clin Immunol 2001;108:871—3.

178. Simons FER, Chan ES, Gu X, Simons KJ. Epinephrine for the out-of-hospital (first-aid) treatment of anaphylaxis in infants: is the ampule/syringe/needle method practical? J Allergy Clin Immunol 2001;108:1040—4.

179. Winbery SL, Lieberman PL. Histamine and antihistamines in anaphylaxis. Clin Allergy Immunol 2002;17:287—317.

180. Kill C, Wranze E, Wulf H. Successful treatment of severe anaphylactic shock with vasopressin. Two case reports. Int Arch Allergy Immunol 2004;134:260—1.

181. Williams SR, Denault AY, Pellerin M, Martineau R. Vasopressin for treatment of shock following aprotinin administration. Can J Anaesth 2004;51:169—72.

182. Visscher PK, Vetter RS, Camazine S. Removing bee stings. Lancet 1996;348:301—2.

183. Yocum MW, Butterfield JH, Klein JS, Volcheck GW, Schroeder DR, Silverstein MD. Epidemiology of anaphylaxis in Olmsted County: a population-based study. J Allergy Clin Immunol 1999;104(pt 1):452—6.

184. Ellis AK, Day JH. Diagnosis and management of anaphylaxis. CMAJ 2003;169:307—11.

185. Smith PL, Kagey-Sobotka A, Bleecker ER, et al. Physiologic manifestations of human anaphylaxis. J Clin Invest 1980;66:1072—80.

186. Stark BJ, Sullivan TJ. Biphasic and protracted anaphylaxis. J Allergy Clin Immunol 1986;78:76—83.

187. Brazil E, MacNamara AF. Not so immediate'' hypersensitivity: the danger of biphasic anaphylactic reactions. J Accid Emerg Med 1998;15:252—3.

188. Brady Jr WJ, Luber S, Carter CT, Guertler A, Lindbeck G. Multiphasic anaphylaxis: an uncommon event in the emergency department. Acad Emerg Med 1997;4:193—7.

189. Joint Working Party of the Association of Anaesthetists of Great Britain and Ireland and the British Society for Allergy and Clinical Immunology. Suspected anaphylactic reactions associated with anaesthesia. 3rd ed. London: The Association of Anaesthetists of Great Britain and Ireland and British Society for Allergy and Clinical Immunology; 2003.

190. Payne V, Kam PC. Mast cell tryptase: a review of its physiology and clinical significance. Anaesthesia 2004;59:695—703.

191. Anthi A, Tzelepis GE, Alivizatos P, Michalis A, Palatianos GM, Geroulanos S. Unexpected cardiac arrest after cardiac surgery: incidence, predisposing causes, and outcome of open chest cardiopulmonary resuscitation. Chest 1998;113:15—9.

192. Wahba A, Gotz W, Birnbaum DE. Outcome of cardiopulmonary resuscitation following open heart surgery. Scand Cardiovasc J 1997;31:147—9.

193. Rhodes JF, Blaufox AD, Seiden HS, et al. Cardiac arrest in infants after congenital heart surgery. Circulation 1999;100:II194—9.

194. Dimopoulou I, Anthi A, Michalis A, Tzelepis GE. Functional status and quality of life in long-term survivors of cardiac arrest after cardiac surgery. Crit Care Med 2001;29:1408—11.

195. Mackay JH, Powell SJ, Osgathorp J, Rozario CJ. Six-year prospective audit of chest reopening after cardiac arrest. Eur J Cardiothorac Surg 2002;22:421—5.

196. Pottle A, Bullock I, Thomas J, Scott L. Survival to discharge following open chest cardiac compression (OCCC). A 4-year retrospective audit in a cardiothoracic specialist centre— Royal Brompton and Harefield NHS Trust, United Kingdom. Resuscitation 2002;52:269—72.

197. Raman J, Saldanha RF, Branch JM, et al. Open cardiac compression in the postoperative cardiac intensive care unit. Anaesth Intensive Care 1989;17:129—35.

198. Birdi I, Chaudhuri N, Lenthall K, Reddy S, Nashef SA. Emergency reinstitution of cardiopulmonary bypass following cardiac surgery: outcome justifies the cost. Eur J Cardiothorac Surg 2000;17:743—6.

199. Rousou JA, Engelman RM, Flack III JE, Deaton DW, Owen SG. Emergency cardiopulmonary bypass in the cardiac surgical unit can be a lifesaving measure in postoperative cardiac arrest. Circulation 1994;90:II280—4.

200. Schwarz B, Bowdle TA, Jett GK, et al. Biphasic shocks compared with monophasic damped sine wave shocks for direct ventricular defibrillation during open heart surgery. Anesthesiology 2003;98:1063—9.

201. Rosemurgy AS, Norris PA, Olson SM, Hurst JM, Albrink MH. Prehospital traumatic cardiac arrest: the cost of futility. J Trauma 1993;35:468—73.

202. Battistella FD, Nugent W, Owings JT, Anderson JT. Field triage of the pulseless trauma patient. Arch Surg 1999;134:742—5.

203. Shimazu S, Shatney CH. Outcomes of trauma patients with no vital signs on hospital admission. J Trauma 1983;23:213—6.

204. Stockinger ZT, McSwain Jr NE. Additional evidence in support of withholding or terminating cardiopulmonary resuscitation for trauma patients in the field. J Am Coll Surg 2004;198:227—31.

205. Fulton RL, Voigt WJ, Hilakos AS. Confusion surrounding the treatment of traumatic cardiac arrest. J Am Coll Surg 1995;181:209—14.

206. Pasquale MD, Rhodes M, Cipolle MD, Hanley T, Wasser T. Defining ''dead on arrival'': impact on a level I trauma center. J Trauma 1996;41:726—30.

207. Stratton SJ, Brickett K, Crammer T. Prehospital pulseless, unconscious penetrating trauma victims: field assessments associated with survival. J Trauma 1998;45:96—100.

208. Maron BJ, Gohman TE, Kyle SB, Estes III NA, Link MS. Clinical profile and spectrum of commotio cordis. JAMA 2002;287:1142—6.

209. Maron BJ, Estes III NA, Link MS. Task Force 11: commotio cordis. J Am Coll Cardiol 2005;45:1371—3.

210. Nesbitt AD, Cooper PJ, Kohl P. Rediscovering commotio cordis. Lancet 2001;357:1195—7.

211. Link MS, Estes M, Maron BJ. Sudden death caused by chest wall trauma (commotio cordis). In: Kohl P, Sachs F, Franz MR, editors. Cardiac mechano-electric feedback and arrhythmias: from pipette to patient. Philadelphia: Elsevier Saunders; 2005. p. 270—6.

212. Bouillon B, Walther T, Kramer M, Neugebauer E. Trauma and circulatory arrest: 224 preclinical resuscitations in Cologne in 1990 [in German]. Anaesthesist 1994;43:786—90.

213. Fisher B, Worthen M. Cardiac arrest induced by blunt trauma in children. Pediatr Emerg Care 1999;15: 274—6.

214. Hazinski MF, Chahine AA, Holcomb III GW, Morris Jr JA. Outcome of cardiovascular collapse in pediatric blunt trauma. Ann Emerg Med 1994;23:1229—35.

215. Calkins CM, Bensard DD, Partrick DA, Karrer FM. A critical analysis of outcome for children sustaining cardiac arrest after blunt trauma. J Pediatr Surg 2002;37:180—4.

216. Yanagawa Y, Saitoh D, Takasu A, Kaneko N, Sakamoto T, Okada Y. Experience of treatment for blunt traumatic out-of-hospital cardiopulmonary arrest patients over 24 years: head injury vs. non-head injury. No Shinkei Geka 2004;32:231—5.

217. Cera SM, Mostafa G, Sing RF, Sarafin JL, Matthews BD, Heniford BT. Physiologic predictors of survival in post-traumatic arrest. Am Surg 2003;69:140—4.

218. Esposito TJ, Jurkovich GJ, Rice CL, Maier RV, Copass MK, Ashbaugh DG. Reappraisal of emergency room thoracotomy in a changing environment. J Trauma 1991;31:881—5, discussion 5—7.

219. Martin SK, Shatney CH, Sherck JP, et al. Blunt trauma patients with prehospital pulseless electrical activity (PEA): poor ending assured. J Trauma 2002;53:876—80, discussion 80—81.

220. Domeier RM, McSwain Jr NE, Hopson LR, et al. Guidelines for withholding or termination of resuscitation in prehospital traumatic cardiopulmonary arrest. J Am Coll Surg 2003;196:475—81.

221. Pickens JJ, Copass MK, Bulger EM. Trauma patients receiving CPR: predictors of survival. J Trauma 2005;58: 951—8.

222. Gervin AS, Fischer RP. The importance of prompt transport of salvage of patients with penetrating heart wounds. J Trauma 1982;22:443—8.

223. Branney SW, Moore EE, Feldhaus KM, Wolfe RE. Critical analysis of two decades of experience with postinjury emergency department thoracotomy in a regional trauma center. J Trauma 1998;45:87—94, discussion -5.

224. Durham III LA, Richardson RJ, Wall Jr MJ, Pepe PE, Mattox KL. Emergency center thoracotomy: impact of prehospital resuscitation. J Trauma 1992;32:775—9.

225. Frezza EE, Mezghebe H. Is 30 min the golden period to perform emergency room thoratomy (ERT) in penetrating chest injuries? J Cardiovasc Surg 1999;40:147—51.

226. Powell DW, Moore EE, Cothren CC, et al. Is emergency department resuscitative thoracotomy futile care for the critically injured patient requiring prehospital cardiopulmonary resuscitation? J Am Coll Surg 2004;199:211—5.

227. Coats TJ, Keogh S, Clark H, Neal M. Prehospital resuscitative thoracotomy for cardiac arrest after penetrating trauma: rationale and case series. J Trauma 2001;50:670—3.

228. Wise D, Davies G, Coats T, Lockey D, Hyde J, Good A. Emergency thoracotomy: "how to do it". Emerg Med J 2005;22:22—4.

229. Kwan I, Bunn F, Roberts I. Spinal immobilisation for trauma patients. Cochrane Database Syst Rev 2001. CD002803.

230. Voiglio EJ, Coats TJ, Baudoin YP, Davies GD, Wilson AW. Resuscitative transverse thoracotomy. Ann Chir 2003;128:728—33.

231. Practice management guidelines for emergency department thoracotomy. Working Group, Ad Hoc Subcommittee on Outcomes, American College of Surgeons-Committee on Trauma. J Am Coll Surg 2001;193:303—9.

232. Jones JH, Murphy MP, Dickson RL, Somerville GG, Brizendine EJ. Emergency physician-verified out-of-hospital intubation: miss rates by paramedics. Acad Emerg Med 2004;11:707—9.

233. Jemmett ME, Kendal KM, Fourre MW, Burton JH. Unrecognized misplacement of endotracheal tubes in a mixed urban to rural emergency medical services setting. Acad Emerg Med 2003;10:961—5.

234. Katz SH, Falk JL. Misplaced endotracheal tubes by paramedics in an urban emergency medical services system. Ann Emerg Med 2001;37:32—7.

235. Deakin CD, Peters R, Tomlinson P, Cassidy M. Securing the prehospital airway: a comparison of laryngeal mask insertion and endotracheal intubation by UK paramedics. Emerg Med J 2005;22:64—7.

236. Pepe PE, Roppolo LP, Fowler RL. The detrimental effects of ventilation during low-blood-flow states. Curr Opin Crit Care 2005;11:212—8.

237. Deakin CD, Davies G, Wilson A. Simple thoracostomy avoids chest drain insertion in prehospital trauma. J Trauma 1995;39:373—4.

238. Luna GK, Pavlin EG, Kirkman T, Copass MK, Rice CL. Hemodynamic effects of external cardiac massage in trauma shock. J Trauma 1989;29:1430—3.

239. Gao JM, Gao YH, Wei GB, et al. Penetrating cardiac wounds: principles for surgical management. World J Surg 2004;28:1025—9.

240. Kwan I, Bunn F, Roberts I. Timing and volume of fluid administration for patients with bleeding. Cochrane Database Syst Rev 2003. CD002245.

241. Pepe PE, Mosesso VN, Falk JL. Prehospital fluid resuscitation of the patient with major trauma. Prehosp Emerg Care 2002;6:81—91.

242. Bickell WH, Wall Jr MJ, Pepe PE, et al. Immediate versus delayed fluid resuscitation for hypotensive patients with penetrating torso injuries. N Engl J Med 1994;331:1105—9.

243. National Institute for Clinical Excellence. Prehospital initiation of fluid replacement therapy for trauma. London: National Institute for Clinical Excellence; 2004.

244. Sumida MP, Quinn K, Lewis PL, et al. Prehospital blood transfusion versus crystalloid alone in the air medical transport of trauma patients. Air Med J 2000;19:140—3.

245. Barkana Y, Stein M, Maor R, Lynn M, Eldad A. Prehospital blood transfusion in prolonged evacuation. J Trauma 1999;46:176—80.

246. Walcher F, Kortum S, Kirschning T, Weihgold N, Marzi I. Optimized management of polytraumatized patients by prehospital ultrasound. Unfallchirurg 2002;105:986—94.

247. Krismer AC, Wenzel V, Voelckel WG, et al. Employing vasopressin as an adjunct vasopressor in uncontrolled traumatic hemorrhagic shock. Three cases and a brief analysis of the literature. Anaesthesist 2005;54:220—4.

248. Department of Health, Welsh Office, Scottish Office Department of Health, Department of Health and Social Services, Northern Ireland. Why mothers die. Report on confidential enquiries into maternal deaths in the United Kingdom, 2000—2002. London: The Stationery Office; 2004.

249. Page-Rodriguez A, Gonzalez-Sanchez JA. Perimortem cesarean section of twin pregnancy: case report and review of the literature. Acad Emerg Med 1999;6:1072—4.

250. Cardosi RJ, Porter KB. Cesarean delivery of twins during maternal cardiopulmonary arrest. Obstet Gynecol 1998;92:695—7.

251. Kinsella SM. Lateral tilt for pregnant women: why 15 degrees? Anaesthesia 2003;58:835—6.

252. Nanson J, Elcock D, Williams M, Deakin CD. Do physiological changes in pregnancy change defibrillation energy requirements? Br J Anaesth 2001;87:237—9.

253. Johnson MD, Luppi CJ, Over DC. Cardiopulmonary resuscitation. In: Gambling DR, Douglas MJ, editors. Obstetric anesthesia and uncommon disorders. Philadelphia: W.B. Saunders; 1998. p. 51—74.

254. Rahman K, Jenkins JG. Failed tracheal intubation in obstetrics: no more frequent but still managed badly. Anaesthesia 2005;60:168—71.

255. Henderson JJ, Popat MT, Latto IP, Pearce AC. Difficult airway society guidelines for management of the unanticipated difficult intubation. Anaesthesia 2004;59:675—94.

256. Catling S, Joels L. Cell salvage in obstetrics: the time has come. Br J Obstet Gynaecol 2005;112:131—2.

257. Ahonen J, Jokela R. Recombinant factor VIIa for life-threatening post-partum haemorrhage. Br J Anaesth 2005;94:592—5.

258. Bouwmeester FW, Bolte AC, van Geijn HP. Pharmacological and surgical therapy for primary postpartum hemorrhage. Curr Pharm Des 2005;11:759—73.

259. El-Hamamy E, CBL. A worldwide review of the uses of the uterine compression suture techniques as alternative to hysterectomy in the management of severe post-partum haemorrhage. J Obstet Gynaecol 2005;25:143—9.

260. Hong TM, Tseng HS, Lee RC, Wang JH, Chang CY. Uterine artery embolization: an effective treatment for intractable obstetric haemorrhage. Clin Radiol 2004;59:96—101.

261. Yu S, Pennisi JA, Moukhtar M, Friedman EA. Placental abruption in association with advanced abdominal pregnancy. A case report. J Reprod Med 1995;40:731—5.

262. Wlody D. Complications of regional anesthesia in obstetrics. Clin Obstet Gynecol 2003;46:667—78.

263. Ray P, Murphy GJ, Shutt LE. Recognition and management of maternal cardiac disease in pregnancy. Br J Anaesth 2004;93:428—39.

264. Abbas AE, Lester SJ, Connolly H. Pregnancy and the cardiovascular system. Int J Cardiol 2005;98:179—89.

265. Doan-Wiggins L. Resuscitation of the pregnant patient suffering sudden death. In: Paradis NA, Halperin HR, Nowak RM, editors. Cardiac arrest: the science and practice of resuscitation medicine. Baltimore: Williams & Wilkins; 1997. p. 812—9.

266. Sibai B, Dekker G, Kupferminc M. Pre-eclampsia. Lancet 2005;365:785—99.

267. Sibai BM. Diagnosis, prevention, and management of eclampsia. Obstet Gynecol 2005;105:402—10.

268. Dapprich M, Boessenecker W. Fibrinolysis with alteplase in a pregnant woman with stroke. Cerebrovasc Dis 2002;13:290.

269. Turrentine MA, Braems G, Ramirez MM. Use of thrombolytics for the treatment of thromboembolic disease during pregnancy. Obstet Gynecol Surv 1995;50:534—11.

270. Thabut G, Thabut D, Myers RP, et al. Thrombolytic therapy of pulmonary embolism: a meta-analysis. J Am Coll Cardiol 2002;40:1660—7.

271. Patel RK, Fasan O, Arya R. Thrombolysis in pregnancy. Thromb Haemost 2003;90:1216—7.

272. Tuffnell DJ. Amniotic fluid embolism. Curr Opin Obstet Gynecol 2003;15:119—22.

273. Stanten RD, Iverson LI, Daugharty TM, Lovett SM, Terry C, Blumenstock E. Amniotic fluid embolism causing catastrophic pulmonary vasoconstriction: diagnosis by transesophageal echocardiogram and treatment by cardiopulmonary bypass. Obstet Gynecol 2003;102:496—8.

274. Katz VL, Dotters DJ, Droegemueller W. Perimortem cesarean delivery. Obstet Gynecol 1986;68:571—6.

275. Guidelines 2000 for Cardiopulmonary Resuscitation and Emergency Cardiovascular Care: International Consensus on Science. Part 8: advanced challenges in resuscitation. Section 3. Special challenges in ECC. 3F: cardiac arrest associated with pregnancy. Resuscitation 2000;46:293—5.

276. Cummins RO, Hazinski MF, Zelop CM. Chapter 4, Part 6: cardiac arrest associated with pregnancy. In: Cummins R, Hazinski M, Field J, editors. ACLS—the reference textbook. Dallas: American Heart Association; 2003, p. 143—158.

277. Oates S, Williams GL, Rees GA. Cardiopulmonary resuscitation in late pregnancy. BMJ 1988;297:404—5.

278. Strong THJ, Lowe RA. Perimortem cesarean section. Am J Emerg Med 1989;7:489—94.

279. Boyd R, Teece S. Towards evidence based emergency medicine: best BETs from the Manchester Royal Infirmary. Perimortem caesarean section. Emerg Med J 2002;19:324—5.

280. Moore C, Promes SB. Ultrasound in pregnancy. Emerg Med Clin N Am 2004;22:697—722.

281. Budnick LD. Bathtub-related electrocutions in the United States, 1979 to 1982. JAMA 1984;252:918—20.

282. Lightning-associated deaths—United States, 1980—1995. MMWR Morb Mortal Wkly Rep 1998;47:391—4.

283. Geddes LA, Bourland JD, Ford G. The mechanism underlying sudden death from electric shock. Med Instrum 1986;20:303—15.

284. Zafren K, Durrer B, Herry JP, Brugger H. Lightning injuries: prevention and on-site treatment in mountains and remote areas. Official guidelines of the International Commission for Mountain Emergency Medicine and the Medical Commission of the International Mountaineering and Climbing Federation (ICAR and UIAA MEDCOM). Resuscitation 2005;65:369—72.

285. Cherington M. Lightning injuries. Ann Emerg Med 1995;25:517—9.

286. Fahmy FS, Brinsden MD, Smith J, Frame JD. Lightning: the multisystem group injuries. J Trauma 1999;46:937—40.

287. Patten BM. Lightning and electrical injuries. Neurol Clin 1992;10:1047—58.

288. Browne BJ, Gaasch WR. Electrical injuries and lightning. Emerg Med Clin North Am 1992;10:211—29.

289. Kleiner JP, Wilkin JH. Cardiac effects of lightning stroke. JAMA 1978;240:2757—9.

290. Lichtenberg R, Dries D, Ward K, Marshall W, Scanlon P. Cardiovascular effects of lightning strikes. J Am Coll Cardiol 1993;21:531—6.

291. Cooper MA. Emergent care of lightning and electrical injuries. Semin Neurol 1995;15:268—78.

292. Milzman DP, Moskowitz L, Hardel M. Lightning strikes at a mass gathering. S Med J 1999;92:708—10.

293. Cooper MA. Lightning injuries: prognostic signs for death. Ann Emerg Med 1980;9:134—8.

294. Kleinschmidt-DeMasters BK. Neuropathology of lightning strike injuries. Semin Neurol 1995;15:323—8.

295. Stewart CE. When lightning strikes. Emerg Med Serv 2000;29:57—67, quiz 103.

296. Duclos PJ, Sanderson LM. An epidemiological description of lightning-related deaths in the United States. Int J Epidemiol 1990;19:673—9.

297. Epperly TD, Stewart JR. The physical effects of lightning injury. J Fam Pract 1989;29:267—72.

298. Whitcomb D, Martinez JA, Daberkow D. Lightning injuries. S Med J 2002;95:1331—4.

299. Goldman RD, Einarson A, Koren G. Electric shock during pregnancy. Can Fam Physician 2003;49:297—8.

Resuscitation (2005) **67S1**, S171—S180

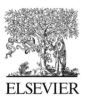

ELSEVIER

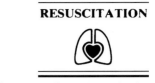

RESUSCITATION

www.elsevier.com/locate/resuscitation

European Resuscitation Council Guidelines for Resuscitation 2005
Section 8. The ethics of resuscitation and end-of-life decisions

Peter J.F. Baskett, Petter A. Steen, Leo Bossaert

Introduction

Successful resuscitation attempts have brought extended, useful and precious life to many, and happiness and relief to their relatives and loved ones. And yet, there are occasions when resuscitation attempts have merely prolonged suffering and the process of dying. In few cases resuscitation has resulted in the ultimate tragedy—the patient in a persistent vegetative state. Resuscitation attempts are unsuccessful in 70—95% of cases and death ultimately is inevitable. All would wish to die with dignity.

Several ethical decisions are required to ensure that the decisions to attempt or withhold cardiopulmonary resuscitation (CPR) are appropriate, and that patients and their loved ones are treated with dignity. These decisions may be influenced by individual, international and local cultural, legal, traditional, religious, social and economic factors.[1—10] Sometimes the decisions can be made in advance, but often they have to be made in a matter of seconds at the time of the emergency. Therefore, it is important that healthcare providers understand the principles involved before they are put in a situation where a resuscitation decision must be made.

This section of the guidelines deals with ethical aspects and decisions, including

- advance directives, sometimes known as living wills;
- when not to start resuscitation attempts;
- when to stop resuscitation attempts;
- decision making by non-physicians;
- when to withdraw treatment from those in a persistent vegetative state following resuscitation;
- decisions about family members or loved ones who wish to be present during resuscitation;
- decisions about research and training on the recently dead;
- the breaking of bad news to relatives and loved ones;
- staff support.

Principles

The four key principles are beneficence, non-maleficence, justice and autonomy.[11]

Beneficence implies that healthcare providers must provide benefit while balancing benefit and risks. Commonly this will involve attempting resuscitation, but on occasion it will mean withholding

doi:10.1016/j.resuscitation.2005.10.005

cardiopulmonary resuscitation (CPR). Beneficence may also include responding to the overall needs of the community, e.g. establishing a programme of public access to defibrillation.

Non maleficence means doing no harm. Resuscitation should not be attempted in futile cases, nor when it is against the patient's wishes (expressed when the individual is in a mentally competent state).

Justice implies a duty to spread benefits and risks equally within a society. If resuscitation is provided, it should be made available to all who will benefit from it within the available resources.

Autonomy relates to patients being able to make informed decisions on their own behalf, rather than being subjected to paternalistic decisions being made for them by the medical or nursing professions. This principle has been introduced particularly during the past 30 years, arising from legislature such as the Helsinki Declaration of Human Rights and its subsequent modifications and amendments.[12] Autonomy requires that the patient is adequately informed, competent, free from undue pressure and that there is consistency in the patient's preferences.

Advance directives

Advance directives have been introduced in many countries, emphasising the importance of patient autonomy. Advance directives are a method of communicating the patient's wishes concerning future care, particularly towards the end of life, and must be expressed while the patient is mentally competent and not under duress. Advance directives are likely to specify limitations concerning terminal care, including the withholding of CPR.

The term advance directive applies to any expression of patient preferences, including mere dialogue between patient and/or close relatives and loved ones and/or medical or nursing attendants. This may help healthcare attendants in assessing the patient's wishes should the patient become mentally incompetent. However, problems can arise. The relative may misinterpret the wishes of the patient, or may have a vested interest in the death (or continued existence) of the patient. Healthcare providers tend to underestimate sick patients' desire to live.

Written directions by the patient, legally administered living wills or powers of attorney may eliminate some of these problems but are not without limitations. The patient should describe as precisely as possible the situation envisaged when life

support should be withheld or discontinued. This may be aided by a medical adviser. For instance, many would prefer not to undergo the indignity of futile CPR in the presence of end-stage multi-organ failure with no reversible cause, but would welcome the attempt at resuscitation should ventricular fibrillation (VF) occur in association with a remediable primary cardiac cause. Patients often change their minds with change in circumstances, and therefore the advanced directive should be as recent as possible and take into account any change of circumstances.

In sudden out-of-hospital cardiac arrest, the attendants usually do not know the patient's situation and wishes, and an advance directive is often not readily available. In these circumstances, resuscitation is begun immediately and questions addressed later. There is no ethical difference in stopping the resuscitation attempt that has started if the healthcare providers are later presented with an advance directive limiting care. The family doctor can provide an invaluable link in these situations.

There is considerable international variation in the medical attitude to written advance directives.[1] In some countries, the written advanced directive is considered to be legally binding and disobedience is considered an assault; in others, the advance directive is flagrantly ignored if the doctor does not agree with the contents. However, in recent years, there has been a growing tendency towards compliance with patient autonomy and a reduction in patronising attitudes by the medical profession.[1]

When to withhold a resuscitation attempt

Whereas patients have a right to refuse treatment, they do not have an automatic right to demand treatment; they cannot insist that resuscitation must be attempted in any circumstance. A doctor is required only to provide treatment that is likely to benefit the patient, and is not required to provide treatment that would be futile. However, it would be wise to seek a second opinion in making this momentous decision, for fear that the doctor's own personal values, or the question of available resources, might influence his or her opinion.[13]

The decision to withhold a resuscitation attempt raises several ethical and moral questions. What constitutes futility? What exactly is being withheld? Who should decide? Who should be consulted? Who should be informed? Is informed consent required?

When should the decision be reviewed? What religious and cultural factors should be taken into consideration?

What constitutes futility?

Futility exists if resuscitation will be of no benefit in terms of prolonging life of acceptable quality. It is problematic that, although predictors for non-survival after attempted resuscitation have been published,[14–17] none has been tested on an independent patient sample with sufficient predictive value, apart from end-stage multi-organ failure with no reversible cause. Furthermore, studies on resuscitation are particularly dependent on system factors such as time to CPR, time to defibrillation, etc. These may be prolonged in any study but not applicable to an individual case.

Inevitably, judgements will have to be made, and there will be grey areas where subjective opinions are required in patients with heart failure and severe respiratory compromise, asphyxia, major trauma, head injury and neurological disease. The age of the patient may feature in the decision but is only a relatively weak independent predictor of outcome[18,19]; however, age is frequently associated with a prevalence of comorbidity, which does have an influence on prognosis. At the other end of the scale, most doctors will err on the side of intervention in children for emotional reasons, even though the overall prognosis is often worse in children than in adults. It is therefore important that clinicians understand the factors which influence resuscitation success.

What exactly should be withheld?

Do not attempt resuscitation (DNAR) means that, in the event of cardiac or respiratory arrest, CPR should not be performed; DNAR means nothing more than that. Other treatment should be continued, particularly pain relief and sedation, as required. Ventilation and oxygen therapy, nutrition, antibiotics, fluid and vasopressors, etc., are continued as indicated, if they are considered to be contributing to the quality of life. If not, orders not to continue or initiate any such treatments should be specified independently of DNAR orders.

DNAR orders for many years in many countries were written by single doctors, often without consulting the patient, relatives or other health personnel, but there are now clear procedural requirements in many countries such as the USA, UK and Norway.

Who should decide not to attempt resuscitation?

This very grave decision is usually made by the senior doctor in charge of the patient after appropriate consultations. Decisions by committee are impractical and have not been shown to work, and hospital management personnel lack the training and experience on which to base a judgement. Decisions by legal authorities are fraught with delays and uncertainties, particularly if there is an adversarial legal system, and should be sought only if there are irreconcilable differences between the parties involved. In especially difficult cases, the senior doctor may wish to consult his or her own medical defence society for a legal opinion.

Medical emergency teams (METs), acting in response to concern about a patient's condition from ward staff, can assist in initiating the decision-making process concerning DNAR (see Section 4a).[20,21]

Who should be consulted?

Although the ultimate decision for DNAR should be made by the senior doctor in charge of the patient, it is wise for this individual to consult others before making the decision. Following the principle of patient autonomy it is prudent, if possible, to ascertain the patient's wishes about a resuscitation attempt. This must be done in advance, when the patient is able to make an informed choice. Opinions vary as to whether such discussions should occur routinely for every hospital admission (which might cause undue alarm in the majority of cases) or only if the diagnosis of a potentially life-threatening condition is made (when there is a danger that the patient may be too ill to make a balanced judgement). In presenting the facts to the patient, the doctor must be as certain as possible of the diagnosis and the prognosis and may seek a second or third medical opinion in this matter. It is vital that the doctor should not allow personal life values to distort the discussion—in matters of acceptability of a certain quality of life, the patient's opinion should prevail.

It is considered essential for the doctor to have discussions with close relatives and loved ones if at all possible. Whereas they may influence the doctor's decision, it should be made clear to them that the ultimate decision will be that of the doctor. It is unfair and unreasonable to place the burden of decision on the relative.

The doctor would also be wise to discuss the matter with the nursing and junior medical personnel, who are often closer to the patient and more likely to be given personal information. The patient's family doctor may have very close and long-term insight into the patient's wishes and the family relationships, based on years of knowledge of the particular situation.

Who should be informed?

Once the decision has been made it must be communicated clearly to all who may be involved, including patient and relatives. The decision and the reasons for it, and a record of who has been involved in the discussions should be written down, ideally on a special DNAR form that should be placed in a place of prominence in the patient's notes, and should be recorded in the nursing records. Sadly, there is evidence of a reluctance to commit such decisions to writing by doctors in some centres in some countries.[22]

When to abandon the resuscitation attempt

The vast majority of resuscitation attempts do not succeed and have to be abandoned. Several factors will influence the decision to stop the resuscitative effort. These will include the medical history and anticipated prognosis, the period between cardiac arrest and start of CPR, the interval to defibrillation and the period of advanced life support (ALS) with continuing asystole and no reversible cause.

In many cases, particularly in out-of-hospital cardiac arrest, the underlying cause of arrest may be unknown or merely surmised, and the decision is made to start resuscitation while further information is gathered. If it becomes clear that the underlying cause renders the situation to be futile, then resuscitation should be abandoned if the patient remains in asystole with all ALS measures in place. Additional information (such as an advance directive) may become available and may render discontinuation of the resuscitation attempt ethically correct.

In general, resuscitation should be continued as long as VF persists. It is generally accepted that ongoing asystole for more than 20 min in the absence of a reversible cause, and with all ALS measures in place, constitutes grounds for abandoning the resuscitation attempt.[23] There are, of course, reports of exceptional cases that prove the general rule, and each case must be assessed individually.

In out-of-hospital cardiac arrest of cardiac origin, if recovery is going to occur, a return of spontaneous circulation usually takes place on site. Patients with primary cardiac arrest, who require ongoing CPR without any return of a pulse during transport to hospital, rarely survive neurologically intact.[24]

Many will persist with the resuscitation attempt for longer if the patient is a child. This decision is not generally justified on scientific grounds, for the prognosis after cardiac arrest in children is certainly no better, and probably worse, than in adults. Nevertheless, the decision to persist in the distressing circumstances of the death of a child is quite understandable, and the potential enhanced recruitment of cerebral cells in children after an ischaemic insult is an as yet unknown factor to be reckoned with.

The decision to abandon the resuscitation attempt is made by the team leader, but after consultation with the other team members, who may have valid points to contribute. Ultimately, the decision is based on the clinical judgement that the patient's arrest is unresponsive to ALS. The final conclusion should be reached by the team leader taking all facts and views into consideration and dealing sympathetically, but firmly, with any dissenter.

When considering abandoning the resuscitation attempt, a factor that may need to be taken into account is the possibility of prolonging CPR and other resuscitative measures to enable organ donation to take place. Mechanical chest compressions may be valuable in these circumstances,[25] but this has not been studied. The issue of initiating life-prolonging treatment with the sole purpose of harvesting organs is debated by ethicists, and there is variation between the different countries of Europe as to the ethics of this process; at present no consensus exists.

Decision-making by non-physicians

Many cases of out-of-hospital cardiac arrest are attended by emergency medical technicians or paramedics, who face similar dilemmas of when to determine if resuscitation is futile and when it should be abandoned. In general, resuscitation is started in out-of-hospital cardiac arrest unless there is a valid advanced directive to the contrary or it is clear that resuscitation would be futile in cases of a mortal injury, such as decapitation, hemicorporectomy, known prolonged submersion, incineration, rigor mortis, dependent lividity and fetal maceration. In such cases, the non-physician is making a diagnosis of death but is not certifying death (which can be done only by a physician in most countries).

But what of the decision to abandon a resuscitation attempt? Should paramedics trained in ALS be able to declare death after 20 min of asystole in the absence of reversible causes, bearing in mind the very negative results achieved with ongoing CPR during transport? Opinions vary from country to country.[26] In some countries it is routine, and it is surely unreasonable to expect paramedics to continue with resuscitation in the precise circumstances where it would be abandoned by a doctor. In making this recommendation, it is essential that times are recorded very accurately and written guidelines provided.[27] The answer would appear to lie in superior training and thereafter confidence in those who have been trained to make the decision.

Similar decisions and a diagnosis of death may have to be made by nurses in nursing homes for the aged and terminally ill without a resident doctor. It is to be hoped that a decision on the merits of a resuscitation attempt will have been made previously, and the matter of DNAR should always be addressed for all patients in these establishments.

Mitigating circumstances

Certain circumstances, for example hypothermia at the time of cardiac arrest, will enhance the chances of recovery without neurological damage, and the normal prognostic criteria (such as asystole persisting for more than 20 min) are not applicable. Furthermore, sedative and analgesic drugs may obscure the assessment of the level of consciousness in the patient who has a return of spontaneous circulation.

Withdrawal of treatment after a resuscitation attempt

Prediction of the final neurological outcome in patients remaining comatose after regaining a spontaneous circulation is difficult during the first 3 days (see Section 4g). There are no specific clinical signs that can predict outcome in the first few hours after the return of a spontaneous circulation. Use of therapeutic hypothermia after cardiac arrest makes attempts at predicting neurological outcome even more difficult.

In a very small number of distressing cases, patients regain spontaneous circulation but remain in persistent vegetative state (PVS). Continued existence in this state may not be in the patient's best interest compared with the alternative of dying. If remaining alive but in PVS is considered not to be in the patient's best interests, consideration must be given to the potential withdrawal of food and fluids to terminate life. These are profoundly difficult decisions, but generally there is agreement between relatives and the doctors and nurses on the correct course of action. In these cases, decisions can often be made without the need for legal intervention. Difficulties arise if there is a disagreement between the doctors and nurses and the relatives, or between the relatives. In Europe, although there also may be extreme views, it seems that the majority are content to leave the decision to the family and physicians in private.

Family presence during resuscitation

The concept of a family member being present during the resuscitation process was introduced in the 1980s[28] and has become accepted practice in many European countries.[29-38] Many relatives would like to be present during resuscitation attempts and, of those who have had this experience, over 90% would wish to do it again.[33] Most parents would wish to be with their child at this time.[39]

Relatives have considered several benefits from being permitted to be present during a resuscitation attempt, including

- help in coming to terms with the reality of death and easing the bereavement process;
- being able to communicate with, and touch, their loved one in their final moments while they were still warm. Many feel that their loved one appreciated their presence at that moment, and this may be quite possible if consciousness returns during effective CPR (as has been recorded particularly with mechanical CPR on occasions);
- feeling that they had been present during the final moments and that they had been a support to their loved one when needed;
- feeling that they had been there to see that everything that could be done, was done.

Several measures are required to ensure that the experience of the relative is the best under the circumstances.

- The resuscitation should be seen to be conducted competently, under good team leadership, with an open and welcoming attitude to relatives.
- Brief the relatives, in terms that they can understand, before entering; and ensure that continual support is provided by a member of staff (usually a nurse) trained in this subject. Ensure

that relatives understand that the choice to be present is entirely theirs, and do not provoke feelings of guilt, whatever their decision.

- Make the relatives aware of the procedures they are likely to see (e.g., tracheal intubation, insertion of central venous catheters) and the patient's response (e.g., convulsive movements after defibrillation). Emphasise the importance of not interfering with any procedures and explain clearly the dangers of doing so.
- In the majority, of cases it will be necessary to explain that the patient has not responded to the resuscitation attempt and that the attempt has to be abandoned. This decision should be made by the team leader, involving the members of the team. Explain to the relatives that there may be a brief interval while equipment is removed, and that then they will be able to return to be with their loved one at their leisure, alone or supported, as they wish. Certain tubes and cannulae may have to be left in place for medicolegal reasons.
- Finally, there should be an opportunity for the relative to reflect, ask questions about the cause and the process, and be given advice about the procedure for registering the death and the support services available.

In the event of an out-of-hospital arrest, the relatives may already be present, and possibly performing basic life support (BLS). Offer them the option to stay; they may appreciate the opportunity to help and travel in the ambulance to hospital. If death is pronounced at the scene, offer the relatives the help and support of their family doctor or community nurse and bereavement councillor.

For resuscitation staff, both in and out hospital, it is worth offering training in the matter of relatives being present.[40]

With increasing experience of family presence during resuscitation attempts, it is clear that problems rarely, if ever, arise. In the majority of instances, relatives come in and stay for just a few minutes and then leave, satisfied that they have taken the opportunity to be there to support their loved one and say goodbye as they would have wished. Ten years ago most staff would not have countenanced the presence of relatives during resuscitation, but a recent survey has shown an increasingly open attitude and appreciation of the autonomy of both patient and relatives.[1] Perhaps this is related to a generally more permissive and less autocratic attitude. International cultural and social variations still exist, and must be understood and appreciated with sensitivity.

Training and research on the recently dead

Another matter that has raised considerable debate is the ethics, and in some cases the legality, of undertaking training and/or research on the recently dead.

Training

The management of resuscitation can be taught using scenarios with manikins and modern simulators, but training in certain skills required during resuscitation is notoriously difficult. External chest compressions and, to an extent, expired air ventilation and insertion of oropharyngeal and nasopharyngeal airways can be taught using manikins; but despite technological advances in manikins and simulators, many other skills that are needed on a regular basis during resuscitation can be acquired satisfactorily only through practice on humans, dead or alive. These other skills include, for example, central and peripheral venous access, arterial puncture and cannulation, venous cut-down, bag-mask ventilation, tracheal intubation, cricothyroidotomy, needle thoracostomy, chest drainage and open-chest cardiac massage. Some of these skills may be practised during routine clinical work, mostly involving anaesthesia, and to a lesser degree surgery; but others such as cricothyroidotomy, needle thoracostomy and open chest cardiac massage cannot, and are needed only in a life-threatening emergency when it is difficult to justify a teaching exercise. In modern day practice, with practitioners being called increasingly to account and patient autonomy prevailing, it is becoming more and more difficult to obtain permission for student practice of skills in the living. Gone are the days when admission to a 'teaching hospital' implied automatic consent for students to practise procedures on patients under supervision as they wished. And yet the public expect, and are entitled to, competent practitioners for generation after generation.

So the question arises as to whether it is ethically and morally appropriate to undertake training and practice on the living or the dead. There is a wide diversity of opinion on this matter.[41] Many, particularly those in the Islamic nations, find the concept of any skills training and practice on the recently dead completely abhorrent because of an innate respect for the dead body. Others will accept the practice of non-invasive procedures that do not leave a mark, such as tracheal intubation; and some are open and frank enough to accept that any procedure may be learned on the dead body with the justification that the learning of skills is paramount for the well-being of future patients.

One option is to request informed consent for the procedure from the relative of the deceased. However, only some will obtain permission,[1,40] and many find this very difficult to do in the harrowing circumstances of breaking bad news simultaneously to the recently bereaved. As a result, frequently only non-invasive procedures are practised, on the basis that what is not seen will not cause distress. The days of undertaking any procedure without consent are rapidly coming to an end, and perhaps it is now becoming increasingly necessary to mount a publicity campaign to exhort the living to give permission for training on their dead body through an advance directive, in much the same way as permission for transplant of organs may be given. It may be that an 'opt-out' rather than an 'opt-in' arrangement may be adopted, but this will require changes in the law in most countries. It is advised that healthcare professionals learn local and hospital policies regarding this issue and follow the established policy.

Research

There are important ethical issues relating to undertaking randomized clinical trials for patients in cardiac arrest who cannot give informed consent to participate in research studies. Progress in improving the dismal rates of successful resuscitation will only come through the advancement of science through clinical studies. The utilitarian concept in ethics looks to the greatest good for the greatest number of people. This must be balanced with respect for patient autonomy, according to which patients should not be enrolled in research studies without their informed consent. Over the past decade, legal directives have been introduced into the USA and the European Union[42,43] that place significant barriers to research on patients during resuscitation without informed consent from the patient or immediate relative.[44] There are data showing that such regulations deter research progress in resuscitation.[45] It is indeed possible that these directives may in themselves conflict with the basic human right to good medical treatment as set down in the Helsinki Agreement.[12] Research in resuscitation emanating from the USA has fallen dramatically in the last decade,[46] and it appears very likely that the European Union will follow suit as the rules bite there.[47] The US authorities have, to a very limited extent, sought to introduce methods of exemption,[42] but these are still associated with problems and almost insurmountable difficulties.[45]

Research on the recently dead is likely to encounter similar restrictions unless previous permission is granted as part of an advance directive by the patient, or permission can be given immediately by the relative who is next of kin. Legal ownership of the recently dead is established only in a few countries, but in many countries it is at least tacitly agreed that the body 'belongs' to the relatives (unless there are suspicious circumstances or the cause of death is unknown), and permission for any research must be granted by the next of kin unless there is an advance directive giving consent. Obtaining consent from relatives in the stressful circumstances of immediate bereavement is unenviable and potentially damaging to the relationship between doctor and relative.

Research can still be carried out during post-mortem examination, for instance to study the traumatic damage resulting from the use of specific methods of chest compression, but all body parts must be returned to the patient unless specific permission is obtained from relatives to do otherwise.

Breaking bad news and bereavement counselling

Breaking news of the death of a patient to a relative is an unenviable task. It is a moment that the relative will remember for ever, so it is very important to do it as correctly and sensitively as possible. It also places a considerable stress on the healthcare provider who has this difficult duty. Both may need support in the ensuing hours and days. It is salutary that the breaking of bad news is seldom taught in medical school or at postgraduate level.[1]

Contacting the family in the case of death without the relatives being present

If the relatives are not present when the patient dies, they must be contacted as soon as possible. The caller may not be known to the relative and must take great care to ensure that his or her identity is made quite clear to the relative and, in turn, the caller must make sure of the relationship of the call recipient to the deceased. In many cases it is not stated on the telephone that the patient has actually died, unless the distance and travel time are prolonged (e.g., the relative is in another country). Many find that it is better to say that the patient is seriously and critically ill or injured and that the relatives should come to hospital immediately, so that a full explanation can be given face to face. It is wise to request that relatives to ask a friend to drive them to hospital, and to state that nothing will be gained by driving at speed. When the relatives arrive they should be greeted right away by a competent and knowledgeable member of staff, and the situation explained immediately. Delays in being told the facts are agonising.

Who should break the bad news to the relative?

Gone are the days when it was acceptable for the patronising senior doctor to delegate the breaking of bad news to a junior assistant. Nowadays, it is generally agreed that it is the duty of the senior doctor or the team leader to talk to the relatives. Nevertheless, it is wise to be accompanied by an experienced nurse who may be a great comfort for the patient (and indeed the doctor).

Where and how should bad news be given?

The environment where bad news is given is vitally important. There should be a room set aside for relatives of the seriously ill that is tastefully and comfortably furnished, with free access to a telephone, television and fresh flowers daily (which may be provided by the florist who runs the flower shop that is in most hospitals in Europe).

There are some basic principles to be followed when breaking bad news, that should be adhered to if grave errors are to be avoided and the relative is not to be discomforted. It is essential to know the facts of the case and to make quite sure to whom who you are talking. Body language is vital; always sit at the same level as the patient and relative; do not stand up when they are sitting down. Make sure you are cleanly dressed; wearing blood-stained clothing is not good. Do not give the impression that you are busy and in a hurry. Give the news they are anxious to hear immediately, using the words "dead" or "has died", "I am very sorry to have to tell you that your father/husband/son has died". Do not leave any room for doubt by using such phrases as "passed on" or left us" or "gone up above".

Discussing the medical details comprehensively at this stage is not helpful; wait until they are asked for. Touching may be appropriate, such as holding hands or placing an arm on the shoulder, but people and customs vary and the doctor needs to be aware of these. Do not be ashamed if you shed a tear yourself. Allow time for the news to be assimilated by the relative. Reactions may vary, including

- relief ("I am so glad his suffering is over," or "He went suddenly—that is what he would have wished");
- anger with the patient ("I told him to stop smoking," or "He was too fat to play squash," or "Look at the mess he has left me in");
- self-guilt ("If only I had not argued with him this morning before he left for work," or "Why did I not tell the doctor he got chest pain?");
- anger with the medical system ("Why did the ambulance take so long?" or "The doctor was far too young and did not know what he/she was doing");
- uncontrollable wailing and crying and anguish;
- complete expressionless catatonia.

It may be useful to reassure the family that they did everything correctly, such as calling for help and getting to the hospital but, in the vast majority of cases, healthcare providers are unable to restart the heart.

Some time may elapse before conversation can resume and, at this stage, ask relatives if they have any questions about the medical condition and the treatment given. It is wise to be completely open and honest about this, but always say "He did not suffer".

In the majority of cases the relative will wish to see the body. It is important that the body and bedclothes are clean and all tubes and cannulae are removed, unless these are needed for post-mortem examination. The image of the body will leave an impression on the relative that will last for ever. A post-mortem examination may be required, and this should requested with tact and sensitivity, explaining that the procedure will be carried out by a professional pathologist and will help to determine the precise cause of death.

Children

Breaking bad news to children may be perceived to present a special problem, but experience seems to indicate that it is better to be quite open and honest with them, so helping to dispel the nightmarish fantasies that children may concoct about death. It is helpful to contact the school, so that the teachers and fellow pupils can be prepared to receive the child back into the school environment with support and sensitivity.

Closure

In many cases this will be the relative's first experience of death, and help should be offered with the bewildering administration of the official registration of death, funeral arrangements and socioeconomic support by the hospital or community social worker. Depending on religious beliefs, the hospital padre or priest may have a vital role to play. Whenever possible, family physicians should be informed immediately by telephone or e-mail with the essential details of the case, so that they can give full support to the relatives. A follow-up telephone call to the relative a day or two later from a member of the hospital staff who was involved, offering to be of help and to answer any questions that the relative may have forgotten about at the time, is always appreciated.

Staff debrief

Although many members of staff seem, and often are, little affected by death in the course of their work, this should not be assumed. Their sense of accomplishment and job satisfaction may be affected adversely, and there may be feelings of guilt, inadequacy and failure. This may be particularly apparent in, but not restricted to, very junior members of staff. A team debrief of the event using positive and constructive critique techniques should be conducted and personal bereavement counselling offered to those with a particular need. How this is done will vary with the individual and will range from an informal chat in the pub or cafe (which seems to deal effectively with many cases) to professional counselling. It should be explained that distress after a death at work may be a normal reaction to an abnormal situation.

Conclusions

Resuscitation has given many a new lease of life, to the delight of themselves and their relatives, but has the potential to bring misery to a few. This chapter addresses how that misery can be reduced by not attempting resuscitation in inappropriate circumstances or in cases with a valid advanced directive, and when to discontinue the resuscitation attempt in cases of futility or PVS.

Ethical issues such as training and research on the recently dead, and the presence of family members during the resuscitation attempt, place further burdens on the medical profession but must be dealt with sympathetically, and with an appreciation of growing patient autonomy and human rights throughout the world.

Finally, the breaking of bad news is one of the most difficult tasks to be faced by the medical and nursing professions. It requires time, training, compassion and understanding.

References

1. Baskett PJ, Lim A. The varying ethical attitudes towards resuscitation in Europe. Resuscitation 2004;62:267—73.
2. Sprung CL, Cohen SL, Sjokvist P, et al. End-of-life practices in European intensive care units: the Ethicus Study. JAMA 2003;290:790—7.
3. Richter J, Eisemann MR, Bauer B, Kreibeck H, Astrom S. Decision-making in the treatment of elderly people: a cross-cultural comparison between Swedish and German physicians and nurses. Scand J Caring Sci 2002;16:149—56.
4. da Costa DE, Ghazal H, Al Khusaiby S. Do not resuscitate orders and ethical decisions in a neonatal intensive care unit in a Muslim community. Arch Dis Child Fetal Neonatal Ed 2002;86:F115—9.
5. Ho NK. Decision-making: initiation and withdrawing life support in the asphyxiated infants in developing countries. Singapore Med J 2001;42:402—5.
6. Richter J, Eisemann M, Zgonnikova E. Doctors' authoritarianism in end-of-life treatment decisions. A comparison between Russia, Sweden and Germany. J Med Ethics 2001;27:186—91.
7. Cuttini M, Nadai M, Kaminski M, et al. End-of-life decisions in neonatal intensive care: physicians' self-reported practices in seven European countries. EURONIC Study Group. Lancet 2000;355:2112—8.
8. Konishi E. Nurses' attitudes towards developing a do not resuscitate policy in Japan. Nurs Ethics 1998;5:218—27.
9. Muller JH, Desmond B. Ethical dilemmas in a cross-cultural context. A Chinese example. West J Med 1992;157:323—7.
10. Edgren E. The ethics of resuscitation; differences between Europe and the USA-Europe should not adopt American guidelines without debate. Resuscitation 1992;23:85—9.
11. Beauchamp TL, Childress J, editors. Principles of biomedical ethics. 3rd ed. Oxford: Oxford University Press; 1994.
12. Declaration of Helsinki. Ethical principles for medical research involving human subjects adopted by the 18th WMA General Assembly, Helsinki, Finland, June 1964 and amended at the 29th, 35th, 41st, 48th, and 52nd WMA Assemblies. Geneva, 1964.
13. Aasland OG, Forde R, Steen PA. Medical end-of-life decisions in Norway. Resuscitation 2003;57:312—3.
14. Danciu SC, Klein L, Hosseini MM, Ibrahim L, Coyle BW, Kehoe RF. A predictive model for survival after in-hospital cardiopulmonary arrest. Resuscitation 2004;62:35—42.
15. Dautzenberg PL, Broekman TC, Hooyer C, Schonwetter RS, Duursma SA. Review: patient-related predictors of cardiopulmonary resuscitation of hospitalized patients. Age Ageing 1993;22:464—75.
16. Haukoos JS, Lewis RJ, Niemann JT. Prediction rules for estimating neurologic outcome following out-of-hospital cardiac arrest. Resuscitation 2004;63:145—55.
17. Herlitz J, Engdahl J, Svensson L, Young M, Angquist KA, Holmberg S. Can we define patients with no chance of survival after out-of-hospital cardiac arrest? Heart 2004;90:1114—8.
18. Herlitz J, Engdahl J, Svensson L, Angquist KA, Young M, Holmberg S. Factors associated with an increased chance of survival among patients suffering from an out-of-hospital cardiac arrest in a national perspective in Sweden. Am Heart J 2005;149:61—6.
19. Ebell MH. Prearrest predictors of survival following in-hospital cardiopulmonary resuscitation: a meta-analysis. J Fam Pract 1992;34:551—8.
20. Hillman K, Parr M, Flabouris A, Bishop G, Stewart A. Redefining in-hospital resuscitation: the concept of the medical emergency team. Resuscitation 2001;48:105—10.

21. The MERIT study investigators. Introduction of the medical emergency team (MET) system: a cluster-randomised controlled trial. Lancet 2005;365:2091—7.

22. Sovik O, Naess AC. Incidence and content of written guidelines for "do not resuscitate" orders. Survey at six different somatic hospitals in Oslo. Tidsskr Nor Laegeforen 1997;117:4206—9.

23. Bonnin MJ, Pepe PE, Kimball KT, Clark Jr PS. Distinct criteria for termination of resuscitation in the out-of-hospital setting. JAMA 1993;270:1457—62.

24. Kellermann AL, Hackman BB, Somes G. Predicting the outcome of unsuccessful prehospital advanced cardiac life support. JAMA 1993;270:1433—6.

25. Steen S, Liao Q, Pierre L, Paskevicius A, Sjoberg T. Evaluation of LUCAS, a new device for automatic mechanical compression and active decompression resuscitation. Resuscitation 2002;55:285—99.

26. Naess A, Steen E, Steen P. Ethics in treatment decisions during out-of-hospital resuscitation. Resuscitation 1997;35:245—56.

27. Joint Royal Colleges Ambulance Liaison Committee. Newsletter 1996 and 2001. Royal College of Physicians: London.

28. Doyle CJ, Post H, Burney RE, Maino J, Keefe M, Rhee KJ. Family participation during resuscitation: an option. Ann Emerg Med 1987;16:673—5.

29. Adams S, Whitlock M, Higgs R, Bloomfield P, Baskett PJ. Should relatives be allowed to watch resuscitation? BMJ 1994;308:1687—92.

30. Hanson C, Strawser D. Family presence during cardiopulmonary resuscitation: Foote Hospital emergency department's nine-year perspective. J Emerg Nurs 1992;18:104—6.

31. Cooke MW. I desperately needed to see my son. BMJ 1991;302:1023.

32. Gregory CM. I should have been with Lisa as she died. Accid Emerg Nurs 1995;3:136—8.

33. Boie ET, Moore GP, Brummett C, Nelson DR. Do parents want to be present during invasive procedures performed on their children in the emergency department? A survey of 400 parents. Ann Emerg Med 1999;34:70—4.

34. Boudreaux ED, Francis JL, Loyacano T. Family presence during invasive procedures and resuscitations in the emergency department: a critical review and suggestions for future research. Ann Emerg Med 2002;40:193—205.

35. Martin J. Rethinking traditional thoughts. J Emerg Nurs 1991;17:67—8.

36. Robinson SM, Mackenzie-Ross S, Campbell Hewson GL, Egleston CV, Prevost AT. Psychological effect of witnessed resuscitation on bereaved relatives. Lancet 1998;352:614—7 [comment].

37. Baskett PJF. The ethics of resuscitation. In: Colquhoun MC, Handley AJ, Evans TR, editors. The ABC of resuscitation. 5th ed. London: BMJ Publishing Group; 2004.

38. Azoulay E, Sprung CL. Family-physician interactions in the intensive care unit. Crit Care Med 2004;32:2323—8.

39. Bouchner H, Vinci R, Waring C. Pediatric procedures: do parents want to watch? Pediatrics 1989;84:907—9.

40. Resuscitation Council (UK) Project Team. Should relatives witness resuscitation? London, UK: Resuscitation Council; 1996.

41. Morag RM, DeSouza S, Steen PA, et al. Performing procedures on the newly deceased for teaching purposes: what if we were to ask? Arch Intern Med 2005;165:92—6.

42. US Department of Health and Human Services. Protection of human subjects: informed consent and waiver of informed consent requirements in certain emergency circumstances. In: 61 Federal Register 51528 (1996) codified at CFR #50.24 and #46.408; 1996.

43. Fontaine N, Rosengren B. Directive/20/EC of the European Parliament and Council of 4th April 2001 on the approximation of the laws, regulations and administrative provisions of the Member States relating to the implementation of good clinical practice in the conduct of trials on medical products for human use. Off J Eur Commun 2001;121:34—44.

44. Lemaire F, Bion J, Blanco J, et al. The European Union Directive on Clinical Research: present status of implementation in EU member states' legislations with regard to the incompetent patient. Intensive Care Med 2005;31:476—9.

45. Nichol G, Huszti E, Rokosh J, Dumbrell A, McGowan J, Becker L. Impact of informed consent requirements on cardiac arrest research in the United States: exception from consent or from research? Resuscitation 2004;62:3—23.

46. Mosesso Jr VN, Brown LH, Greene HL, et al. Conducting research using the emergency exception from informed consent: the public access defibrillation (PAD) trial experience. Resuscitation 2004;61:29—36.

47. Sterz F, Singer EA, Bottiger B, et al. A serious threat to evidence based resuscitation within the European Union. Resuscitation 2002;53:237—8.

Resuscitation (2005) **67S1**, S181—S189

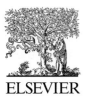

RESUSCITATION

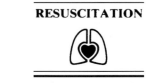

ELSEVIER

www.elsevier.com/locate/resuscitation

European Resuscitation Council Guidelines for Resuscitation 2005
Section 9. Principles of training in resuscitation

Peter J. F. Baskett, Jerry P. Nolan, Anthony Handley, Jasmeet Soar, Dominique Biarent, Sam Richmond

Introduction

There are a variety of methods used for training in resuscitation. None are perfect and, in the absence of frequent practice, retention of knowledge and skills is suboptimal. The optimal interval for retraining has not been established, but repeated refresher training at intervals of less than 6 months seems to be needed for most individuals who are not undertaking resuscitation on a regular basis.[1—12]

Objectives

The objective of training is to equip the learner with the ability to be able to undertake resuscitation in a real clinical situation at the level at which they would be expected to perform, be they be lay bystander, first responder in the community or hospital, a healthcare professional working in an acute area, or a member of the medical emergency or cardiac arrest response team.

Methods

Training should follow the principles of adult education and learning. Generally this will mean an established European Resuscitation Council (ERC) course with small-group (four to eight members) participation using interactive discussion and hands-on practice for skills and clinical scenarios for problem-solving and team leadership.[13] The ratio of instructors to candidates should range from 1:3 to 1:6, depending on the type of course.

Core knowledge should be acquired by candidates before the course by study of the course manual or an interactive CD designed for the purpose. The course should aim to produce an improvement in competence in the learner, and there should be a test of core knowledge and an ongoing assessment of practical skills and scenario management. Sophisticated manikins, simulators and virtual reality techniques may be incorporated into the scenario-based training.[14]

For basic life support (BLS) by lay people or first responders, home-based learning using a video or interactive CD with a simple manikin may offer a valuable alternative to traditional instructor-based courses.[15—19] This method minimises candidate disruption and instructor time and finances. However, the role of the instructor should not be underestimated and, in addition to explaining situations that were unforeseen on the original video or CD, the instructor can act as a role model and provide invaluable enthusiasm and motivation.

0300-9572/$ — see front matter © 2005 European Resuscitation Council. All Rights Reserved. Published by Elsevier Ireland Ltd.
doi:10.1016/j.resuscitation.2005.10.006

Group participation has also been demonstrated to enhance the overall learning process.

Ethos

The course should be taught by trained instructors who have undertaken the relevant specific ERC course in teaching and assessment. Teaching should be conducted by encouragement with constructive feedback on performance rather than humiliation. First names are encouraged among both faculty and candidates to reduce apprehension, and the mentor/mentee system is used to enhance feedback and support for the candidate. Stress is inevitable,[20] particularly during assessment, but the aim of the instructors is to enable the candidates to do their best.

Language

Initially, the ERC courses were taught in English by an international faculty.[13] As local instructors have been trained, and manuals and course materials have been translated into different languages, the courses, particularly the provider courses, are now taught increasingly in the candidates' native language.

Instructors

A tried and tested method has evolved for identifying and training instructors.

Identification of instructor potentials

Instructors will be individuals who, in the opinion of the faculty, have demonstrated good competence in the subjects at a provider course and, importantly, have shown qualities of leadership and clinical credibility and skills that involve being articulate, supportive and motivated. These individuals will be invited to take part in an instructor course called the Generic Instructor Course (GIC) in the case of Advanced Life Support (ALS) and European Paediatric Life Support (EPLS) courses, or Basic Life Support (BLS)/Automated External Defibrillation (AED) Instructor Course in the BLS and AED courses. An instructor course for Immediate Life Support (ILS) is under development.

The instructor courses

These are conducted for instructor potentials (IPs) by experienced instructors and, in the case of the GIC, include an educator who has undertaken specific training in medical educational practice and the principles of adult learning. Details of these instructor courses are given below. There are no formal tests for candidates during the course, but assessment is done by the faculty and feedback is given as appropriate.

Instructor candidate stage

Following successful completion of an instructor course, the individual is designated as an instructor candidate (IC), normally taught on two separate courses under supervision, and is given constructive feedback on performance. After experience of two courses, the IC normally progresses to full instructor status, but occasionally the faculty decides that a further course is required or, rarely, that the candidate is not suitable to progress to be an instructor. An appeal can be lodged with the relevant International Course Committee, which makes the final decision.

Course director status

Selected individuals may progress to the status of the course director. They will be selected by their peers and approved by the relevant committee of the National Resuscitation Council or the relevant International Course Committee. Course directors must be relatively senior individuals with considerable clinical credibility, good judgement and impeccable powers of assessment and fairness. They will have embraced the educational principles inherent in the instructor course. Normally, individuals will have had experience of teaching on at least six courses and will have been appointed course codirector on at least one occasion.

Interchange of instructors

Interchange between instructors of different disciplines is possible. For instance, an ALS instructor may proceed directly to be an IC on an EPLS course, provided that he or she has passed the EPLS course and has been identified as an IP and vice versa. There is no need to repeat the GIC. Similarly, current instructors in the Advanced Trauma Life Support (ATLS) Course of the American College of Surgeons, having been identified as an IP in the relevant provider course, may proceed directly to being an IC in ALS or EPLS. Current American Heart Association Advanced Cardiac Life Support (ACLS) or Paediatric Advanced Life Support (PALS) instructors may proceed directly to IC status in the relevant course.

Code of conduct

All instructors must adhere to the code of conduct for the instructors, which is set out in Appendix A.

The Basic Life Support (BLS) and Automated External Defibrillator (AED) courses

BLS and AED courses are appropriate for a wide range of providers. These may include clinical and non-clinical healthcare professionals (particularly those who are less likely to be faced with having to manage a cardiac arrest), general practitioners, dentists, medical students, first-aid workers, lifeguards, those with a duty of care for others (such as school teachers and care workers), and members of first-responder schemes, as well as members of the general public.

Provider course format

The aim of these provider courses is to enable each candidate to gain competency in BLS or the use of AED. Details of appropriate competencies have been published by the ERC BLS Working Group and may be found on http://www.erc.edu. BLS and AED courses are developed and managed by the ERC International BLS Course Committee (ICC).

Each BLS or AED provider course lasts approximately half a day and consists of skill demonstrations and hands-on practice, with a minimum number of lectures. The recommended ratio of instructors to candidates is 1:6, with at least one manikin and one AED for each group of six candidates. Formal assessment is not usually undertaken, but each candidate receives individual feedback on performance. Those who need a certificate of competency for professional or personal use may be assessed continuously during the course or definitively at the end.

BLS provider and AED provider manuals, together with certificates, may be purchased from the ERC. Approved alternative manuals, translated if necessary into the local language, may also be used.

Instructor course

Many of the candidates attending a BLS or AED provider course are lay people, and some subsequently want to become instructors themselves. For this reason, the ERC has developed a 1-day BLS/AED instructor course. Candidates for this course must be healthcare professionals, or lay people who hold the ERC BLS or AED provider certificate and are des-ignated as IP. The aim is to be as inclusive as possible regarding the course attendance, the over-riding criterion being that all candidates should have the potential and knowledge to teach the subject.

The BLS/AED instructor course follows the principles of the GIC, with an emphasis on teaching lay people. Following successful completion of the course, each candidate becomes an IC and teaches two BLS or AED courses before becoming a full instructor.

Introducing courses into a country

Many ERC BLS and AED provider courses are run by, or under the control of, the National Resuscitation Council. The normal procedure for introducing ERC BLS/AED courses into a country is that ERC international instructors visit that country to run a 2-day combined BLS provider, AED provider and BLS/AED instructor course. If there are local instructors (e.g., those who have passed an ERC course successfully, or who are ERC ALS instructors), they teach on the course in a 1:1 ratio of international to local instructor, with the course director (an international instructor) as an additional person who can support local instructors. After a successful course the local instructors become full ERC instructors, and the outstanding local instructors are selected to become instructor trainers. Subsequent courses are normally held in the language of the country concerned, and training materials are translated into that language. The candidates who are on the combined course qualify, hopefully, as ERC BLS/AED ICs. They then need to teach on one or two provider courses, under the supervision of full instructors, before becoming full instructors themselves.

The Immediate Life Support (ILS) course

The ILS course is for the majority of healthcare professionals who attend cardiac arrests rarely but have the potential to be first responders or cardiac-arrest team members.[21] The course teaches the healthcare professionals the skills that are most likely to result in successful resuscitation while awaiting the arrival of the resuscitation team.[22] Importantly, the ILS course also includes a section on preventing cardiac arrest, and complements other short courses that focus on managing sick patients in the first 24 h of critical illness when critical care expertise is not immediately available.[23–25] There is a large group of potential candidates including nurses, nursing students, doctors, medical students, dentists, physiotherapists, radiographers and cardiac technicians.

Current ALS instructors and ICs can teach and assess on ILS courses. There is also a pilot project underway to develop specific ILS instructors. There must be at least 1 instructor for every 6 candidates, with a maximum of 30 candidates on a course.

Course format

The ILS course is delivered over 1 day and comprises lectures, hands-on skills teaching and cardiac-arrest scenario teaching (CASTeach) using manikins. The programme includes a number of options that allow instructors to tailor the course to their candidate group.

Course content

The course covers those skills that are most likely to result in successful resuscitation: causes and prevention of cardiac arrest, starting CPR, basic airway skills and defibrillation (AED or manual). There are options to include the teaching of the laryngeal mask airway and drug treatments during cardiac arrest. Once all the skills have been covered, there is a cardiac arrest demonstration by the instructors that outlines the first-responder role to the candidates. This is followed by the CASTeach station where candidates practise. ILS candidates are not usually expected to undertake the role of the team leader. Candidates should be able to start a resuscitation attempt and continue until more experienced help arrives. When appropriate, the instructor takes over as a resuscitation team leader. This is not always necessary, as in some scenarios resuscitation may be successful before more experienced help arrives. Set scenarios are used that are adapted to the workplace and the clinical role of the candidate.

Assessment

Candidate's performances are assessed continuously and they must show their competence throughout the ILS course. There are no formal testing stations, removing the threat associated with spot testing at the end of the course. Candidates are sent the assessment forms with the pre-course materials. The forms indicate clearly how their performance will be measured against a pre-determined criteria. Assessment on the ILS course enables the candidate to see what is expected and frame learning around achievement of these outcomes. The following practical skills are assessed on the ILS course: airway management, BLS and defib-

rillation. With a supportive approach, the majority of candidates achieve the course learning outcomes.

Equipment

The ILS course is designed to be straightforward to run. Most courses are conducted in hospitals with small groups of candidates (average 12 candidates). The course requires lecture facilities and a skills teaching area for each group of six candidates. There needs to be at least one ALS manikin for every six candidates. The course should be suitable for local needs. Course centres should try as far as possible to train candidates to use the equipment (e.g., defibrillator type) that is available locally.

Course report and results sheet

A course report and the results sheet are compiled by the course director and filed with the National Resuscitation Council and the ERC.

The Advanced Life Support (ALS) course

The target candidates for this course are doctors and senior nurses working in emergency areas of the hospital and those who may be members of the medical emergency or cardiac arrest teams.[26] The course is also suitable for senior paramedics and certain hospital technicians. The ILS course is more suitable for first-responder nurses, doctors who rarely encounter cardiac arrest in their practice, and emergency medical technicians. Up to 32 candidates can be accommodated on the course, with a ratio of at least 1 instructor for every 3 candidates. Up to a maximum of 50% of the instructors may be ICs. Groups for teaching should not exceed eight candidates and should be six ideally. Each instructor acts as a mentor for a small group of candidates. The course normally lasts for two to two and a half days.

Course format

The course format has very few formal lectures (four), and teaching concentrates on hands-on skills, clinically based scenarios in small groups with emphasis on the team leader approach and interactive group discussions. Mentor/mentee sessions are included, to allow candidates to give and receive feedback. Faculty meetings are held at the beginning of the course and at the end of each day of the course. Social occasions, such as course and faculty dinners, add greatly to the course interaction and enjoyment.

Course content

The course content is based on the current ERC guidelines for resuscitation. Candidates are expected to have studied the ALS course manual carefully before the course.

The course aims to train candidates to highlight the causes of cardiac arrest, identify sick patients in danger of deterioration and manage cardiac arrest and the immediate periarrest problems encountered in and around the first hour or so of the event. It is not a course in advanced intensive care or cardiology. Competence in BLS is expected before the candidate enrols for the course.

Emphasis is placed on the techniques of safe defibrillation and ECG interpretation, the management of the airway and ventilation, the management of periarrest rhythms, simple acid/base balance and special circumstances relating to cardiac arrest. Post-resuscitation care, ethical aspects related to resuscitation and care of the bereaved are included in the course.

Assessment and testing

Each candidate is assessed individually and reviewed at the end of each day by the faculty at their meeting. Feedback is given as required. There is a testing scenario towards the end of the course, and an on going assessment of the management of the sick patient and the need to be able to defibrillate effectively and safely. There is a multiple-choice question paper taken at the end of the course to test core knowledge. Candidates are required to achieve 75% to pass this test.

Course venue and equipment

The course requires four practical rooms, a lecture room, a faculty room and facilities for lunches and refreshments. At least two digital projectors and computers and up to four flip charts are needed. The practical rooms each should have an adult ALS manikin with ECG simulator and a defibrillator. Four adult airway manikins are required, together with the equipment for simple airway care and ventilation, tracheal intubation and placing a supraglottic airway, such as the laryngeal mask. Intravenous cannulae, syringes, infusion fluids and simulated drugs make up the list.

Course report and results sheet

A course report and the results sheet are compiled by the course director and filed with the national resuscitation council and the ERC.

The European Paediatric Life Support (EPLS) course

The EPLS course is designed for healthcare workers who are involved in the resuscitation of a newborn, an infant or a child whether in or out of hospital The course aims at providing caregivers with the knowledge and skills for the management of the critically ill child during the first hour of illness and to prevent progression of diseases to cardiac arrest.

Competence in basic paediatric life support is a prerequisite, although a 90-min refresher course on BLS and relief of foreign-body airway obstruction is included. The EPLS course is suitable for doctors, nurses, emergency medical technicians and paramedics, etc., who have a duty to respond to sick newborns, infants and children in their practice.[27,28] EPLS is not a course in neonatal or paediatric intensive care aimed at the advanced providers.

The course can accommodate 24 candidates with a ratio of at least 1 instructor for every 4 candidates. In exceptional circumstances, 28 candidates may be accepted with extra instructors. Experience in paediatrics is necessary to keep scenarios realistic and to answer candidates' questions, so a minimum of 50% of the faculty must have regular experience in neonatal or paediatric practice. Up to a maximum of 50% of the instructors may be ICs. Groups for teaching should not exceed eight candidates and ideally should be five or six; two instructors act as mentors for a group of five to seven candidates. The course normally lasts for two to two and a half days.

Course format

The new course format has fewer formal lectures (three). Teaching of knowledge and skills is given in small groups using clinically based scenarios. The emphasis is on assessment and treatment of the sick child, team working and leadership. Formal mentor/mentee sessions are included, to allow candidates to give and receive feedback. Faculty meetings are held at the beginning of the course and at the end of each day of the course. Feedback is also given to ICs after each series of workshops and after their lectures.

Course content

The course content follows the current ERC guidelines for neonatal and paediatric resuscitation. The course candidates are expected to have studied the manual before attending the course. In the future they also may receive a CD or a DVD for home training in BLS.[15] A precourse MCQ is sent with the manual to candidates 4–6 weeks before the course. It is collected at the beginning and feedback is given during the course.

The EPLS is aimed at training the candidates to understand the causes and mechanisms of cardiorespiratory arrest in neonates and children, to recognise and treat the critically ill neonate, infant or child and to manage cardiac arrest if it occurs. Skills taught include airway management, bag-mask ventilation, log roll and cervical collar placement, oxygen delivery, an introduction to intubation and vascular access, safe defibrillation, cardioversion and AED use.

Each candidate is assessed individually and reviewed by the faculty. Feedback is given as required. A BLS assessment follows the BLS refresher course, and a second scenario-based test at the end of the course emphasises the assessment of the sick child and the core skills. There is a multiple-choice question paper taken at the end of the course to test the core knowledge. Candidates are required to achieve 75% to pass this test.

Course venue and equipment

The course requires four practical rooms, a lecture room, a faculty room and facilities for lunches and refreshments. At least one digital projector and computer and up to four flip charts are needed. Paediatric manikins (infant and child for basic and advanced techniques) and adjuncts must be available in each classroom. One defibrillator, one AED and one rhythms simulator device must also be available.

Course report and results sheet

A course report and the results sheet are compiled by the course director and filed with the national resuscitation council and the ERC.

The Newborn Life Support (NLS) course

This course is designed for health workers likely to be present at the birth of a baby in the course of their job. It aims to give those who may be called upon to start resuscitation at birth the background knowledge and skills to approach the management of the newborn infant during the first 10–20 min in a competent manner. The course is suitable for midwives, nurses and doctors and, like most such courses, works best with candidates from a mixture of specialties.

The course is usually conducted over 1 day and runs best with 24 candidates, though up to 32 may be permitted. There should be one instructor for every three candidates in addition to the course director.

Course format

The NLS manual is sent to each of the candidates 4 weeks before the course. Each candidate receives a multiple-choice questionnaire, with the manual and is asked to complete this and bring it to the course. There are two 30-min and two 15-min lectures. The candidates are then divided into four groups and pass through three workstations before lunch. The afternoon is taken up by a demonstration scenario, followed by 2 h of scenario teaching in small groups and finally a theoretical and practical assessment by an MCQ and an individual practical airway test. The course concentrates on airway management but also covers chest compression, umbilical venous access and drugs.

Course venue and equipment

The venue requires a lecture room, four good-sized practical rooms, a faculty room and facilities for lunch and refreshments. A digital projector is required in the lecture theatre and a flip chart or a black/white board in each practical room. Ideally, one of the practical rooms should have hand-washing facilities. At least four infant BLS and four infant ALS manikins (ideally six of each) should be available, as well as other airway adjuncts. Four Resuscitaires, ideally complete with gas cylinders, should also be available.

Course report and results sheet

A course report and results sheet are compiled by the course director and lodged with the national resuscitation council and the ERC.

The Generic Instructor Course (GIC)

This course is for candidates who have been recommended as IP, emanating from the ALS or EPLS provider courses. In some, the MIMMS course is undertaken under the auspices of the ALSG, and IPs from that course may take the GIC to qualify as ICs for teaching that course. There should be a maximum of 24 candidates, with a ratio of at least 1 instructor to 3 candidates. Instructors must all be fully experienced ERC instructors, not ICs. A key person is the educator. Groups should not exceed six candidates. The emphasis of the course is on developing instruction skills. Core knowledge of the original provider course is assumed. The course lasts for two to two and a half days.

Course format

The course format is largely interactive. The educator plays a key role and leads many of the discussions and feedback. There is one formal lecture on effective teaching and adult learning, conducted by the educator. This lecture is interspersed with group activities. The remainder of the course is conducted in small group discussions and skill- and scenario-based hands-on sessions.

Mentor/mentee sessions are included, and there is a faculty meeting at the beginning of the course and at the end of each day.

Course content

The course concentrates on teaching techniques and skills. Candidates are expected to have studied the GIC manual carefully before the course (reference manual). The theoretical background of adult learning and effective teaching is covered by the educator at the beginning of the course. The features of PowerPoint and the flip chart are demonstrated, and candidates have an opportunity to present a 5-min lecture and are given personal feedback on their performance. The principle of equipment familiarisation, followed by a demonstration by the faculty with subsequent candidate practice, is followed in all aspects of the course.

The teaching of skills is based on the four-stage approach. Scenario-based sessions use scenarios from the candidate's original provider course. Emphasis is placed on the role of the instructor throughout this teaching day, and each candidate has the opportunity to adopt the instructor role. Constructive feedback is a key element of the instructor role.

During the second day, the emphasis moves to assessment and, after demonstrations by the faculty, all candidates are offered the opportunity to act in the instructor assessor role for the assessment of skills and scenario leadership. Further sessions include the conduct of open and closed discussions and the role and qualities of the instructor.

Assessment

Each candidate has ongoing assessment by the faculty throughout the course. Candidates' performances and attitudes are discussed at the daily faculty meetings and feedback is given as required. Successful candidates may proceed to the status of IC.

Course venue and equipment

This is as for the original provider course. If the candidates come from mixed backgrounds, then a variety of equipment is required.

Course report and results sheet

A course report is compiled by the course director and the educator. This and the results sheet are filed with the national resuscitation council and the ERC.

The Educator Master Class (EMC)

This course, normally held annually, is designed for those aspiring to become medical educators for the GIC. Suitable candidates are selected by the faculty, and generally must have a background and qualification in medical education or must have demonstrated a special commitment to educational practice over a number of years. They should have experience of a provider course and a GIC, and should have studied the background reading for the course.

The instructors for the course are experienced educators. A maximum of 18 candidates can be accommodated with 6 instructors. The groups should comprise a maximum of six candidates. The course lasts just under 2 days.

Course format

The course consists mainly of closed discussion groups for the whole course, led by one or two of the instructors, together with break-out small group discussions and problem solving.

Course content

The course covers the theoretical framework for medical educators, assessment and quality control, teaching methodologies, critical appraisal, the role of the mentor, multiprofessional education strategies and continued development of the medical educator.

Assessment

Each candidate has ongoing assessment by the faculty throughout the course. Individual progress is discussed at a faculty meeting at the end of each day, and candidates are given the feedback as appropriate. Successful candidates may proceed to the status of educator candidate (EC), where they will be supervised and assessed by an experienced educator and course director until it is decided whether or not they will be suitable educators to work on their own.

Course venue and equipment

The course venue requires a lecture room and three break-out rooms. A digital projector and three flip charts are needed; no manikins are required.

Course report and results

The course director compiles a course report after consultation with the faculty. This, and the results sheet, are conveyed to the educator's national resuscitation council and the ERC.

Appendix A. European Resuscitation Council Code of Conduct

The Code of Conduct applies to all who instruct, or otherwise assist, at courses held under the auspices of the ERC.

It is essential that these individuals

- fully understand that accreditation, and continuing accreditation, of the individual instructor or assistant is dependent on observing this code as well as completing the necessary requirements for re-certification
- ensure that courses approved by the ERC are run in accordance with the ethos and regulations currently in force using the manuals, slides and other materials to ensure that consistent standards of attitude, knowledge and skills are achieved
- behave at all times while participating in courses or social events related to the courses, which are run under the auspices of the ERC, in a responsible manner and observe and other applicable professional codes of conduct

- cooperate with other instructors, educators and administrators (the faculty) and recognise and respect their individual contributions
- avoid any abuse of their position and maintain confidentiality about candidates' results and performance.

References

1. Makker R, Gray-Siracusa K, Evers M. Evaluation of advanced cardiac life support in a community teaching hospital by use of actual cardiac arrests. Heart Lung 1995;24:116—20.
2. Anthonypillai F. Retention of advanced cardiopulmonary resuscitation knowledge by intensive care trained nurses. Intensive Crit Care Nurs 1992;8:180—4.
3. Azcona LA, Gutierrez GE, Fernandez CJ, Natera OM, Ruiz-Speare O, Ali J. Attrition of advanced trauma life support (ATLS) skills among ATLS instructors and providers in Mexico. J Am Coll Surg 2002;195:372—7.
4. Birnbaum ML, Robinson NE, Kuska BM, Stone HL, Fryback DG, Rose JH. Effect of advanced cardiac life-support training in rural, community hospitals. Crit Care Med 1994;22:741—9.
5. Hammond F, Saba M, Simes T, Cross R. Advanced life support: retention of registered nurses' knowledge 18 months after initial training. Aust Crit Care 2000;13:99—104.
6. Kaye W, Mancini ME, Rallis SF. Advanced cardiac life support refresher course using standardized objective-based mega code testing. Crit Care Med 1987;15:55—60.
7. Kaye W, Wynne G, Marteau T, et al. An advanced resuscitation training course for preregistration house officers. J R Coll Physicians Lond 1990;24:51—4.
8. O'Steen DS, Kee CC, Minick MP. The retention of advanced cardiac life support knowledge among registered nurses. J Nurs Staff Dev 1996;12:66—72.
9. Schwid HA, O'Donnell D. Anesthesiologists' management of simulated critical incidents. Anesthesiology 1992;76:495—501.
10. Young R, King L. An evaluation of knowledge and skill retention following an in-house advanced life support course. Nurs Crit Care 2000;5:7—14.
11. Stross JK. Maintaining competency in advanced cardiac life support skills. JAMA 1983;249:3339—41.
12. Su E, Schmidt TA, Mann NC, Zechnich AD. A randomized controlled trial to assess decay in acquired knowledge among paramedics completing a pediatric resuscitation course. Acad Emerg Med 2000;7:779—86.
13. Baskett P. Progress of the advanced life support courses in Europe and beyond. Resuscitation 2004;62:311—3.
14. Chamberlain DA, Hazinski MF. Education in resuscitation. Resuscitation 2003;59:11—43.
15. Braslow A, Brennan RT, Newman MM, Bircher NG, Batcheller AM, Kaye W. CPR training without an instructor: development and evaluation of a video self-instructional system for effective performance of cardiopulmonary resuscitation. Resuscitation 1997;34:207—20.
16. Todd KH, Braslow A, Brennan RT, et al. Randomized, controlled trial of video self-instruction versus traditional CPR training. Ann Emerg Med 1998;31:364—9.
17. Todd KH, Heron SL, Thompson M, Dennis R, O'Connor J, Kellermann AL. Simple CPR: a randomized, controlled trial of video self-instructional cardiopulmonary resuscitation training in an African American church congregation. Ann Emerg Med 1999;34:730—7.

18. Batcheller AM, Brennan RT, Braslow A, Urrutia A, Kaye W. Cardiopulmonary resuscitation performance of subjects over forty is better following half-hour video self-instruction compared to traditional four-hour classroom training. Resuscitation 2000;43:101—10.

19. Lynch B, Einspruch E, Nichol G, Becker L, Aufderheide T, Idris A. Effectiveness of a 30-minute CPR self-instruction program for lay responders: a controlled randomized study. Resuscitation 2005;67:31—43.

20. Sandroni C, Fenici P, Cavallaro F, Bocci MG, Scapigliati A, Antonelli M. Haemodynamic effects of mental stress during cardiac arrest simulation testing on advanced life support courses. Resuscitation 2005;66:39—44

21. Soar J, Perkins GD, Harris S, Nolan JP. The immediate life support course. Resuscitation 2003;57:21—6.

22. Soar J, McKay U. A revised role for the hospital cardiac arrest team. Resuscitation 1998;38:145—9.

23. Smith GB, Osgood VM, Crane S. ALERT—a multiprofessional training course in the care of the acutely ill adult patient. Resuscitation 2002;52:281—6.

24. Smith GB, Poplett N. Impact of attending a 1-day multiprofessional course (ALERT) on the knowledge of acute care in trainee doctors. Resuscitation 2004;61:117—22.

25. Featherstone P, Smith GB, Linnell M, Easton S, Osgood VM. Impact of a one-day inter-professional course (ALERT^{TM}) on attitudes and confidence in managing critically ill adult patients. Resuscitation 2005;65:329—36.

26. Nolan J. Advanced life support training. Resuscitation 2001;50:9—11.

27. Buss PW, McCabe M, Evans RJ, Davies A, Jenkins H. A survey of basic resuscitation knowledge among resident paediatricians. Arch Dis Child 1993;68:75—8.

28. Carapiet D, Fraser J, Wade A, Buss PW, Bingham R. Changes in paediatric resuscitation knowledge among doctors. Arch Dis Child 2001;84:412—4.